Green Electroni
Green Bottom L

Green Electronics Green Bottom Line

Environmentally Responsible Engineering

Edited by Lee H. Goldberg
and Wendy Middleton

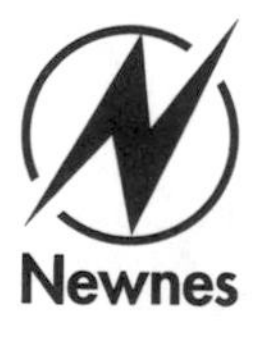

Newnes
Boston Oxford Auckland Johannesburg Melbourne New Delhi

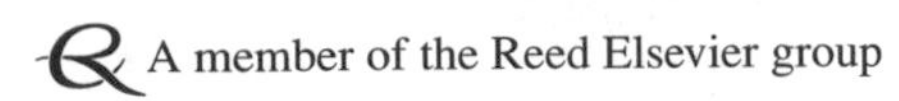

A member of the Reed Elsevier group

Newnes is an imprint of Butterworth–Heinemann.

Recognizing the importance of preserving what has been written, Butterworth–Heinemann prints its books on acid-free paper whenever possible.

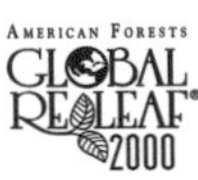

Butterworth–Heinemann supports the efforts of American Forests and the Global ReLeaf program in its campaign for the betterment of trees, forests, and our environment.

Library of Congress Cataloging-in-Publication Data

Goldberg, Lee.
Green electronics/green bottom line : environmentally responsible Engineering / Lee Goldberg.
p. cm.
Includes index.
ISBN 0-7506-9993-0 (alk. paper)
1. Electronic apparatus and appliances-Design and construction-Safety Measures. 2. Electronics. 3. Electronic industries. 4. Green products. 5. Environmental protection. I. Title.
TK7836.G62 1999
621.381-DC21 99-14522
CIP

British Library Cataloguing-in-Publication Data

A catalogue record for this book is available from the British Library.

The publisher offers special discounts on bulk orders of this book.
For information, please contact:
Manager of Special Sales
Butterworth–Heinemann
225 Wildwood Avenue
Woburn, MA 01801-2041
Tel: 781-904-2500
Fax: 781-904-2620

For information on all Newnes publications available, contact our World Wide Web home page at: http://www.newnespress.com

10 9 8 7 6 5 4 3 2 1

Printed in the United States of America

A blessing from the past:

To Martin Kramer and his wife, Esther, who kept faith with me and taught me the power of values and value of dreams.

A blessing for the future:

To my daughter, Anwyn Imara Tonisha Goldberg, whose arrival opened my heart and inspired me to embark on this adventure.

Contents

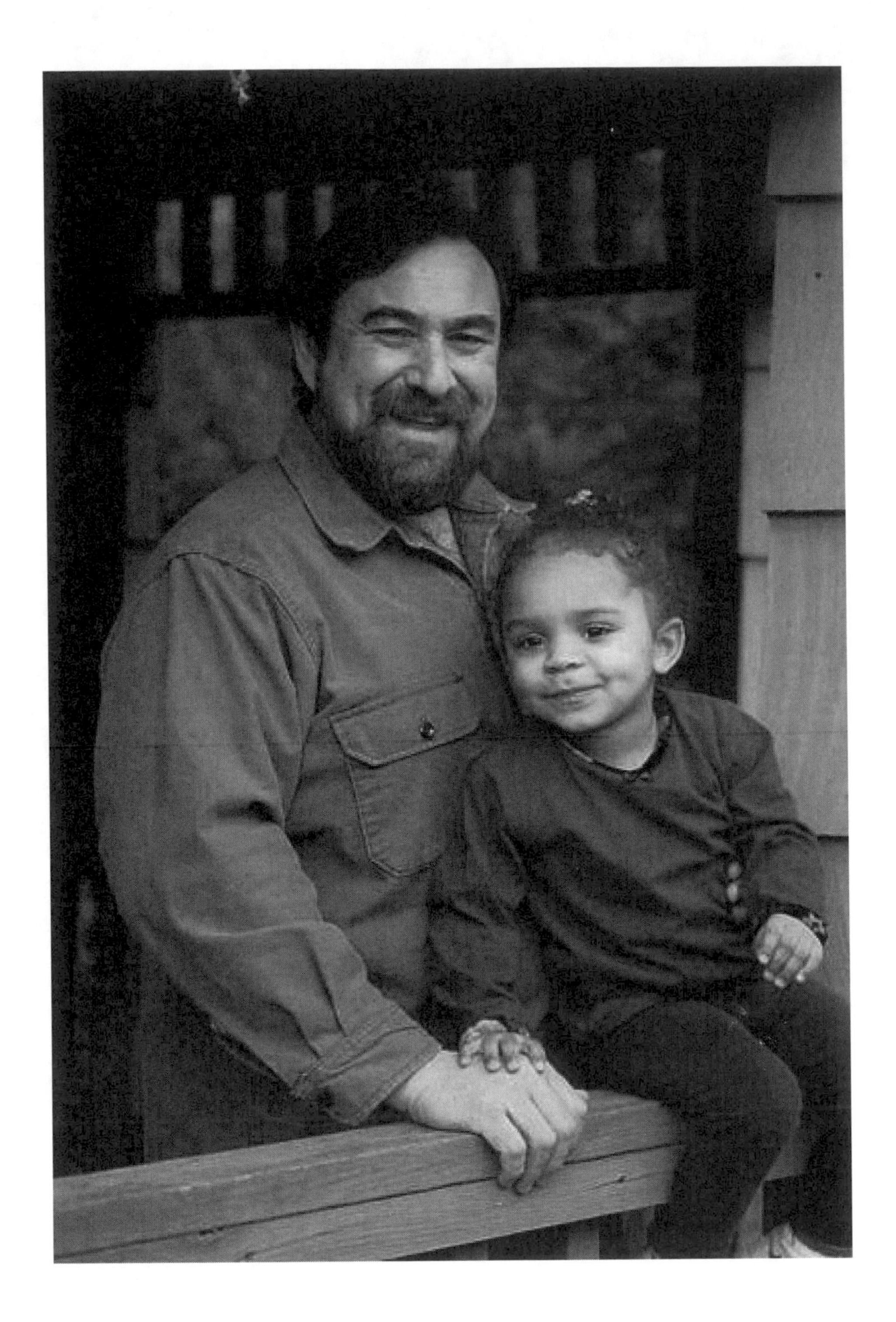

Acknowledgments

Eight years of working on spacecraft taught me that nearly any worthwhile achievement represents both the fruit of individual inspiration and the collective effort of a team of dedicated people. Much like those glorious machines I happily poured my soul into, this book embodies these principles. While my name is on the title page, it was written primarily by other people and supported in countless ways by many more.

I thank my wife, Catherine Beach, who believed in me and put up with being a near-widow for the past six months. She also shouldered the majority of household and childcare duties as the book entered its final, manic stage. Thanks, partner, it's payback time.

Even though it's a terrible cliché, I'm going to thank my mother, Caryll Goldberg, for being a support and inspiration. As well as keeping the faith for this and my other wild projects, she's always set an example for being tough-minded and acting in earnest on one's deeply held principles. Hats off to my sister Annie, who encouraged me by both her heartfelt words and powerful example. Also thanks to my father, Harold Goldberg, who, despite our serious differences and misunderstandings, taught me many things I still value today.

Words cannot fully express my gratitude to Wendy Middleton, one of my oldest and best friends. She served as my assistant editor, research librarian, logistics administrator, secretary, editor, author wrangler, key grip, best boy, foley operator, cheerleader, and coconspirator throughout this wild ride. Special thanks goes to her husband, James Middleton, who provided unswerving support and encouragement for both Wendy and me through even the most difficult parts of this project.

Several people taught me important lessons about technology which led me to this book. My great-uncle Martin Kramer first opened my eyes to its wonders and taught me much about the art of kindness. In high school, my teachers Steve Vedro and Aaron Schneider made me consider the social and political implications of technology. At the same time, another teacher, Steve Futterman, taught us how to subvert technology and use it as a tool for social change. Finally, in college, Professor

Eugene Steiger kept my interest in electronics from being crushed and served as a living lesson on the critical connection between technology and human values.

I also thank my friends Sandy Brainard and Steve Masticola for the insight and inspiration they gave me in the course of our conversations. Although they are only professional acquaintances, the same deep thanks goes to Amory Lovins, Robert Laudise, Ted Polakowski, Jill Matzke, and Greg Pitts. Together, they helped shape the book and keep it from being crippled by my blind spots.

Special thanks go out to all the authors who contributed to this book. In addition to writing their chapters free of charge, they had to endure my incessant corrections and demands for "more technical substance." Without exception, the authors demonstrated the meaning of commitment, which an old friend once defined this way: "When it comes to breakfast, the chicken is involved, but the pig is committed."

However, several people went beyond even my unreasonable expectations. William Trumble spent his vacation writing three critical portions of the book. Jim Lamprecht graciously donated an enormous chunk of material on ISO 14001 and then endured the anguish of two serious rewrites without complaint. The "good sport" award goes to Carsten Nagel, who cheerfully endured my editorial badgering during three major rewrites as we sweated the details of his work. Pitipong Veerakamolmal and Surendra Gupta get the "early bird" award for being first team to deliver a completed manuscript (an excellent one, I might add), while heartfelt thanks also go to Radim Visinka, Ondrej Pauk, Petr Lidik, Joan Williams, and Brian Glazebrook, who filled important gaps in this book with their contributions on ridiculously short notice.

Finally, I extend my gratitude to Jo Gilmore, who got this project started at Newnes, and Pam Chester, Susan Prusak, and Candy Hall, who bravely saw it through to conclusion. Thanks for your enthusiasm, insights, patience, and faith in the project.

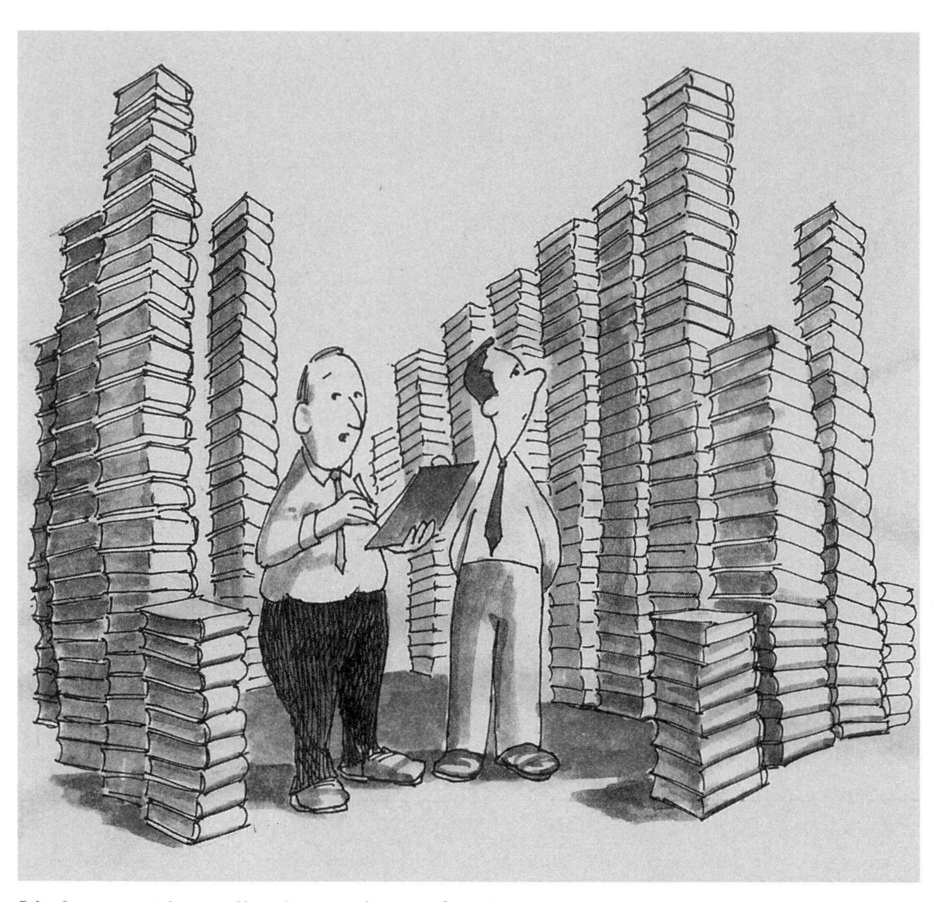

It’s the current best-seller about saving our forests.

Preface: About This Book

Hey, there, thanks for picking up this book. I'm pleasantly surprised that you are taking the time to read this preface, something I didn't start doing regularly until I made the transition from engineer to writer a few years ago. For both of our sakes, I'll try to keep this interesting, with only the obligatory paragraph or two of dreadfully serious, high-minded prose required for all first-time authors of technical books.

Before we begin in earnest, I want to tell you a bit about how Anwyn, my two-and-a-half-year-old daughter, got me started writing this book. She's pretty advanced for her age, so it's no surprise to me that she managed to do this before she was born.

It began about three years ago, just before Anwyn bounced into our lives. I had just checked the assignment sheet at the magazine where I worked and saw I had an editorial due the next day. Since *Electronic Design* is a hard-core engineering magazine for my fellow travelers of the pocket-protector set, it is heavily technical. Consequently, our editorials are supposed to babble on in glowing tones with expert opinions about the subtleties of the next generation of electronic technologies, chips, and widgets.

Unfortunately, it's been five years since I laid down my 'scope probe and picked up a pen, so some of my knowledge on key topics is not as deep as I'd like. Because I find it hard to consider myself an expert on the technology I cover, I usually manage to tap dance around any potentially embarrassing displays of ignorance by writing funny stuff about it instead. Happily for me (and the guy who writes the "Dilbert" comic strip), there is no shortage of funny and downright weird aspects to our profession.

In many of these editorials, I play the straight man for Catherine, my wife, who gets to say all the intelligent things. By letting her do the preaching, she gets to look as smart as she really is, and I don't have to take the heat for any opinions that may really piss off my readers. So, with the arrival of our daughter close at hand, I figured she was fair game too, and tossed off the following.

Death and Children

Wow-there's nothing like the prospect of your first child to make you think about death! At 40, I have been able to pretty much ignore the warning signs of my own mortality as I continue to do most of the stuff I did when I was 20. It just hurts more and takes longer to recover. Even when I married Catherine last year, I was able to mumble through the "till death do us part" stuff without really having to acknowledge that this was a closed-term contract. It is only now that I'm facing the imminent release of Goldberg 2.0 that the concept of having a limited product life cycle is really dawning on me. Uncomfortable as staring old Mr. Bones in the face is, it does make me think hard about what kind of legacy I want to give to the little girl who is waiting for us under the mountain of paperwork that surrounds an adoption.

I hope to leave her a better, more peaceful, and more interesting world than the one I was born into. This puts me in an ugly double bind, as part of me is seized with the urge to join every crusade to clean up the planet, while the other part tries to heed Catherine's wise advice to make more time at home for our family-to-be. I'm also having to face up to the painful fact that most of the things I've worked on for the past 20 years had little or no lasting value, other than giving a paycheck to the folks who made it. I don't get a warm fuzzy feeling when I realize that so many of the products I devoted my blood, sweat, and tears to ended up as next year's landfill. I guess it's time I took some responsibility for not wasting the next couple of decades, too.

For me, acting as a responsible professional breaks down into two separate issues: what we do and how we do it. Both are equally important. I understand that most of us end up doing the necessary but unglamorous chores, making the paper clips, toasters, and the electronic widgets that form the underpinnings of our "civilization," but we can all make a difference by the way we do our jobs. Not all of us get to do cool, important stuff like finding the cure for cancer, sending people to Mars, or inventing Spandex, but the choices we make each day down in the trenches can have just as big an impact on the quality of the world we leave our kids. For example, we can, as I have, make the difficult choices to not participate in projects that undermine, human rights, the environment, and other things that we hold dear to our hearts.

Although we can't all play starring roles in the slow, painful evolution of our species, we all can contribute in some way toward a gentler, funnier, and more hopeful future. Should our professional duties extend beyond delivering designs on time and under budget? Should we be worrying about a product's energy efficiency? And whether it poses an environmental hazard in its manufacture, use, or disposal? Should we care if it contributes to, or erodes, the social fabric? I think so.

As I look into trading in my sports car for a nice Saturn station wagon and begin to install a safety parachute on my ultralight aircraft, the idea of making the world better for all our children begins to look like one of the few things I can do that has any value past the day the Grim Reaper comes calling. What do you think?

Reflection

Somehow, the editorial made it past our copy editors and hit the street. Shortly after, my e-mail account began to overflow with letters from engineers who, like myself, were wrestling with the same dilemmas in their own lives. It was kind of cool to actually have readers agreeing with me for once and, better yet, to see that corporate America had not been able to squeeze the paternal instincts out of some of its hardest working citizens.

Tucked away in the midst of all this was a nice letter from a lady named Jo Gilmore, at Newnes Press. Somehow, she'd gotten hold of my editorial and decided I'd be just the kind of quixotic fool who would take on the task of putting together a book on green engineering. Only half-realizing that our soon-to-arrive child would soak up every available nano-joule of energy that was not devoted to making a paycheck, I accepted her offer.

Two and a half years, two editors (Jo moved on to another firm in the interim), and several thousand diapers later, the book is ready, and my daughter is negotiating the tricky transition between infanthood and personhood. The journey toward the book you hold in your hand started out innocently enough but ended up as a major adventure that consumed a year of nights, weekends, and any remaining bits of sanity that my child might have missed. I'm now an author of sorts and a reasonably competent father.

My hope for this book is much the same as I have for my daughter, I want both of them to go out into the world, enjoy a long and happy life, and do more good than harm. What you have in your hands is a small, incomplete map of an exciting territory I've discovered. While not intended to be a definitive text on the subject, I hope this book will at least be a good introduction to the relatively new field of green engineering. Its real goal is to help convince you and others that environmentally sound practices are not only possible within the electronics industry but, more important, practical-and profitable.

As technologists, we have an enormous influence on the direction humanity takes, because we create the tools that shape and propel our cultures and civilizations forward. Many of the things we have created tend to amplify both our best and dumbest tendencies, leading us to a dangerous crossroads at the end of the 20th century. If we are to keep our grandkids from exhausting the remaining natural resources and prevent the rest of the critters on the planet from choking on their waste, we've got to change the way we do business in a big hurry.

Perhaps the most important thing I've learned while working on this book is that the real trick to inventing a greener future is not simply technological. It lies in developing ways to integrate environmental factors into the design and management cultures where we work and into the consumption patterns and behaviors of the folks who use the stuff we make. I believe that, over the next decade, the high-tech sector can lead the way in making environmental considerations an integral part of industry's culture. Whether or not this happens, in good measure, is up to folks like us. If I've done the job I set out to do, you'll have enough concepts and tools, as well as places to look for more information, to help each one of us begin to clean up his or her small corner of the world.

Finally, I'd like to ask that, if you find something especially useful that should have been in this book, please bring it to my attention. Because this field is just starting to approach the knee of a sharp maturity curve, I'm already starting to contemplate a second edition. If I don't get back to you right away, please be patient. Wendy, my assistant editor, and I are suffering from a serious case of toasted brains from a six-month final push on this book, and I miss being something more than a shadowy figure to my family. Now that the book is done, I'm going to lie down till the urge to do "just one more rewrite" subsides and the world stops looking like one big, mind-sucking computer screen. Once my head clears, my first priority will be to spend a good chunk of time just hanging out with my wife and daughter.

The second edition can wait a little while, they can't.

Section I
Design Issues

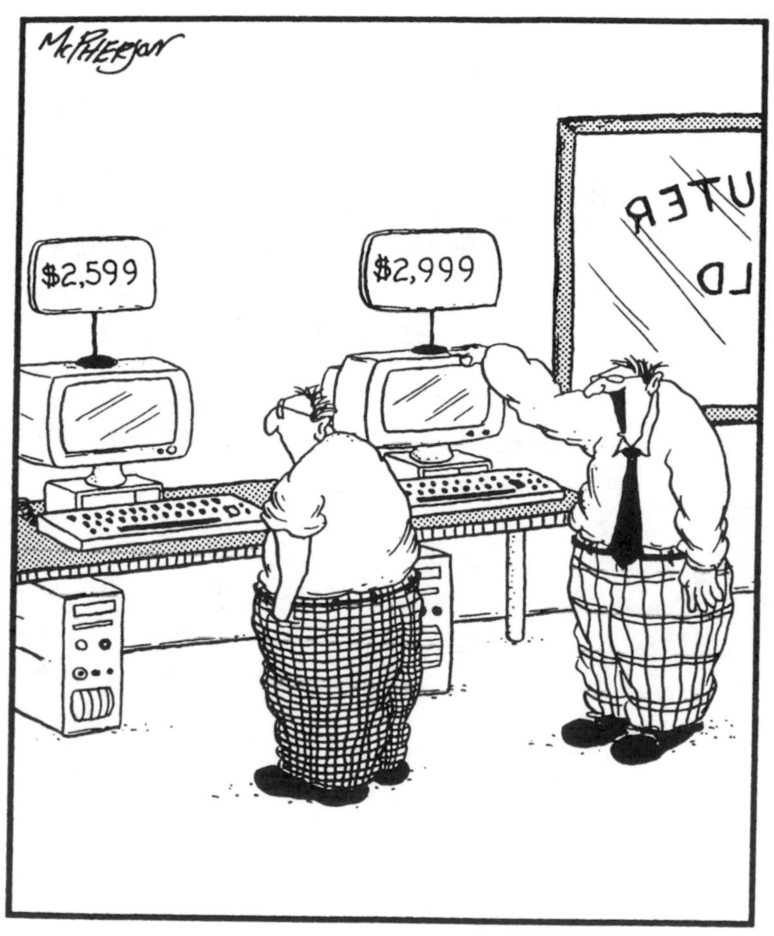

"The main difference is that that system will be obsolete in eight months, whereas, for only $400 more, you can have a system that's guaranteed not to be obsolete for a full year."

Introduction: If You Think Education Is Expensive, Try Ignorance!

An Interview with Dr. Amory Lovins on Technology, the Environment, and the Existential Pleasures of Whole-System Engineering.

LEE H. GOLDBERG
Chip Center Magazine

Dr. Amory Lovins and his wife, Hunter, are a rare breed of visionaries who see a potentially bright future for humanity and the other species we share the world with. Cofounders of Rocky Mountain Institute, a technology-oriented, nonprofit, resource policy center, they believe that technology and capitalism are the source of not just many problems but also many fruitful solutions. A self-described "recovering physicist," Dr. Lovins is a proponent of something he calls *whole-system engineering*—applying knowledge of the entire system to the design and implementation of every element within it and how they fit together.

Time and time again, Lovins and his merry band of techno-ecologists have demonstrated remarkable results in improving the energy efficiency and reducing the environmental impact of everything from factories, office buildings, and private homes to personal computers and automobiles. He claims that the results they achieve come from applying a relatively simple set of concepts and engineering principles to nearly any set of problems. Although he was quite busy with the final details of his latest book, *Natural Capitalism*, which he and Hunter cowrote with Paul Hawken (of Smith & Hawken Garden Supply fame), Lovins was eager to hold this interview, because he feels that helping to educate engineers about whole-systems design is one of the most important missions he has.

Lee Goldberg: So, why is it so important for engineers to practice this whole-systems stuff?

Amory Lovins: Well, aside from the fact that it's a lot more fun than simply solving the same old problems with plug-and-chug solutions, it's critical that engineers understand the vital role they play in both the economy and the ecosystem. Engineers and their immediate management are some of the most influential people on the planet.

LG: How so?

AL: Every decision an engineer makes—good or bad—has the potential to be multiplied a millionfold on a production line or amplified by the magnitude and influence of the project he or she is working on. That's why I keep telling anybody who will listen that investing in an engineer's "mindware" yields the highest return of any capital improvement available.

LG: Mindware? You mean an engineer's education?

AL: Well, formal education is the beginning of the software upload, but it's much more, and more powerful, than that. Think of mindware also as the ways a person learns to see the world, approach problems, and create solutions. Unlike most of what passes for education, mindware doesn't depreciate but rather ripens with age and experience.

LG: So the way an engineer approaches a problem can profoundly affect its outcome? I thought that most engineering tasks were fairly cut and dried, with little room for creativity.

AL: Not at all! The typical engineer wields a level of power and discretionary action that would terrify timid managers if they really understood its implications. Let's take a simple example from my colleague, the mechanical-engineering wizard Mr. Eng Lock Lee in Singapore. Say you're a senior heating, ventilating, and air conditioning (HVAC) engineer somewhere in Asia. On reasonable assumptions, you probably specify nearly $3 million worth of equipment every year—over 50 times your salary—with a total rated cooling capacity of around 1,700 refrigerative tons. Each year, the HVAC equipment you have specified adds around 1 MW of net peak load to the local power grid. This increased load costs the power company around $1–3 million to build the generating capacity and grid infrastructure. Now, suppose you learn how to specify high-efficiency HVAC equipment, which saves (conservatively), 20–50% of the normal power required. Besides lowering your customer's utility bills, you also cut the amount that the utility must spend to upgrade its system by around $1 million or more every year. Over a 30-year engineering career, a modest investment in what goes on in your brain has saved the utility about $6–15 million in present value—several orders of magnitude more than it costs. This doesn't even take into account the saved fuel, the reduced pollution, and other significant benefits to society.

LG: So the primary beneficiary is the power company and not the engineer's customer? Who'd buy that?

AL: We're not done yet. The utility benefits, of course, but the biggest savings are realized in the customer's building itself. In brief, coupling an efficient HVAC system to a properly designed or retrofitted office space can yield 40–90% energy savings while actually improving the comfort, health, and performance of the occupants. Payback on the extra cost of premium systems can run from a few years on the least favorable retrofits to less than zero for many new designs. After that, the building pays dividends for decades to come and yields superior market and financial performance for its owner. Better still, the occupants will do about 6–15% more and better work—a productivity boost that's been well documented when people work in a more comfortable environment. The HVAC systems you design over your career can do this for perhaps 65,000 office workers, whose present-valued salaries total about $36 billion! So the enhanced labor productivity is worth perhaps a million times what it cost to invest in your better engineering practice. A better return is hardly available anywhere!

LG: But this scenario isn't typical. I mean, there are lots of other areas of engineering where this doesn't hold true.

AL: You're right, there is only a potential for a 100 times return to be realized on some engineers' mindware upgrades. But then again, certain industries like semiconductors can allow a single engineer to create savings several orders of magnitude larger than my example. These are empirical numbers. An RMI team recently surveyed a half-dozen typical chip fabs. The low-hanging fruit that hit us in the eye as we walked around—retrofits that would roughly halve the energy to deliver chilled water and clean air—clearly would save $1–2 million per plant per year, with after-tax returns typically upwards of 100% per year. Three more kinds of low-hanging fruit had already rotted and fallen down so they were mushing up underfoot—drive-system retrofits, thermal integration, and tool redesign—and their savings were even bigger and more lucrative.

LG: So, why isn't this whole-system engineering concept being used more widely?

AL: Well, for one thing, it's more difficult than standard practices—both to do and to teach. It requires a meticulous attention to detail not often taught in school or practiced on the job. It's also difficult to justify the extra time it takes to come up with a whole-systems solution if your management simply looks at the up-front engineering charges and ignores the downstream effects. Another problem is that it's a new discipline, with few textbooks or design tools. We're working on that part, though . . .

LG: Sounds like a tough sell . . .

AL: It is a tough sell to shortsighted people, but the benefits are enormous and companies that capture them first will gain decisive competitive advantage. When you stop being blinded by the problem at hand and take the entire system into account, it's relatively easy to tap into synergies that allow very valuable savings in resources and energy. Of course, the secondary benefits, such as improved quality and productivity, often can be even more valuable. For example, retrofitting chip fabs probably yields even more valuable benefits in yield, throughput, setup time, production flexibility, and other operational parameters than in energy savings. In new fabs, the reductions in construction time and cost could be so important that companies that don't adopt the better designs won't be a problem, because ultimately they won't be around.

LG: How do you get a typical engineer who's probably already overworked to take the time and energy to learn these principles and put them into action?

AL: Most engineers are natural self-learners and appreciate elegantly frugal solutions. Besides, as I said before, whole-systems thinking is much more fun. Because of this, the whole-systems approach has a great appeal to folks like engineers, who were originally drawn to their profession because they enjoy solving problems. Who wants to sit around and repeat the mistakes of others when you can go out and make your own? Or better yet, make a difference!

In energy efficiency alone, there are tremendous opportunities for exercising one's creative side to realize order-of-magnitude savings in everything from commercial and residential lighting to home computers. The industrial sector also is an area that's hardly been "mined" for the billions of kilowatt-hours that can be extracted from inefficient processes at a low or negative cost.

LG: So you're talking mostly about energy savings?

AL: That's just the start. Whole-systems engineering uses natural and economic synergies to make savings of water, materials, effort, and other resources multiply like loaves and fishes. But let's start with energy because it simplifies an otherwise complex story.

LG: Could you give me an example?

AL: Sure. A standard industrial pumping loop, supposedly optimized by the top specialist firm in its industry (carpet making), recently was redesigned from 70.8 kW of pumping power to 5.3 kW—a 92% reduction—yet it worked better in all respects and cost less to build. No new technologies were needed—just two changes in design mentality. First, the redesigner used big pipes and small pumps, rather than small pipes and big pumps. Friction in a pipe drops as almost the fifth power of diameter, but engineers buy fatter pipe only up to the point where its extra cost is justified by the pumping energy saved over time. This standard practice is wrong because it omits the *capital* cost of the pumping equipment—the pump, motor, inverter, and electricals that must all be big enough to fight the friction. Such optimization of the pipes in isolation pessimizes the system. Instead, we should optimize the entire system together—pipes and pumping equipment—both up front and over the long run. Then, we find that it's a better deal to make the pipe so much fatter that the equipment becomes very small—so its far lower capital cost more than pays for the fatter pipe, making the entire system cheaper to build.

The second design change was even simpler and therefore more difficult: Lay out the pipes first, then the equipment they connect. Normally, people plunk down the equipment in arbitrary positions, far apart, with stuff in between, and often at the wrong height and facing the wrong way. Then, they call in the pipe fitter and ask that Point A be connected to Point B. The pipes must go through so many curlicues that friction often rises three to six times compared to a straight shot. Wherever practical, it's smarter to use short, straight pipes than long, crooked pipes. Friction drops; both the piping and the pumping systems become cheaper to build. In this case, the greater ease of insulation from short, straight pipes also saved 70 kW of thermal loss, with a three-month payback. An engineer who grasps this example never again will design piping the old way—at least, not without wincing.

LG: How does this thinking play out in motor systems?

AL: It's a much longer and more complicated story, but in short, both RMI and EPRI found in 1989–90 that if you do the right 35 things to retrofit a typical industrial motor system, in the right order, you typically can save around half its energy and earn an after-tax return on investment approaching 200% per year. The reason it's so cheap is that you pay for only 7 kinds of savings, and then you get another 28 as free by-products, because of favorable interactions between different parts of the system. And I'm talking here about savings only in between the electric meter and the input shaft of the driven machine. Savings in and beyond that driven machine are often even bigger and cheaper.

LG: Which of these savings should you pursue first?

AL: Always start downstream. For example, a typical industrial pumping system needs about ten units of fuel at the power plant to deliver one unit of flow in the pipe because of all the compounding losses in between. But savings at the downstream end turn those compounding losses around backward, so they become compounding *savings*. That is, saving one unit of flow or friction in the pipe will save about ten units of fuel, cost, and pollution (global warming, acid rain, nuclear waste, etc.) back upstream at the power station. It's even better than that, because a lot of the losses are in your own equipment right in your facility. For example, saving 1 unit of flow or friction in the pipe typically saves about 2.4 units of sizing, and therefore roughly of capital cost, in the motor—typically saving more capital cost there than a lower-friction pipe might incur. Of course, some downstream savings will be better than free. For example, a profitable lighting retrofit (which also looks better and lets you see better) will reduce cooling loads and hence the pumping needed for chilled water and condenser water, and that lower flow then multiplies back through severalfold smaller pumping equipment and tenfold less power-plant fuel consumption.

LG: I start to see what you mean by loaves and fishes. Do similar principles apply to other areas of design?

AL: It's the same story for industrial lighting except more spectacular, with 70–90% savings in energy alone. In fact, engineer Jim Rogers just retrofitted a warehouse's supposedly efficient metal-halide lighting to an even more efficient occupancy-controlled fluorescent system, saving 92–95% of the energy with a one-year payback. The same sort of opportunity also applies to smaller consumer products. Even the smallest improvement in the design of a television, radio, or computer is multiplied by the tens or hundreds of thousands of times it is produced. Conversely, because of inattentive design, the United States uses about 10 GW to run household and office gadgets that are turned off—1 GW for TVs alone. Good design can provide the same convenient standby features with only 5–10% as much energy and at no extra cost.

Similarly, there is no good reason for desktop computers to consume five to ten times as much juice as their portable counterparts, except that the engineers are driven to make incremental improvements rather than rethink the entire design concept to achieve many kinds of economies at once. Years ago, I was asked to help make a new desktop computer far more energy efficient. One of the first things I suggested was using a slightly more expensive, high-reliability, flat-curve, very-high-efficiency power supply. As you might imagine, the bean counters went nuts until I showed them how these supplies threw off much less heat, eliminating the need for the cooling fan. That saved more manufacturing cost than the excellent power supply added.

The tiny form-factor of the new power supply also reduced the size and cost of the case, improving packaging and customer convenience. Ergonomics got even better because there was no fan noise—a great new marketing feature. As a bonus, the reduced thermal load allowed for a sealed case design, which, along with the lack of fan-forced airflow, eliminated the dust accumulation on chips and circuit boards that cause heat buildup implicated in a majority of premature system failures. So, a single, well-placed improvement ended up yielding multiple benefits that paid back the increased cost of the power supply several times over and yielded a much more marketable and durable product.

LG: So thinking beyond the immediate problem really paid off.

AL: And that was years ago. Much more is possible today, with the aggressive energy management technologies now available and the low-power, flat-panel displays that are becoming so popular. The trick to design excellence is avoiding "infectious repetitis."

LG: What?

AL: Infectious repetitis—the tendency to repeat old mistakes without thinking. It's a common disease among engineers, and quite contagious unless you're inoculated against it. In a normal engineering setting, you're often taking designs and procedures that have been developed previously and are directed to make incremental changes to them using rule-of-thumb design practices. Typically, these practices are based on old information that was not well thought out in the first place and leads to extremely suboptimal designs. Often, a local cost savings, such as a cheap power supply or a bargain-basement motor, a commodity window or a skinny pipe, can lead to a much larger overall system cost.

LG: So, what's the cure, Doctor?

AL: Breaking free of rule-of-thumb engineering requires rethinking most of the design process. A good place to start is to identify and correct the negative or perverse incentives that are encouraging poor design.

LG: Perverse incentives?

AL: Most engineering organizations reward certain kinds of inefficiencies. After all, a manager typically is evaluated on the initial cost of the system his or her team produces, not the cost of its operation. Engineering time also is rationed carefully, so few people are given the time to study really carefully the problem they're solving. This results in things like copying the plans for a cooling system, lighting plan, or other design that sort of worked on another project and making the minimal changes needed to shoehorn it into the next job. This yields grossly missized systems that often are working against each other because nobody stopped to think about how they all fit together. And then, if performance isn't carefully measured, there's no feedback to improve the next design.

Another prime area to look for perverse incentives is the rules of thumb that are used to specify components and select materials. Often, the engineering manuals that specify wire gauges, pipe diameters, valve types and sizes, thermal insulation levels, heat-exchanger areas, and other things that we'd rather not bother thinking about are terribly out of date. The "common wisdom" only looked at the cost of the component, not the cost of the resources it carries—yet it got passed down as gospel!

LG: So, I guess there are all kinds of silly rules of thumb hobbling us today? From what you say, saving a few dollars on each component, and bringing the job in under cost, can force the owner to live with a bunch of badly designed, poorly coordinated systems that will break down too often and cost much more than they should to operate.

AL: When the National Electrical Code specifies a certain gauge wire, it gives you the smallest gauge that will not pose a fire hazard at a given amperage, not the gauge that gives you the lowest life-cycle costs. That is, the NEC is meant to prevent fires, not to save money. If you want to save money, you often should double the wire diameter, cutting resistive losses by 75%. If, instead, a designer were rewarded not just for delivering a product or building to a certain price but also for things like life-cycle cost or operational longevity, we'd see many more people interested in whole-system engineering! For example, on a fully loaded commercial lighting circuit, using one-size-fatter wire yields about a 169%-per-year after-tax return. Why wasn't it so specified? Because the wire size is chosen by the low-bid electrician who's told to meet code. An electrician altruistic enough to buy fatter wire to cut your future electric bills wouldn't be the low bidder any more and hence wouldn't be chosen by the general contractor. So optimal wire size won't be chosen unless the owner or developer requires and rewards that choice.

Rewarding engineers for measured savings also would start to focus their attention on empirical costs rather than theoretical assumptions. For example, we all assume that premium-efficiency industrial motors cost more to purchase—as they should, because they use more and better copper and iron. Surprise! In fact, there is no correlation whatever between efficiency and price for 1800-rpm

NEMA Type B machines up to at least 200 hp (and probably for lots of other kinds, too—that's just one we happen to have examined). In God we trust; all others bring data . . . a good principle to apply to any area of engineering!

LG: Well, it can be applied to any area of engineering that your management allows you to. There's no way that most engineering groups can convince management to take the risks and invest in the kind of effort it takes to do a whole-systems design.

AL: Managing management may be the toughest part of an engineer's job, but it can be done. Actually, selling your organization on new ideas can be a very constructive part of the design process. The trick is to get outside your very comfortable engineering head space and try to understand the motivations of the rest of the members of your team. Once you have a sense of what's important to these folks, it's easy to frame a new engineering approach in a way that makes sense to them—to speak to them where they're at, not where you're at.

LG: So you pitch an idea with a strong emphasis on the bottom line?

AL: That's a good start, but be sure to use whole-systems accounting to identify the many categories of savings that would result. Don't just talk about energy savings, give a detailed accounting of things like reduced maintenance or service calls, improved productivity, reduced downtime, improved customer satisfaction, extended service life, and all the other factors that your solution will yield. Wherever possible, use dollars-and-cents estimates. Speak to managers' concerns in their language.

You also can couch environmental issues in ways that are easy to appreciate. When you talk about pollution prevention, it's always good to show how simple upstream measures can avoid embroilment with complex and costly regulatory issues. Environmental performance also is becoming a strategic marketing issue—a big plus for you. Power efficiency, recyclability, nontoxicity, and other design features are becoming key differentiating factors in certain markets, such as governments and several large companies with emerging "green purchasing" policies. As soon as you can get management to recognize that efficient design is a strategic resource that makes them look good, you've got their attention!

LG: Everything you've talked about sounds really great in theory, but has anybody applied all of this stuff in the real world? Are there any results an engineer can learn from, and point to as an example?

AL: Yes and yes. Rocky Mountain Institute and its affiliated organizations have conducted numerous real-world projects over the past 20 years and produced results that often surprised even us. These have ranged from consulting on the retrofitting of office buildings and factories to achieve severalfold energy savings to designing composite-bodied, computerized, 100+ mile-per-gallon, mid-sized, uncompromised cars that should go into production in the next few years. Other projects have addressed problems with water and wastewater, urban design, land-use planning, and electric power generation and distribution. No matter what engineering discipline you're involved with, we've probably done some work relevant to it.

If any of your readers want to know more about what we're up to, we have a fun-to-visit Web site at www.rmi.org, which offers diverse publications detailing our nonproprietary work. If you are not "wired" you can call or write the institute's outreach specialists at 1739 Snowmass Creek Road, Snowmass, CO 81654-9199, 970/927-3851, fax -4510, outreach@rmi.org. Excellent technical design tools are available from RMI's E SOURCE subsidiary at www.esource.com, 4755 Walnut Street, Boulder, CO 80301, 303/440-8500, fax -8502. Recent RMI publications posted on the Web include "Putting Central Power Plants Out of Business," at http://redtail.stanford.edu/seminar/presentations/lovins1/sld001.htm; "Negawatts for Fabs," at http://redtail.stanford.edu/seminar/presentations/lovins3/index.htm; and "Climate: Making Sense *and* Making Money," at www.rmi.org/catalog/climate.htm.

Part I

Designing for Energy Efficiency

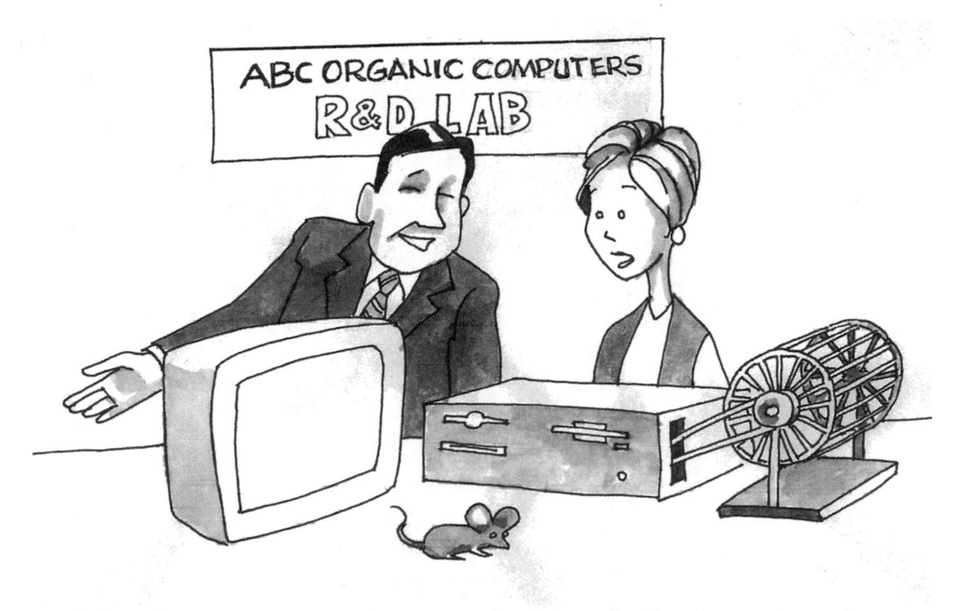

And as a bonus, our new organic power pack generates fertilizer for your houseplants.

CHAPTER 1

Designing Energy-Efficient PCs Using Integrated Power Management

GARY SMERDON

Marketing Director AMD, Network Products Division, Sunnyvale, California

Considering the growing number of personal computers and workstations at use throughout the world, the current trend to make them as energy efficient as possible can translate into significant savings in electricity and the fossil fuel required to generate power. Studies performed by the U.S. Energy Information Administration determined that, in 1995, U.S. office PCs consumed approximately 250 trillion BTU (around 65 billion kilowatt-hours) of energy (Goldberg, 1998). This figure is expected to increase by 15% or more by 2015. On a similar note, a study by the Microelectronics and Computer Corporation, Austin, Texas, revealed that computers will account for around 10% of the projected electrical consumption in the United States by the year 2000 (Goldberg, 1998). Clearly then, improvements in computer power efficiency can have a significant positive effect on the environment.

Among the many important aspects to PC power conservation (power supply efficiency, low-power displays, low-power processors, etc.), one of the most promising areas to affect energy conservation is in changing the power consumption of computers when they are not in use. Often, the average corporate or domestic computer user is at the keyboard only 3–4 hours a day but leaves the machine on continuously. This means that a savings of 70% or more can be realized by implementing a means to put the machine into a low-power idle, or "sleep," mode while it awaits its next task. As corporate and institutional computer purchasers become more environmentally aware and energy conscious, market forces are making the emerging discipline of power management an important aspect of computer design.

A Brief History of the Green PC

The power management features of the PC architecture have evolved to high levels of sophistication and standardization to meet the diverse needs of the business, home, and portable computing segments. The OnNow Initiative, first supported in Windows 98, finally brought integrated power management to the next generation of PCs. This industry standard embraces a diverse collection of hardware and software standards that provide system designers the opportunity to design computers that not only manage their own energy consumption but also work in concert with peripherals and other networked devices.

The early efforts in power management technology began as a natural outgrowth of the short battery life of portable computers in the late 1980s. Rudimentary power management then came to desktop PC architectures in phases as a result of government regulation to stimulate energy conservation in the early 1990s. In 1992, the U.S. Environmental Protection Agency (EPA) created a set of regulations that gave birth to the Energy Star Program. Energy Star requirements encompass many types of consumer products, including PCs (www.epa.gov/energystar.html).

The 1993 executive order, which required that all PCs, monitors, and printers purchased by U.S. federal government agencies meet Energy Star requirements, helped create the first wave of "Green PCs." These machines were designed using a mix of proprietary techniques and industry standards to meet the Energy Star requirement that, after 15–30 minutes of inactivity, the PC enter a low-power sleep mode where it draws 30 W or less.

Many solutions developed for portable systems were adapted for desktops. For the relatively simple 486-class units, the 25 W limit could be met simply by spinning down the hard disk drive. With the proliferation of the Intel Pentium processor, meeting the 25 W limit involved slowing or stopping the processor clock.

Since CRT monitors make up a major portion of a PC system's overall power usage, they too incorporate power savings modes. Energy Star monitors have a 30 W limit and must support the display power management signaling standard or equivalent, which put the monitor into a sleep mode after 15–30 minutes and into its lowest power mode within 70 minutes.

Power Management Evolution

The advanced power management (APM) technique was the first ad hoc industry standard. Devised by Microsoft and Intel to work in DOS and Windows portables environments, APM was a simple scheme with two different power states, known as *suspend* and *resume*. After a period of inactivity, the system entered the suspend state through a special software interrupt that was implemented in the APM BIOS in ROM.

Special hardware also could be used to turn off a laptop's LCD display and spin down the hard disk. Since portables generally were self-contained, the BIOS had to be aware of only the hardware components integrated in the system. Specialized keyboard controllers remained active when the processor was stopped and were responsible for beginning the resume process when the keyboard or mouse was touched.

APM was applied to desktop systems, but with some limitations. In general, desktops were not self-contained, and therefore, some components could not be power managed. Desktops controlled the factory-installed hard disk and slowed the processor but left the expansion bus (e.g., ISA, VL, PCI) powered on to respond to interrupts.

Reducing CRT Power

Outside the PC system enclosure lurks one very power-hungry component, the CRT. While PCs became more efficient, color CRT monitors became larger and began to consume as much, or more, power than the PC itself. In addition, the only connection between the monitor and the PC was the standard VGA connector with no specialized auxiliary connectors.

The Video Electronics Standards Association (www.vesa.org) solved many of these problems with the introduction of the Display Power Management Signaling Standard 1.0 (DPMS). DPMS uses a simple signaling scheme on the existing horizontal sync and vertical sync signals to support four unique states. Since most monitors are so-called multisync monitors supporting various scanning rates, they already have some intelligence to interpret the sync signals. The DPMS states correspond to APM states as follows.

State switching is achieved simply through the presence or absence of horizontal or vertical sync pulses. Since some existing display controllers were not capable of turning off sync pulses altogether, the "no pulses" state is defined as less than 10 Hz with a less than 25% duty cycle rather than a 0 Hz display rate. To avoid accidental state changes during resolution or mode changes, it is recommended that the display wait at least five seconds before entering a power saving state from the on state. In addition, video should be blanked in all power-saving states. Under the Windows 3.1 operating system, the display would enter DPMS suspend at the same time as the rest of the system enters APMS suspend via a software interface defined in the VESA BIOS power management (VBE/PM) specification. Under the Windows 95 operating system, display power management is integrated in the standard screen saver accessible through the Control Panel. Windows 95 bypasses the video BIOS and communicates directly with a DPMS-aware video driver. The screen saver supports both standby and suspend modes, allowing multiple levels of power savings. Note that the Display Control Panel describes the suspend mode as shut off monitor even though the DPMS Off state is not used.

Green PCs vs. Network PCs

Over the last few years, network technology and green PC technology have evolved in parallel, and occasionally antagonistic, directions. Often, they seem to be competing rather than complementing each other at the PC desktop. As companies and institutions have shifted more of their operational capabilities onto desktop computers, it has become critical for network managers to have remote access to the PCs.

Unfortunately, green PCs are not inherently network friendly. That is, if the machine is asleep (in a low-powered state), it cannot be addressed from the network. A computer in sleep mode cannot be used by network administrators and MIS personnel to perform tasks, such as backups or installation of software upgrades at remote sites. These tasks normally are performed during evenings and off hours to minimize the impact of system downtime on the users.

Powered-down green PCs frustrated corporate IS departments, which were primarily interested in keeping their networks available. To maintain control of the network, many system administrators were forced to disable the power management features, causing the computers to consume twice as much electricity overnight than their actual daytime usage. This issue was the impetus for the development of magic packet technology, which provides the intelligence required to awaken a sleeping PC across the network.

Several network protocol stacks have evolved to address the problem of lost network connections on corporate networks. A mechanism is required to wake these sleeping systems during off hours. Taking this idea one step further, the mechanism could be developed to remotely turn on systems powered off by the user, so that users did not have to leave their systems on when not in use.

Hewlett-Packard's PC division recognized these problems and developed the concept of a special packet that the network controller could recognize and use to signal the system. Working together, AMD and Hewlett Packard (HP) came up with a silicon solution to this problem in mid-1995. Since power generally is on inside a green machine, the network side of the machine could be left in a state in which it could continue to scan every packet coming in from the network.

The two companies developed a scheme to wake remote PCs that employed a special, or "magic," Ethernet frame that did not occur in normal network traffic. Known as the *magic packet* frame, this "awaken" message consists of the PC's node address repeated 16 times. Embedding the necessary circuitry to recognize and respond to a magic packet frame requires only a small amount of additional logic in standard 10BASE-T or 100BASE-T Ethernet controller and uses only one signal connected to the power management logic.

When magic packet-capable PCs are powered down, they go into a sleep mode but leave a small portion of their network interface circuitry active and connected to the LAN, monitoring the link for the transmission of a magic packet frame. When another PC sends the magic packet frame, the Ethernet media access controller (MAC) in the receiving system creates a system interrupt that activates the automatic power-up sequence for the rest of the system.

To promote a standardized energy management method, AMD licensed the magic packet technology to many leading network silicon vendors such as Intel and Digital Equipment at minimal cost, on a royalty-free basis. Since magic packet-capable controllers debuted in PCs from Hewlett-Packard's Performance Desktop

Company, it has been widely utilized and accepted in the industry. Subsequently, PC makers Toshiba and Unisys announced systems that utilize the technology.

Based on this technology, remote desktop management has reduced the total cost of ownership (TCO) of PCs by simplifying network maintenance and enabling desktop PCs to be managed and administered remotely. Activities including asset management, driver and application updates, file backups, and BIOS updates can be accomplished remotely.

Magic packet technology gives network administrators the ability to power up a PC from across the network. Once a magic packet frame awakens a PC, it can be managed through normal means. Standards-based software solutions use the desktop management interface (DMI) to accomplish a variety of end-to-end enterprise network management functions, such as remotely running PC diagnostics or distributing software updates.

While magic packet technology is a solid solution for large LANs controlled by enterprise management tools, it does not work as effectively in the many clusters of smaller peer-to-peer networks found in smaller offices and home environments today. Implementing power management in this environment requires an even more sophisticated wake-up scheme that is integrated within the existing installed base of applications and management solutions and does not require special packets. This led to the development of the OnNow initiative from Microsoft, envisioned as a wake-up scheme based on the concept of "virtual connections." As we shall see, this capability is possible but requires embedding more intelligence in the network controller to filter packets while the rest of the system is sleeping.

The OnNow Initiative

The OnNow design initiative is a comprehensive, systemwide approach to system and device power control that puts the operating system in control of power management. OnNow describes a PC that is always on but appears to be off. OnNow systems respond immediately to requests from both local and remote users.

OnNow involves changes in the Microsoft Windows 98 and Windows NT operating systems, device drivers, hardware subsystems, and software applications themselves. The latest information and specifications concerning the OnNow initiative are posted at www.microsoft.com/hwdev/onnow.htm. As a part of the OnNow initiative, AMD and Microsoft jointly developed a specification defining the requirements for such a network controller. Together with Microsoft, AMD wrote the networking class power management reference specification for the OnNow 1.0 version.

The OnNow initiative represents the first time that power management is fully integrated into an operating system. The operating system views the hardware platform as made up of a motherboard and peripherals and adapters. The operating system interface to the motherboard is defined by a new specification known as the *advanced configuration and power interface* (ACPI).

ACPI Specification

ACPI is implemented by leading chip vendors and PC companies in conjunction with Microsoft. ACPI is a foundation technology that enables the operating system to intelligently control the amount of power used by each device attached to the computer.

Beyond moving the locus of control from the BIOS into the operating system, OnNow specifications bring about other important improvements. First, individual devices now will be managed separately instead of having one system power state applied to all devices. The ACPI controls when the operating system goes to sleep, when it wakes up, and when it enables functionality. With ACPI support, the operating system can turn off peripheral devices, such as CD-ROM players and modems, when they are not in use.

Second, with ACPI support, applications could be made power-management aware so that they enhance rather than prevent power savings. This will enable manufacturers to produce computers that automatically power up as they are needed.

The ACPI is a fairly complex architecture with multiple layers of hardware and software specifications and interfaces. The ACPI specification defines a standard register interface for functions such as system events, processor power and thermal management, clock control, and resume handling. The ACPI specification, implementers guide, and a listing of frequently asked questions is listed at the ACPI Web site (www.teleport.com/~acpi/).

Device Class Specifications

Different devices have varying constraints and capabilities with regard to power management. In addition, the OS already has different classes of devices operating through different control stacks. To maximize power savings and functionality, a series of different specifications for different device classes were defined as audio, communications, display, input, network, PC card, and storage. Each class has its own specification detailing how these devices should behave.

All device classes share four defined power states, D0–D3. These power states are independent of the system power state, enabling devices not in use to be put to sleep even when the system appears fully operational to the user. D0 is the fully on state, with maximum power consumption and full performance and functionality available. D3 is the lowest-power state, where in some cases power may be removed from the device altogether. D3 with power is called *D3hot*, while the powered-off state is called *D3cold*. The primary difference is that devices in D3hot must still respond to configuration space accesses so that they can be returned to D0 without the need for a reset.

Devices supporting power management in D3cold must preserve information about their earlier state during the transition back to D0. This, of course, implies that some type of auxiliary power is available to the device. Recovery from D3 is slow, since device context may be lost and must be restored. The D1 and D2 states fall in between D0 and D3 and are useful for devices that can support intermediate levels of power consumption and functionality. For example, in the display class, D1 represents the DPMS standby state, with a typical recovery time of less than 5 seconds. D2 takes the CRT to the DPMS suspend state and enables a typical recovery time less than 10 seconds.

One of the most challenging classes was the network device, due to the unique requirements associated with the virtual connection concept discussed earlier. The network device class specification includes a new wake-up mechanism that enables a virtual connection by filtering incoming packets. The protocol stack recognizes the types of packets important to maintaining the network connection. The device driver is told by the protocol stack what packets to look for in the filters. Two other wake-up sources are magic packet frames and link status changes (cable connect/disconnect). The controller signals the system through a bus specific wake-up signal. For desktop applications, most controllers will use the PME# signal on the PCI bus (discussed later).

PCI Bus Power Management

The PCI bus has been extended to support power management through the PCI bus power management interface specification, which was completed in June 1997. This specification defines the bus states (B0, B3) and mechanisms for controlling the bus power and clock. It also defines the function of a new PCI bus signal called power management event (PME#).

Since this is an extension to the PCI bus, changes to the PCI configuration space were required to allow discovery of a device's capabilities. Two changes were made to the original 40H bytes of configuration space header. First, Bit 4 of the status register (offset 06H) indicates extended capabilities. If Bit 4 is set, there is a linked list of extended capabilities. This linked list is pointed to by a byte in a previously reserved location (offset 34H) known as the *capabilities pointer*.

This pointer simply is the offset into the PCI configuration space where the first extended item can be found. The item then begins with a capability ID field and next item pointer, so that other extensions can be linked in the future. The capability ID is an 8-bit field with a value of 01H for the PCI power management type. The next item pointer also is 8 bits and set to 00H if this is the last or only item in the list. The rest of the item consists of a 16-bit read-only power management capabilities register, a 16-bit power management control/status register, and an option 8-bit read-only data register. The capabilities register provides information on what states are supported (specifically D1 and D2) as well as which states support assertion of PME#.

The control/status register handles control of the PME# signal, power state query and setting, clock control, and power requirement reporting. For PCI chip designers, further details can be found in Chapter 3 of the PCI bus power management interface specification.

As with devices, four bus power states are defined for the PCI bus. B0 is the fully on state capable of any legal PCI bus transaction. Data transactions can take place only in this state. B1 is an idle state where Vcc is maintained to all devices on the bus and all bus signals are required to be held at valid logic states. Unlike B0, no transactions are allowed. B2 is identical to B1 except that the clock is stopped and held low. B3 is the off state, where power is removed. When recovering from B3, RST# must be asserted and the bus returned to an idle state. Therefore, this is the same as a cold boot situation with any PCI revision 2.1 compliant implementation.

The new PME# signal is an optional open drain, active low signal assigned to pin A19 of the standard PCI connector. This signal is asynchronous to the PCI clock. When asserted, it should be driven low until software clears the PME status bit in the status/control register. The system will typically wire-OR the PME# signal from all slots together. It also must provide a pull-up resistor on the signal.

Add-in card design for this signal is more complex than for a simple open drain driver, because the signal is shared between devices that may be in different power states. A device in D3cold must not assert PME#, while a device with power must not cause damage to a device in D3cold. Refer to Chapter 7 of the specification for add-in card implementation details.

A PCI engineering change request (ECR) was approved by the PCI SIG Steering Committee to add a 3.3V auxiliary power pin on the bus. This provides a standardized way for devices supporting wake-up events (through PME#) in D3cold to get auxiliary power. Without this specification, ECR power had to be provided by special connectors, fly wires, wall transformers, and the like. The ECR assigns pin 14A as 3.3Vaux. The maximum current available to an enabled device is 375 mA. System designers should refer to the ECR (Addition of 3.3Vaux Signal to Connector) for a more detailed description of power requirements.

PC 98 Requirements

The *PC 98 System Design Guide* specifies power management requirements for designed for Windows 98 logo compliance. In general, the system must support ACPI 1.0 or higher but some ACPI options are mandatory for PC 98. A real-time clock alarm that supports wake-up due to a scheduled time and day of the month is required. At least one of the S1, S2, or S3 sleep states is required in addition to S5 (soft off). The USB host controller must be able to wake the system from at least one sleeping state (S1, S2, or S3). Implementing the ACPI thermal model and fan control is recommended to reduce fan noise but is not mandatory. Finally, the system should not provide any capability to disable ACPI support.

In addition to the ACPI requirements are requirements related to the OnNow user experience. For instance, the PC must appear to be off when it is in a sleep state. The user should hear no noise and see no lights coming from disk drives, fans, the display, and so forth. There also should be an LED sleep indicator, so the user can tell whether the PC is working or sleeping. A message waiting indicator is recommended for systems with telephone answering machine capabilities.

Power states must be controllable through both switches and software. The system can have either a power button or a sleep button, but having both is recommended. The sleep button should be the user's primary switch and the power button should be hidden. There also must be an override mechanism in case a hardware or software failure prevents normal operation of the software-controlled buttons. The recommended implementation is to override the software controls and turn off the PC when the sleep button is held down for 4 seconds.

Beyond ACPI, integrated buses and devices must support their relevant power management specifications. This includes the PCI, USB, 1394, and PC card buses. Integrated devices must support the specification for their class. It is recommended that they support the D1 or D2 states and wake-up events as defined for their class. Additional OnNow BIOS requirements are detailed in Chapter 3 of the *PC 98 System Design Guide*.

Developing Remote Wake and Power-on Systems

The magic packet technology enables better working networks within the corporate environment and easily can be added to a green-enabled computer at little or no cost above the standard system cost.

PC vendors and embedded system users who implement magic packet technology have a variety of hardware options, including different interfaces for three different hardware models. To bring a complete solution to the market, designers also must understand how the DOS-level magic packet software driver interfaces both with the operating system and the hardware. These technical issues are described in detail in the application note "Magic Packet Technology Application in Hardware and Software" (www.amd.com/products/npd/techdocs/20381a.pdf). Highlights of the application note are summarized here for convenience.

Hardware Options

In the competitive PC environment, *green* has become the byword for the next new standard system feature. The original targets by the Department of Energy (DOE) in its green recommendations were 30 W for the system box and 30 W for the monitor in a low-power state. Since these values were relatively easy to obtain in current technology, the market has shifted to asking the question, "How deep a shade of green is your system?"

At least three different solutions to obtaining green status are now in the market. The following solutions are ordered from most power used to least power used:

1. Simply lower the clock speed on the motherboard to a slow speed, usually 8 MHz. Shut down all disks and stop all synch signals at the video controller.
2. Stop the processor clock, putting the DRAM in slow refresh, in addition to solution 1.
3. Suspend to disk all DRAM and control registers, and then power off the entire system, leaving a small auxiliary power supply to some circuits to allow them to awaken the sleeping machine.

In examining each option, next, an increasing level of complexity will be found in the hardware solutions to implement the magic packet technology. In time, some system vendors may use each of these levels in the orderly shutdown of the box to meet the needs of the green PC market.

Hardware Model 1

Hardware Model 1 requires no hardware, software, or even magic packet technology for implementation, because nothing in the system box, except the disks, is shut down. All network activity is fully alive and the speed of the CPU can be varied with the interrupt rate being handled. The CPU is not stopped and the network controller is not required to do anything differently.

Hardware Model 2

Hardware Model 2 requires some level of interface. Since clocks are stopped in this implementation, something must be used to return the system to normal operating mode. Without the network card installed in the system box, either a keystroke or mouse movement could repower the system to full power. In reality, either of these actions could cause an interrupt on the backplane. This model contains a circuit added by chip set vendors to monitor specifically designated interrupts for activity and then return the clock to the CPU, signaling this event through a technique known as *system management interrupt* (SMI).

Since most controllers already use an interrupt line to signal that the driver's service is needed for network-related activities, this same interrupt line can be used to wake the system as well. The waking interrupt can be added to the designated interrupt list in the main system board setup menu. However, with the PCI clock stopped, neither direct memory access (DMA) activity nor magic packet interrupt generation by the controller on the PCI bus can take place.

Since normal operation of most network controllers requires DMA activity, they must be placed in magic packet mode. In this mode, the controller will initiate no DMA activity. All incoming data are scanned by the address recognition logic until a magic packet is received. When this occurs, magic packet interrupt (MPINT) is set in CSR 5 (bit 4) and reported through the interrupt pin if MPINTE is set in CSR 5 (bit 3).

This level of compliance, required for both green and network specifications, can be achieved on any current card or motherboard implementation on the open market, with no need for hardware additions or modifications.[1] However, one issue must be considered for PCI-based designs. If the PCI clock is stopped when in standby mode, a PCI interrupt cannot be generated, requiring the use of an LED pin to perform the interrupt operation.

Hardware Model 3

Achieving Hardware Model 3 compliance involves solving several hardware implementation issues. Currently, computer systems that have a deep sleep mode rely on the modem ring detect input signal to wake thc sleeping unit. When the modem is called for the first time, the ring detector pulses a logic input to the system box. Because the serial port lacks the data set ready (DSR) true line, the modem does not answer. However, the system starts up its power. The calling party times out and calls again; and by this time, the system is powered up and ready. This is the model to be emulated in a network adapter card using magic packet technology.

Since the network card is plugged into the backplane, which will be powered down, the power for the network card must come from an alternate source. This power is usually supplied by an auxiliary power supply connection. The normal +5 volt connection to the ISA or PCI bus connector is an open circuit. This auxiliary supply would have to be able to supply an additional 100 milliamperes.

The next issue that must be addressed is that of reset. Since the power on the backplane will be cycling, a reset will occur on the first power up and then on the power down and yet a third reset on the subsequent power up. Since a reset to the controller would take the magic packet detection logic off line, at least the second reset has to be blocked, or the MAC will be taken off line and the magic packet frame will not be seen.

Magic Packet DOS Interface

Software is used to interface the network drivers and magic packet code with the operating system. Originally, Microsoft and Intel established a power management standard for DOS systems called the *advanced power management* (APM) specification. In the APM specification, some system interrupts were established to inform the necessary drivers needing the information that the system is preparing for power down or going to resume from a power down state.

Unfortunately, by the time the APM specification was created, all the interrupts used within DOS already were assigned. Therefore, interrupt 2F was chosen to be the APM interrupt. Interrupt 2F had been the catchall for miscellaneous interrupts, so that any driver associating with this interrupt has to check whether this interrupt is even available for its use. Therefore, this interrupt will be used in the DOS-based terminate stay resident (TSR) driver.

A DOS TSR was developed to form the interface between DOS, the PCI controller, and the network driver. Because of the way the operating system and the network drivers work, the APM is unknown to the network stack. This may change in the future, but for now the real interface will be between the operating system and the hardware itself. Once loaded, the network driver operates strictly via interrupts, so that if there are no interrupts the system is asleep and waiting. The hardware is set up by the driver to generate interrupts only for the receive activity.

Transmit activity is initiated by a system call to the disk redirector, which eventually filters down to a call to the transmit routine. Therefore, if the system goes to sleep, no redirection effort will be made because no programs will be running. If the PCI controller hardware is put into its suspend mode before being put into magic packet mode, then any receive activity will be used for magic packet detection only.

Because of this independence between the magic packet TSR driver and the network driver, it was decided to treat them as separate entities. The advantage is that both programs can be revised independently as needed. In addition, the TSR is written so that it can be loaded in any order with respect to the network driver, and both can coexist. If the TSR is loaded without the network driver, the MAC is never initialized and enabled, thereby disabling magic packet functionality.

Developing Magic Packet-Ready Motherboards

If a manufacturer already employs a motherboard-mounted Ethernet connection, magic packet technology can be added at a very small extra cost. The main requirements are the power management circuit, which is popular in many computers, a standby power supply, and one extra connector and cable. This relatively small investment can yield large returns by providing manufacturers with a strategic marketing advantage and users with large energy savings.

The application note "Implementation of Magic Packet-Ready Motherboards" (www.amd.com/products/npd/techdocs/21383a.pdf) provides a description of building a magic packet-ready motherboard for network adapter applications. It also presents the standard signals and connectors that are used in a motherboard. Highlights of the application note are summarized here for convenience.

Magic packet technology is implemented, as a system solution composed of the motherboard, network adapter card, standby supply, BIOS, and network management software. The motherboard-based Ethernet controller accepts the wake-up signal and generates a wake-up signal that will wake the motherboard either from its standby or suspend mode. In the standby mode, the computer is alive and kicking, with power to the entire motherboard. The low power consumption in this mode is accomplished by slowing down the processor clock, spinning down the hard drives, and putting the monitor in a low power consumption state.

In the suspend mode, the computer usually is brought to a complete halt. The CPU is stopped and the power even may be removed. The entire system is powered down, except the power management circuit, which in many cases is a Super I/O or a keyboard controller chip, and the Ethernet controller, which receives the magic packet that wakes up the system.

Power Management and Power Supply

Many PCs already implement a remote wake-up from standby mode via modem ring. When a modem is called for an incoming fax or e-mail, the RI (ring input) signal of COM1 port is asserted. The RI signal is an input to a super I/O chip.

The support for power management circuit requires the incorporation of a standby supply with built-in soft power on. The standby supply will enable the power management circuit and the Ethernet controller circuit. The power requirement for a typical power management circuit is 100 mA, and the Ethernet circuit is 450 mA (in magic packet mode). Therefore, the recommended capacity is at least 550 mA.

Designing Magic Packet Adapter Cards

Some designers may choose to use an adapter card for their network connection instead of the motherboard. To support magic packet protocols in a bus-based adapter, one needs to implement the complete system solution; that is, motherboard, network interface card (NIC), BIOS, standby power supply, and desktop management software.

The application note "Magic Packet Adapter Cards Implementation" (www.amd.com/products/npd/techdocs/21385a.pdf) discusses the various aspects of magic packet adapter card design. To familiarize you with some key concepts, selected portions of the app note follow.

> In this scenario, the motherboard accepts the wakeup signal from the Magic Packet capable NIC and performs the power management protocol. The wakeup signal will wake the motherboard from either standby or suspend mode. In standby mode, the computer is alive, with power to the entire motherboard, with low power consumption accomplished by slowing down the processor clock, spinning down the hard drives, and putting the monitor into a low power consumption state. In suspend mode, the computer is usually brought to a complete halt. The CPU is stopped and the main power supply is turned off, leaving the standby power supply to support the components. The entire system is powered down, except the power management circuit (often a Super I/O or a keyboard controller chip) and the Ethernet components that receive the Magic Packet frame that wakes up the system.

Managing Energy Managers

Much attention has been paid to the hardware portion of the system implementation, but several important software aspects must be noted. On the desktop management software side, a magic packet generation utility such as MPWAKE, can run in conjunction with any existing desktop management software package. IBM Infinity and HP OpenView already integrate this support into their current offerings. Several popular vendor software packages, such as LANDesk from Intel and Unicenter TNG from Computer Associates also integrate support for the magic packet technology.

Note

1. AMD has designed magic packet technology into two of its network controllers, the PCnet ISA II (79C961A) and the PCnet PCI II (79C970A). Both controllers are available and in production today. For further information, refer to the following AMD data sheets: Am79C961A Data Sheet (PID 19364) and Am79C970A Data Sheet (PID 19436).

Reference

Goldberg, Lee. "The Advent of Green Computer Design." *IEEE Computer Magazine* (September 1998), pp. 16–19.

CHAPTER 2

Energy Efficient Three-Phase AC Motor Drives for Appliance and Industrial Applications

RADIM VISINKA

System Application Engineer, Motorola Inc.

Benefits of Microcontrollers in Motor Drives

Electrical energy conservation has become an important part of the overall trend toward protecting the natural environment. Electrical motors that drive systems in both appliances and industry consume a significant part of the produced energy. Most of these motors are AC induction machines that usually operate uncontrolled and thus with low efficiency. Recent progress in the semiconductor industry, especially in power electronics and microcontrollers, has made variable-speed drives more practical and much less expensive. Today, adjustable-speed AC motor drives are required not only for highly professional and high power/performance industrial applications, like tool machines or cranes, but more and more for home appliances, like washing machines, compressors, small pumps, and air conditioning. These drives, controlled by sophisticated algorithms within microcontrollers, bring a number of advantages to an application:

- *System efficiency increases.* Variable-speed controls reduce wasted power in motors.
- *Performance improvements.* Digital control can add features like a smart digital control loop, variable-frequency wave shaping, fault tolerance, and the ability to communicate with other systems.
- *Simpler electromechanical conversion.* Variable-speed drives can help avoid the need for transmissions and gear boxes.
- *Simple software updates.* A microcontroller-based system with flash memory can have its algorithms and control variables quickly changed as needed.

With the introduction of variable-speed drives, the complexity of the system often is increased. The basic condition of its application is that the total cost of the system must stay within reasonable limits. For a number of systems, especially in appliances, the total cost must be equivalent to the uncontrolled ones.

This chapter presents the basic analysis of a three-phase AC motor control together with a practical design of a low cost three-phase AC drive.

Three-Phase AC Induction Motors Drives

The AC induction motor is the workhorse in adjustable-speed drive systems. The most popular type is a three-phase squirrel-cage AC induction motor that is a low-cost, maintenance-free, low-noise motor. Each phase of the stator winding of the motor consists of a coil and the squirrel-cage rotor consists of short-circuited bars. The stator is supplied by a balanced three-phase AC voltage that induces current in the rotor and thus produces a torque.

The synchronous speed n_s of the motor is given by

$$n_s = \frac{120 \times f_s}{p} \text{ [rpm]} \qquad (1\text{–}1)$$

where f_s is the synchronous stator frequency in Hz, and p is the number of stator poles. The AC induction motor produces zero torque at the synchronous frequency and therefore must run at the speed determined by a load torque. The motor speed is characterized by a slip factor, s_r:

$$s_r = \frac{(n_s - n_r)}{n_s} = \frac{n_{sl}}{n_s} \qquad (1\text{–}2)$$

where n_r is the rotor mechanical speed and n_{sl} is the slip speed (both in rpm). Figure 2–1 illustrates the torque characteristics and corresponding slip for the working point of the motor. As can be seen from equations (1–1) and (1–2), the motor speed is controlled by variation of a stator frequency with influence of the load torque.

In applications requiring adjustable speed, inverters drive the AC motors. The inverters convert DC power to AC power of the required frequency and amplitude. A typical three-phase voltage source inverter is illustrated in Figure 2–2.

The inverter consists of three half-bridge units, where the upper and lower switch is controlled complementarily—meaning, when the upper circuit is turned on, the lower one is turned off and vice versa. The simultaneous turn-on of both switches in the half-bridge unit is prohibited because it short-circuits the power supply. Because of limited switching speed of the power devices, some dead time must be inserted between the turn-off of one transistor of the half-bridge and turn-on of its complementary device. Thus, the power devices are protected. The output voltage usually is created using a pulse width modulation (PWM) technique, where an isosceles triangle carrier wave is compared with a fundamental-frequency sine modulat-

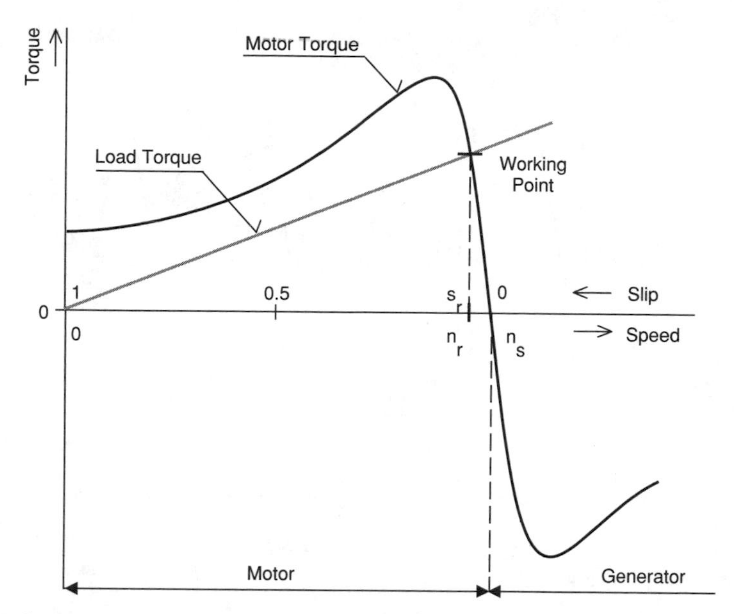

FIGURE 2–1 Torque-speed characteristic at constant voltage and frequency.

ing wave and the natural points of intersection determine the switching points of the power devices of a half-bridge inverter. This technique is shown in Figure 2–3. The three-phase voltage waves are shifted 120° to each other and thus a three-phase motor can be supplied.

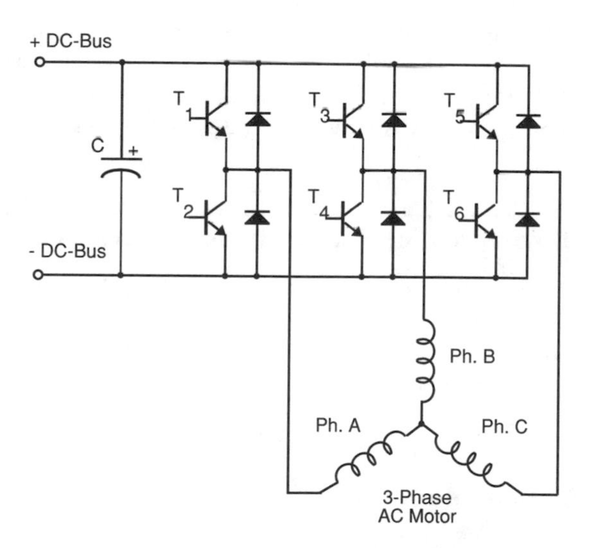

FIGURE 2–2 Three-phase inverter.

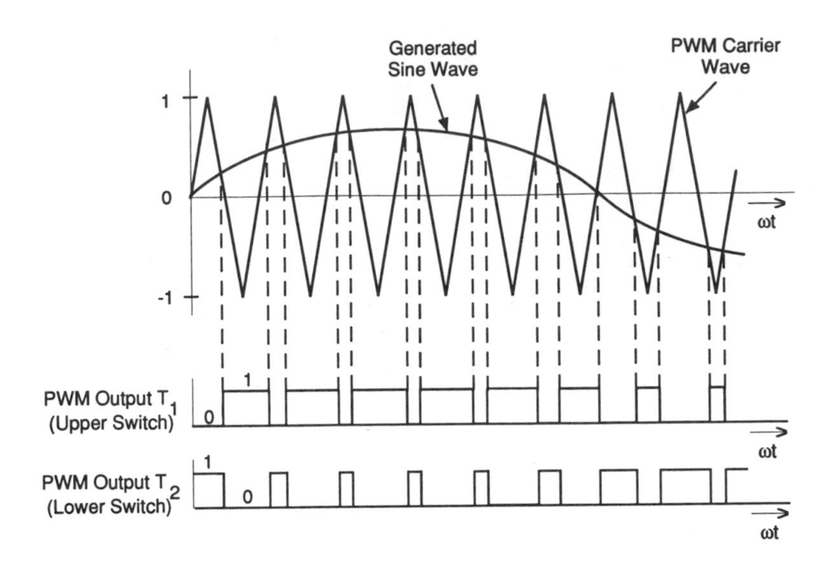

FIGURE 2–3 Pulse width modulation.

Power devices of the inverter are the key components of the motor control. The most popular devices for motor control applications are power MOSFETs and IGBTs.

A *power MOSFET* is a voltage-controlled transistor. Designed for high frequency operation, it has a low voltage drop that results in low power loss. Problems arise, however; the device's low saturation point and its temperature sensitivity limit the MOSFET application in power circuits.

An *insulated gate bipolar transistor* (IGBT) is a bipolar transistor controlled by a MOSFET on its base. The IGBT requires low drive current, has fast switching time, and is suitable for high switching frequencies. Its disadvantage is the higher voltage drop of the bipolar transistor, which causes higher conduction losses.

Control Strategies for Three-Phase AC Drives

A large number of control strategies for three-phase AC motor have been successfully implemented, allowing the motor to be used in a large variety of applications. The methods for control of three-phase AC induction motor mainly fall into the following groups: scalar control methods, vector control methods, adaptive control principles.

Scalar Control Methods

Scalar control methods adjust the magnitude of a variable like frequency, voltage, or current. The command and feedback signals are DC quantities proportional

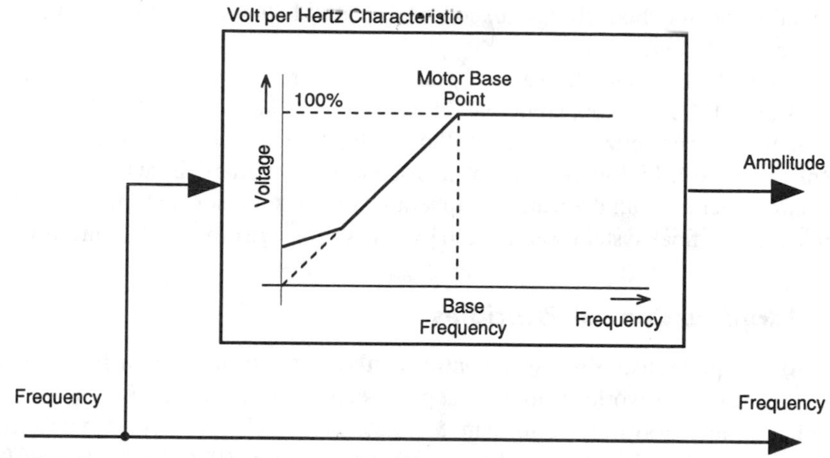

FIGURE 2–4 Volts per hertz control method.

to the respective variables. The most popular method within this group is the volts per hertz control technique, which will be described further.

In volts per hertz control, the voltage applied command is calculated directly from the applied frequency to maintain a constant air-gap flux in the machine. In steady-state operation, the machine air-gap flux is approximately related to the ratio V_s/f_s, where V_s is the amplitude of motor phase voltage and f_s is the synchronous electrical frequency applied to the motor. A typical volts per hertz control system is illustrated in Figure 2–4. The base point of the motor defines the controller's characteristics. Below its base point, the motor operates at optimum excitation because of the constant V_s/f_s ratio. Above this point, the motor operates underexcited because of the DC-bus voltage limit.

A simple open-loop volts per hertz speed control is the technique often used for low-performance drives. This basic scheme is unsatisfactory for more demanding applications, where precision speed control is required.

To improve the basic open-loop system, a closed-loop volts per hertz control was introduced. This method uses a speed sensor to measure the actual motor speed and uses it as a variable in the control loop. A number of applications use the closed-loop volts per hertz method because of its simplicity and relatively good speed accuracy, but it is unsuitable for systems that require servo performance or excellent response to highly dynamic torque or speed variations.

Vector Control Methods

In the vector, or field-oriented, control method, both the magnitude and phase of a vector variable are controlled. Therefore, the AC motor is controlled like a separately excited DC machine. The method takes into consideration not only successive steady states but real mathematical equations that describe the motor itself.

The control results obtained have excellent dynamic behavior for torque variations in a wide speed range.

Although the motor has a very simple structure, its mathematical model is complex (Vas 1992). It is apparent that this technique requires more calculations than a standard volts per hertz control algorithm. One practical way to implement such a system is to use a high-performance microcontroller, perhaps based on a DSP or RISC core together with dedicated peripherals. Such a sophisticated microcontroller often makes the final system solution too expensive for most low-end applications.

Adaptive Control Principles

All the previously discussed control methods are systems with fixed control parameters. In a real-world system, most parameters can vary with different working conditions, causing system performance to deteriorate. The problem can be solved by adaptive control (Rajashekara, Kawamura, and Matuse, 1996; Michels, 1997). In this system, the control parameters are changed according to the current working conditions. Unfortunately, this method demands high computing power and therefore requires the use of high-performance DSP- or RISC-based systems.

Microcontroller Requirements for Motor Control Application

One way to reduce the overall cost of a smart motor controller system is to integrate as many of the essential elements into the controller chip as is economically feasible. The motor control system usually demands a dedicated microcontroller (MCU) that creates the brain of the drive. The motor control microcontroller integrates a central processor unit (CPU) together with special on-chip peripherals that allow one to build the drive most effectively. The main features of the microcontroller required by a low-cost application are as follows:

A 8-bit or 16-bit CPU.
An on-chip memory RAM and ROM; EEPROM or FLASH are the options.
A six-channel motor control PWM unit.
One or more analog-to-digital converters (ADCs).
Timers.
A serial communication interface (SCI), serial peripheral interface (SPI).
A low-voltage reset (LVR).
A computer operating properly (COP).
General purpose input/output (I/O) pins.

The motor control PWM unit is a special peripheral that creates a dedicated motor control part from a more or less standard MCU. This PWM module generates six PWM signals for a three-phase inverter. Key features of the six-channel PWM module include center- or edge-aligned PWM modes, a mode that configures the six outputs as complementary pairs for coherent updates, dead-time generation to prevent short-circuit currents in the motor drive inverter, and fault detect inputs for fast shut down of the PWM outputs. The hardware contained in the PWM module eliminates the need for several external components (i.e., dead-time generation, fault handling, output polarity handling). A microcontroller that lacks these features can be used for the motor control application, but these functions must be built externally with an increase in price and complexity and a decrease in reliability of the system. Therefore, a dedicated device is desirable.

A typical example of the dedicated motor control microcontroller is the Motorola MC68HC908MR24, a HC08-based 8-bit MCU designed for single- or three-phase motor drive applications, including AC, brushless DC, or switched reluctance motors. General features include 24K bytes of FLASH, 768 bytes of RAM, two 16-bit timers, SPI, SCI, 13 general-purpose I/O pins, COP, and a LVR module in a 64-pin QFP package. The internal bus frequency is 8 MHz. The "MR24" also has specific features that target AC induction motor applications, including a six-channel, 12-bit PWM module, a high-current sink port, and a ten-channel 10-bit A/D module.

Design of Low-Cost Three-Phase AC Drive

This section presents a practical design of low-cost three-phase AC drive based on the volts per hertz control technique and a Motorola MC68HC908MR24 microcontroller. The design can be used as a good starting point for an individual drive.

The applications considered are fans, compressors, pumps, air conditioning, or other similar systems, where the total cost of the system is the driving requirement while excellent dynamic performance is not mandatory.

System Requirements

The three-phase AC drive is designed as a low-cost system that meets the general performance requirements listed in Table 2–1.

System Concept

The system is designed to drive a three-phase AC induction motor in a speed closed loop. Based on the requirements stated in Table 2–1, the volts per hertz control algorithm is the best choice, while most of the other methods are out of our scope for the targeted low-cost AC drive. The speed sensor allows us to build a system that improves the speed precision of the drive.

For the drive a standard system concept is chosen (see Figure 2–5), the system incorporates the following parts:

A microcontroller board.
A three-phase inverter.
Feedback sensors: motor speed, DC-bus voltage, DC-bus current, overcurrent.
Opto-isolation between the power stage and the microcontroller.
A power supply.

TABLE 2–1 General Requirements

Motor Characteristics	
Motor type:	4-pole, 3-phase, star-connected, squirrel cage AC induction motor
Speed range:	< 3000 rpm
Base electrical frequency:	50 Hz
Maximum output power:	500 W
Drive Characteristics	
Drive type:	Microcontroller driven 3-phase inverter
Transducer:	16-pole AC tacho-generator
Output frequency range:	< 100 Hz
Line input:	230V/50Hz
Maximum DC-bus voltage:	400 V
Opto-isolation:	Included
Control algorithm:	Speed closed-loop volts per hertz

Hardware Design

Microcontroller Board The microcontroller Motorola MC68HC908MR24 controls the entire drive by reading the speed command together with feedback signals and, according to a preprogrammed algorithm, generating the PWM signals for power devices and status signals for the user interface. Figure 2–6 illustrates the schematic of

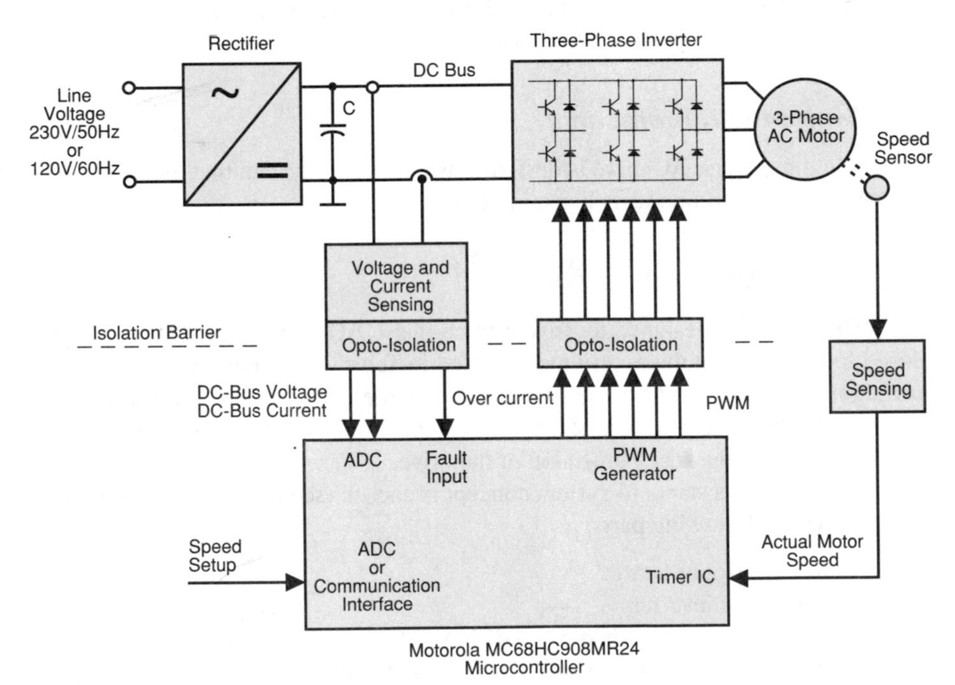

FIGURE 2–5 System concept.

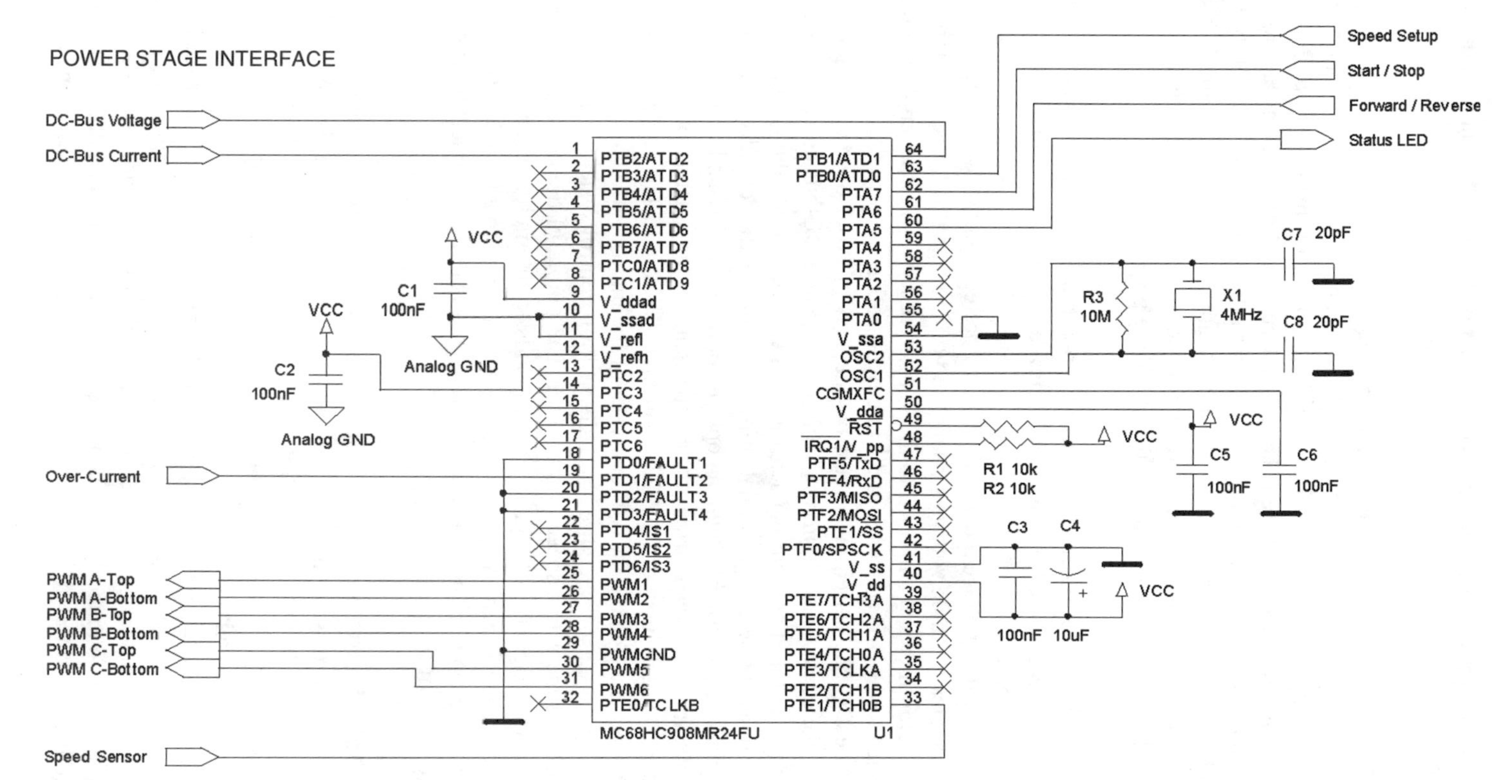

FIGURE 2–6 Microcontroller board accommodating the Motorola MC68HC908MR24.

the microcontroller board. The microcontroller requires only a minimum of external components.

Three-Phase Inverter A three-phase inverter forms the system's power stage. Its function is to convert the 5 V PWM signals from the microcontroller into the high-voltage control pulses that power the motor. In this design, IGBTs with a free-wheeling diode were chosen. Their good current characteristics and relatively high frequency response enable the designer to drive the motor efficiently with a 16–20 kHz PWM frequency that is above the audible noise limit. Figure 2–2 shows a basic schematic of the inverter. Except for the described devices, the power stage includes high-voltage IGBT drivers that drive the power devices.

Feedback Sensors The proper operation of the control system requires collection of feedback signals that are accurate representations of DC-bus voltage, DC-bus current, and motor speed.

The DC-bus voltage must be checked to protect against overvoltage. A resistor divider creates a simple voltage sensor. The voltage signal is transferred through an isolation amplifier and amplified to the 5 V reference level. The amplifier output is connected to the A/D converter of the microcontroller.

The DC-bus current also must be checked to avoid overcurrent production. Further, the control algorithm may require the analog DC-bus current amount. The current is measured by a current-sensing resistor inserted into the ground path of the DC-bus lines, while an operational amplifier amplifies the sensed voltage. The voltage signal is transferred through an opto-isolation amplifier and compared with the threshold. In case of overcurrent, the comparison circuit generates a fault signal connected to the fault input of the microcontroller PWM unit. The analog value of DC-bus current also is fed to the A/D converter of the microcontroller.

A speed sensor is required by a closed-loop control system. An AC tacho-generator senses the actual speed of the motor. The output of the tacho-generator is an AC sine wave signal; its frequency corresponds to the motor speed. The sinusoidal signal of the tacho-generator is filtered and transformed to a logic level square wave by a squaring circuit. The generated square signal is fed to the microcontroller input capture block of the timer.

Opto-Isolation Opto-isolation provides galvanic isolation between the power and control sections of the system. Six opto-couplers isolate motor control PWM signals. To ensure reliability, safety, and avoid ground path noise, all the feedback signals (voltage and current) must be isolated using opto-couplers or opto-isolation amplifiers.

Although opto-isolation implies a hardware complication and added devices (including an additional power supply output), the security of the system is highly improved. For motor control drives where cost is a driving factor of the design, opto-isolation can be omitted and the control signals of the microcontroller can be connected directly to the high-voltage drivers. Caution must be taken to avoid damage to the system and human injury. In this case, galvanic isolation of the human interface is highly recommended.

Power Supply The power supply board provides a high-voltage DC-bus power supply for the drive and +5 V, +15 V, and isolated +5 V auxiliary power supply for microcontroller; opto-isolation; high-voltage drivers; and operational amplifiers.

Typical designs of the high-voltage DC power supply incorporate a simple one- or three-phase diode bridge rectifier with a bulk capacitor that creates a DC-bus voltage directly from the line. It is followed by an in-rush current limiter, which affords protection during the switch-on operation.

Because the system has to meet EMC/EMI regulations, the RF filter and power factor correction (PFC) have to be included. The PFC can be controlled by a dedicated integrated circuit. Another possibility is to use microcontroller PFC control. In this case, the microcontroller Motorola MC68MC908MR24 handles both tasks—motor control and PFC control.

Software Design

Figure 2–7 illustrates a block diagram of control software for a three-phase AC drive implemented on a Motorola MC68HC908MR24. This block maps to the microcontroller block of the system structure illustrated in Figure 2–5. The input to the control algorithm is the speed command and the actual motor speed. The speed

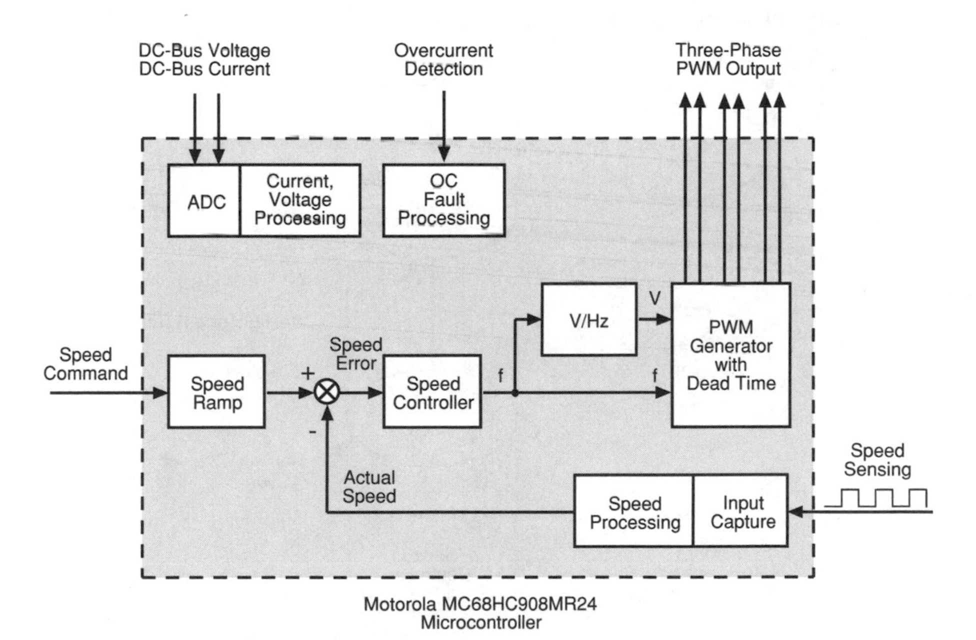

FIGURE 2–7 Software block diagram.

controller generates a motor frequency based on the speed error signal to eliminate motor slip. Thus, under steady-state conditions, the actual motor speed equals the required one. The volts per hertz function generates the voltage that corresponds to the frequency. Then, the PWM block generates six output signals for the power stage.

Figure 2–8 illustrates the actual software implementation. As can be seen, the program structure consists of an initialization routine and running routines that include the background processing and the interrupt service routines (ISR).

The initialization routine provides overall initialization of the microcontroller and is the first piece of code entered after a reset state. For three-phase AC motor control, the PWM module setup is set as follows:

- Set center-aligned PWM in a complementary mode with dead time inserted (MOR register).
- Select negative or positive PWM output polarity according to the power hardware configuration (MOR register).
- Enable COP and LVI (MOR register).
- Set PWM modulus; this defines the PWM frequency (PMOD register).
- Program dead time (DEADTM register) according to the power devices.
- Perform PWM interrupt reload for PWM update (PCTL2 register).
- Enable FAULT interrupt (FCR register).

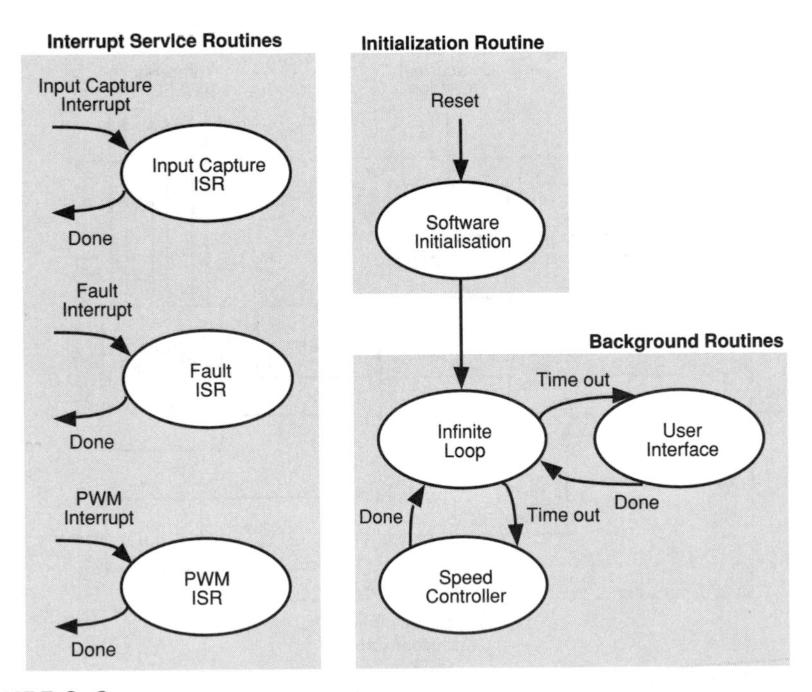

FIGURE 2–8 Structure of the control program.

TABLE 2–2 Memory Usage on the MC68HC908MR24

MEMORY	AVAILABLE	USED
FLASH	24K bytes	3.7K bytes
RAM	768 bytes	82 bytes

After the initialization is finished, the program enters a background routine. This part of the program is an infinite loop that enters and executes the non-time-critical background tasks in preprogrammed intervals. These tasks include the speed ramp and speed controller functions, volts per hertz ramp calculation, communication interface, user interface, and so on. All the time-critical routines are performed in the ISR.

Of these real-time tasks, the PWM generation ISR is the most critical and demanding of the processor's time. In the routine, new values of three-phase PWM output are calculated using a sinusoidal table stored in the memory of the microcontroller. Then, the microcontroller's PWM generator generates corresponding PWM pulses. The process is accessed regularly at the rate given by the set PWM frequency and the selected PWM interrupt prescaler (register PCTL2). The process must happen frequently enough (compared to the controller's output wave frequency) to ensure enough sample points to generate the correct wave shape with no significant PWM distortion. Therefore, for a 16 kHz PWM frequency, the routine is called every fourth PWM pulse, allowing the PWM registers to be updated at a 4 kHz rate (each 250 microsec). The "MR24" can perform this operation in approximately 33 microsec.

The input capture ISR performs the actual motor speed measurements. It filters an input square-wave signal and reads the time between two subsequent rising edges of the generated square wave. The measured time corresponds to the actual speed of the motor.

The fault ISR is the highest-priority interrupt implemented in the software. If an overcurrent fault is detected, the external hardware circuit generates a fault signal that is detected on the fault input pin of the microcontroller. The signal disables the motor control PWM output to protect the power stage and generates a fault interrupt, during which the fault condition is handled.

Microcontroller Usage

Table 2–2 shows how much memory is needed to run the three-phase AC drive in a speed closed loop. A significant part of the microcontroller memory remains available for other tasks.

Conclusion

The general trend of introducing electronically controlled motor drives started relatively recently. Today, motor and semiconductor companies are working hard on replacing constant-speed motors with variable-speed drives. The use of carefully designed AC motor drives and low-cost control systems can enhance a product's performance and marketability, as well as contribute toward the worldwide trend of total electrical energy savings.

References

Bose, Bimal K. *Power Electronic and AC Drives*, pp. 28–40, 129–145. Englewood Cliffs, NJ: Prentice-Hall 1986.

Michels, K. "Fuzzy Logic for Electrical Drives?" Proceedings of the Seventh European EPE Conference, vol. 1, Trondheim, Norway, 1997.

Mohad, N., T. M. Undeland, and W. P. Robins. *Power Electronics*, pp. 399–434. New York: John Wiley and Sons, 1995.

Motorola. *MC68HC908MR24 General Release Specifications*. Motorola Inc., April 1, 1998.

Rajashekara, K., A. Kawamura, and K. Matuse. *Sensorless Control of AC Motor Drives*, pp. 1–19. New York: IEEE Press, 1996.

Vas, P. *Electrical Machines and Drives—A Space-Vector Theory Approach*. New York: Oxford University Press, 1992.

Visinka, R. "Low Cost Three-Phase AC Motor Control System Based on MC68HC908MR24." Motorola Semiconductor Application Note AN1664, 1998.

Wilson, D. "'Get Your Motor Running' with the MC68HC908MP16." Motorola Semiconductor Application Note AN1712, 1997a.

Wilson, D. "Making Low-Distortion Waveforms with the MC68HC908MP16." Motorola Semiconductor Application Note AN1728, 1997b.

CHAPTER 3

A High-Voltage Power Factor Controller Helps Improve Power Quality

Ondrej Pauk and Petr Lidik
Motorola, Inc., Czech Republic

Introduction

Since European and international standards limit current harmonic content, the power factor is becoming an important feature for electrical line-supplied equipment, and for good reason. Adding more generating capacity to the world's electrical pool is very costly and would consume additional resources. Using AC power more efficiently through the broad use of a power-factor correction can create up to 30% excess generating capacity. Currently, motors, electronic power supplies, and fluorescent lighting consume the majority of power in the world, and each of these would benefit from a power-factor correction. The added circuitry will add about 20–30% to the cost of power supplies, but the near-term energy savings will greatly outweigh the initial cost.

Moreover, a power factor correction (PFC) may be required to receive the CE mark for the equipment. The IEC 1000-3-2 standard, published in 1995, sets requirements for harmonic currents.

The Importance of a Power Factor Correction

As just stated, several reasons support implementing PFC in the design of electronic equipment. Switching power supplies, motor control frequency inverters, and lighting electronics pull current in narrow, high-amplitude pulses rather than sinusoidally from the AC lines, see Figure 3–1.

Charging the bulk capacitor, C_{bulk}, causes power disturbances at the AC power source. Current pulses with significant harmonic content can cause a product not only to fail to meet international regulatory standards for harmonic content but, even

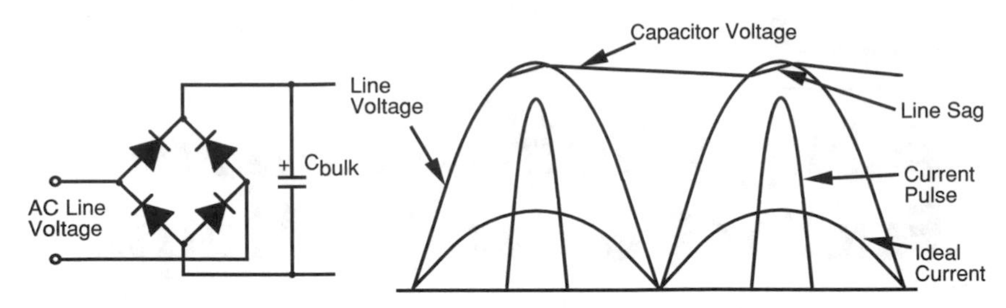

FIGURE 3–1 Capacitive input filter and its waveforms.

worse, actually to fail, sometimes with catastrophic consequences: fire in an office, industrial facility, or hospital.

The odd order harmonics that an uncorrected power supply generates are particularly problematic to three-phase systems with single-phase loads. In an ideally balanced three-phase load, the currents in the neutral line cancel, yielding zero current. If the phased load is switching supply, like the frequency inverter in modern motor control systems, for example, there is no cancellation and third-order high-level neutral currents can overheat of the neutral wire, which is a dangerous safety hazard. This situation is shown in Figure 3–2.

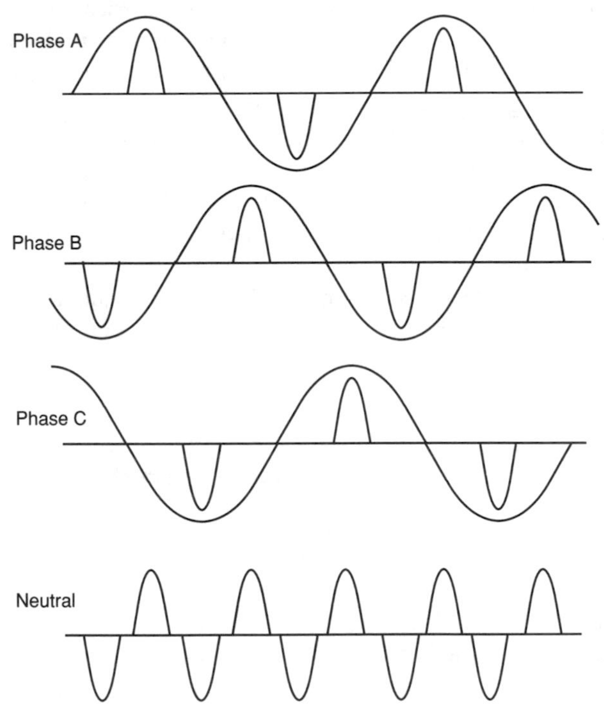

FIGURE 3–2 Unbalanced three-phase system.

International Regulatory Standards

The international community addresses the harmonic-current problems in the IEC 1000-3-2 standard (the successor of IEC 555-2), which establishes requirements that limit harmonic-current injection into the public supply system. IEC 1000-3-2 addresses equipment with nominal line-to-neutral voltages of 220 V and higher. The aim of the standard is to prevent power-control devices from generating low-frequency harmonics.

IEC 1000-3-2 categorizes devices into four classes, each with unique limits. Class A covers balanced three-phase equipment and all others except those defined in specialized classes B, C, and D. Class B covers portable tools. Class C sets the limits for lighting equipment. Those devices that have a special "wave shape" (see Figure 3–3) and are not motor driven or do not fit into Class A, B, or C are considered Class D.

Benefits to the Power Distribution Network

The benefits to power distribution network show up in a number of areas. The first and the most obvious improvement that may be gained by implementing a PFC is the ability to make maximum use of standard circuit breakers, which are rated in rms current. Underwriters Laboratories (UL) requirements will allow a user to draw only 80% or 12 amps from a 15 A/120 V AC circuit breaker, which, with a low line voltage of 90 V AC, will provide ~1.08 kW to a resistive load. With a power factor

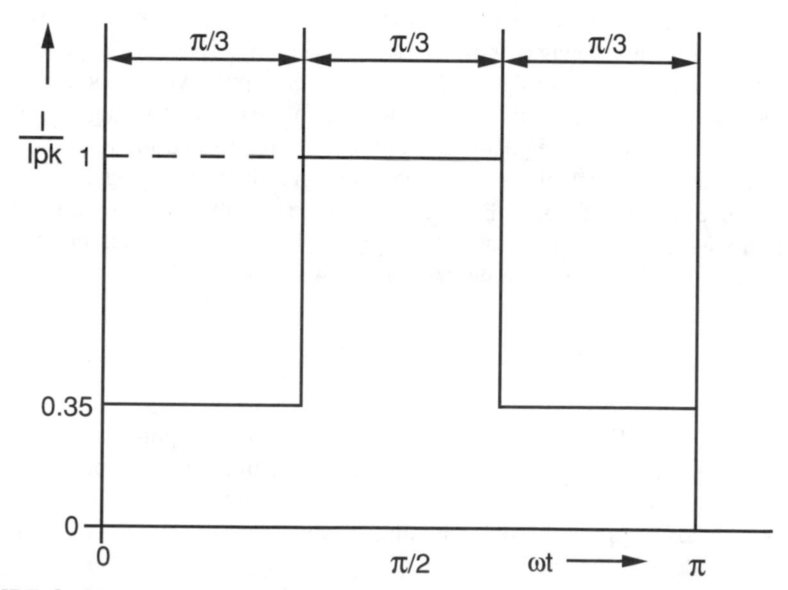

FIGURE 3–3 Class D defines a "special waveshape" of the envelope of the input current.

of only 0.65, which is the typical value for uncorrected power supplies, this power limit drops to less than 700 W—a number easily exceeded by many sophisticated computer terminals, servers, and workstations. To operate such equipment, the user has two alternatives, and both of them are costly: either use a special high-power outlet, which still must be derated by the same way, or switch to the three-phase power system.

The power factor also is important at levels much lower than 1 kW for an office environment with a PC or workstation on almost every desk. Even though each unit may draw less than 300 W, the combined total power supply causes problems for building designers responsible for power distribution networks.

Many systems today require an uninterruptable power supply (UPS) backup. The UPS usually is a battery-powered DC-to-AC converter that supplies the system when the AC line fails. These UPS systems normally are designed with a peak current limitation. If that peak represents a very narrow pulse, the rms power is substantially reduced. That is, with a poor power factor, the user must buy a UPS unit three to five times larger than otherwise would be needed. Consequently, the cost of UPS equipment also is a strong motivating factor in PFC implementation.

Benefits to the Power Supply Design

Using an active PFC circuit in the power supply offers a number of secondary benefits to the supply design itself. First, the lower peak line currents allow some downsizing of the chokes used in the EMI filter. Second, the peak current in the AC input rectifiers and line filter capacitor is reduced. Furthermore, an active power factor correction system can be configured to preregulate the bulk DC voltage, which offers several significant advantages. Foremost among these is the ability to operate from worldwide line voltages without range switching. Even within one voltage range, it is challenging to design a cascaded power supply which operates at peak efficiency across the entire range of potential variations in line voltage. A properly designed power factor preregulator can convert a three-to-one input voltage variation to a relatively constant bulk voltage level, greatly simplifying further power processing. Some of the specific benefits gained by the downstream converter include allowing a higher minimum duty cycle, which in turn results in lower peak current stress and less dissipation in the power switches.

What Is the Power Factor?

Ideally, the AC current provided by local utilities are purely sinusoidal and free of surges, transients, and electrical noise. As mentioned in the previous examples, nonlinear electronic loads are connected to the electrical line. These nonlinear electronic loads, represented by switching power supplies, motor drives, lighting ballast, and the like, degrade power quality because, among other things, they reduce the power factor and introduce harmonic currents into power lines.

In switching power supplies, the problem lies in the input rectification and filter network. The typical input circuit and its associated waveforms are shown in Figure 3–1. The input rectifiers can conduct current only when the AC line voltage exceeds the voltage on the bulk input filter capacitor. This typically occurs within 15° of the crest of the AC voltage waveform. The resulting current pulses can be five to ten times higher than the expected average current draw. This also can lead to distortion of the AC voltage waveform and an imbalance in the three-phase power lines feeding the circuits, which causes a current to flow within the neutral line when no current is expected. Another drawback is that no current is drawn when the rectifiers are not conducting, thus throwing away a significant portion of the power system energy capability.

PFC circuits are intended to increase the conduction angle of the rectifiers and make the AC input current waveform sinusoidal and in phase with the voltage waveform (see Figure 3–4). This means that all the power drawn from the power line is real power and not reactive. The net result is that the peak and rms current drawn from the line are much lower than that drawn by the capacitive input filter traditionally used.

The power factor, PF, is defined by the ratio of the real power, P_R, to total apparent power, P_A:

$$PF = \frac{P_R}{P_A} \tag{3–1}$$

The real power, P_R, can be calculated as the average of the instantaneous product of voltage and current taken at each instance in time over the full period, T:

$$P_R = \frac{1}{T}\int_0^T e \bullet i\,dt \tag{3–2}$$

where e = voltage and i = current.

The apparent power, a sum of the real power and reactive power, is calculated as the product of the rms current measured over the full period and the rms voltage measured over the same full period:

$$P_A = V_{rms} \bullet I_{rms} \tag{3–3}$$

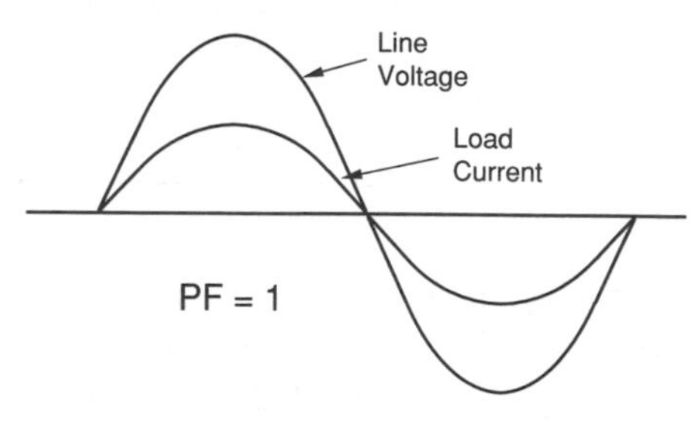

FIGURE 3–4 The AC input current is sinusoidal and in phase with the voltage waveform. The power factor = 1.0.

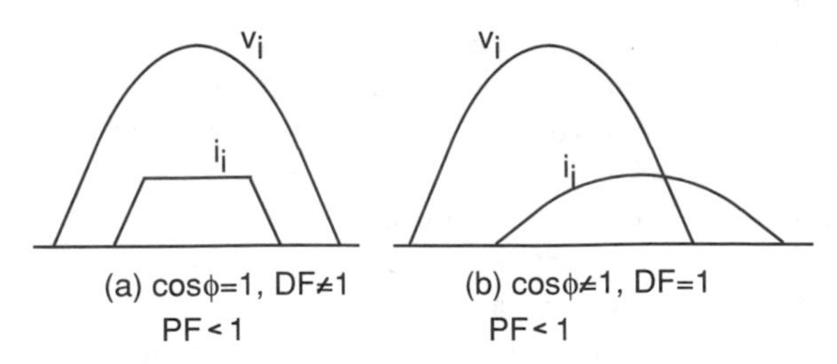

FIGURE 3–5 A comparison of waveforms in an uncorrected power supply as a function of the distortion factor.

In the case of an uncorrected switching power supply, the current and voltage can be nearly in phase due to the capacitor charging near the peak of the voltage waveform, see Figure 3–5. Therefore, using the definition PF = $\cos\phi$ would misleadingly yield a PF of 1.0 when the PF may be very low.

Probably the clearest definition of the power factor can be made in the following way. For sinusoidal input voltage,

$$PF = \frac{P_R}{P_A} = \frac{P_{\text{INPUT}}}{V_{rms} \bullet I_{rms}} = \frac{V_1 I_1 \cos\phi}{V_1 \bullet I_{i,\,rms}} \tag{3–4}$$

where $\frac{I_1}{I_{i,\,rms}} = DF$ is the distortion factor, I_1 = first harmonic of the input current, $I_{i,\,rms}$ = total harmonic current, and $\cos\phi$ = displacement factor.

Then, the distortion factor, DF, can be defined as follows:

$$DF = \frac{1}{\sqrt{1 + (THD)^2}} \tag{3–5}$$

where the total harmonic distortion, THD, equals

$$THD = \sqrt{\frac{I^2_{i,\,rms} - I^2_1}{I_1}} \tag{3–6}$$

The situation is even more clearly seen in Figure 3–5a and b. In both cases power factor is not equal 1.0.

Power Factor Correction Methods

To improve power quality, the main power source should see a sinusoidal load current that appears resistive. Therefore, an ideal power-factor-correction stage should appear as a resistive load to the AC line, pulling current sinusoidally and storing the power for the main converter so that the regulated voltage remains stable while the line voltage varies sinusoidally. This can be approached actively or passively.

Passive PFC

Passive PFC designs are suitable for applications with low power levels. A common method of filtering the harmonic currents is to use a passive LC filter, see Figure 3–6. Since both the inductor and capacitor must filter low-frequency harmonics and allow 50 Hz/60 Hz current to pass, these components suffer from growing bulk, weight, and cost as the power level increases. Moreover, the power factor can be only 0.9 for an LC filter. At higher power levels, a more sophisticated passive component solution, such as a ferroresonant input transformer or a tuned input filter, may be possible. However, these passive solutions are effective over only a limited range of operating frequencies, voltages, and power levels. For all of these reasons, the passive approach is common in small power supplies, where power factor of 0.95 or less is acceptable and where the passive components are not excessively large.

Active PFC Techniques

A more effective solution can be achieved by implementing active power-factor-correction circuits, which take the form of non-transformer-isolated switching power supply. There are three basic PFC circuit topologies: buck, boost, and flyback sometimes called *buck/boost*.

The *buck topology*, shown in Figure 3–6a, produces an output DC voltage lower than the voltage at its input whenever the PFC stage is operating. When the instantaneous input voltage is less than the output DC level, the preregulator is inoperable. This can present a problem for higher-powered power supplies, which would than draw a large amount of current from the PFC circuit. Because of this, buck topology is not well suited for this application.

The *flyback* or *buck/boost topology*, shown in Figure 3–6b, has the distinction of being able to provide an output voltage greater or less than the instantaneous input voltage. This feature makes it possible to provide a 300 V output voltage from a 230 V AC line. Another big advantage is the ability to control the startup current and load current due to the series location of the active element. This topology is better suited for low-power designs due to the high breakdown voltage requirements for the semiconductors. Since the output voltage is negative with respect to the input ground, the cascaded power supply and the PFC voltage sensing networks must work with a negative voltage. Another major disadvantage is the need for a high side power switch.

The *boost topology*, depicted in Figure 3–6c, has become the most popular one due in part to the inherently high efficiency of the boost converter. The output voltage in the boost configuration always is higher than the peak input voltage, which allows the circuit to operate over the full line-voltage range. By setting the output DC voltage level to about 380–400 V, both 120 V and 230 V rms inputs (90 V/260 V) can be handled without range switch.

The location of the inductor makes this topology very popular because the inductor current is the line current and actually provides line filtering, minimizes

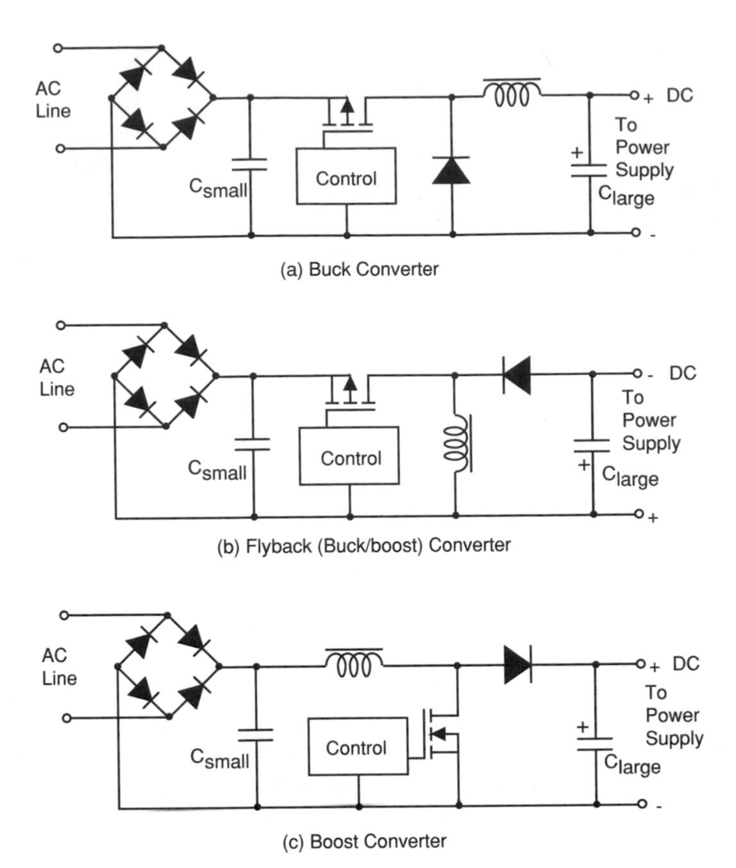

FIGURE 3–6 Three basic power factor correction circuits.

line noise and EMI, and allows an easy implementation of current mode control to program the input current.

The power switch in this circuit controls the inductor charge and discharge time, forcing the current to conform to a sinusoidal shape. The low-side power switch makes it is easy to drive the gate. Nonetheless, this power switch location has one drawback: Overload or startup overcurrent cannot be controlled because there is no series switch between input and output as in the buck and buck/boost topologies.

There are several main implementations in the control of PFC circuits:

- The fixed-frequency average current sensing method widely implemented by Unitrode under the Pioneer Magnetics patent (UC3854 control integrated circuit).
- The fixed-frequency, peak current sensing method by Micro Linear (ML4812).
- The hysteretic control used by Cherry Semiconductor (CS3810).
- The borderline or critical conduction, peak current sensing method used by Siemens (TDA4818), Silicon General (SG3561), and Motorola (MC34262, MC33368).

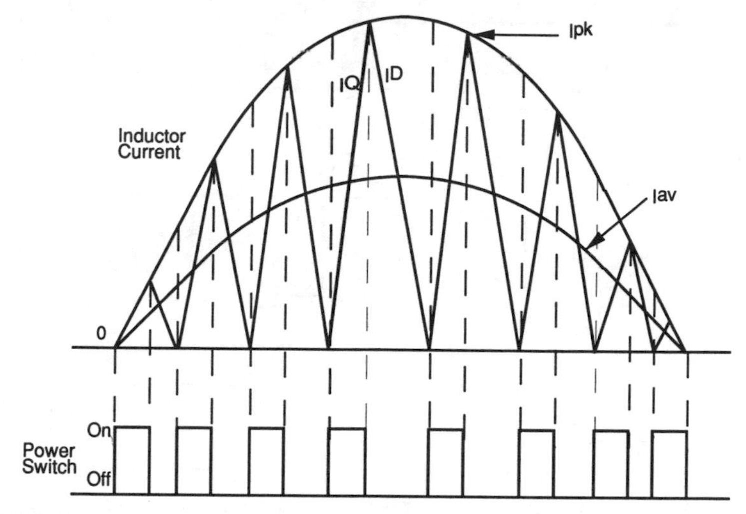

FIGURE 3–7 Critical conduction mode current waveform and power switch gate voltage.

The last two methods are variable frequency methods of control. All the methods produce acceptable power factors as specified by regulatory agencies. Figure 3–7 shows current waveforms of the critical conduction mode control method.

The inductor operating mode is a major consideration in designing a PFC circuit. A discontinuous mode of operation typically is used for power levels less than 500 W. It has high peak currents, which limits its use at the higher input power levels. For greater power levels, the continuous mode of operation is used. This lowers the peak currents seen by the power switch and output rectifier and makes it much easier to filter in the EMI filter, since there are no rapid transitions in the input switched current waveforms. The disadvantage is that the switching losses rise significantly because the power switch must force off the output rectifier at the beginning of each "on" time period. Therefore, a larger heat sink, to cool the output rectifier, must be used. Another disadvantage is that the output rectifier reverse recovery action is a source of significant noise.

Practical PFC Design

As already mentioned, more and more often, the PFC circuits find their use in lower-power applications, where overall system cost is critical factor. Motorola's MC33368 high-voltage PFC controller integrated circuit offers a practical, cost-effective solution for power factor correction design.

The MC33368 functions as a boost to the preconverter in off-line power supply applications. This power factor controller is optimized for lower-power, high-density power supplies requiring a minimum board area, reduced component count, low power dissipation, and relatively low noise.

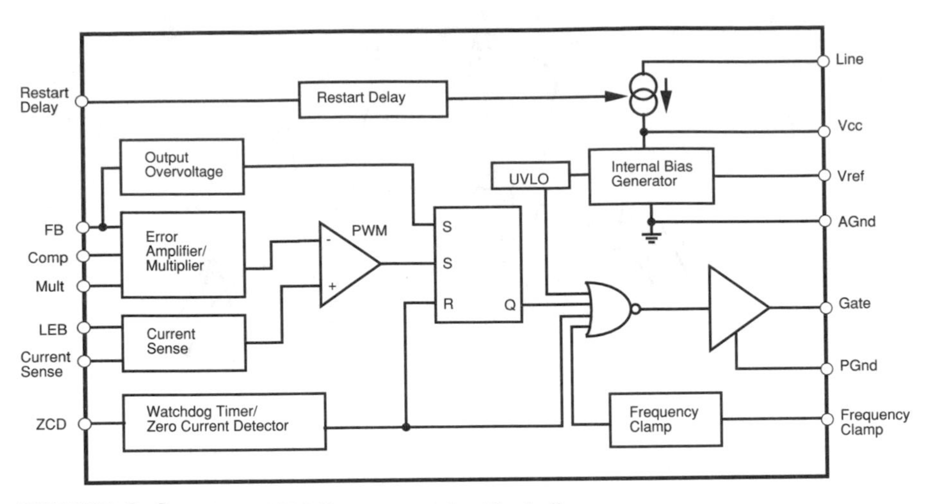

FIGURE 3–8 The MC33368 representative block diagram.

The MC33368 contains many of the building blocks and protection features employed in modern high-performance power supply controllers. Figure 3–8 shows its representative block diagram.The major difference between this controller and a general boost controller is that a multiplier has been added to the current sense loop and this device contains no oscillator. Figure 3–9 shows some of the specifics involved with using the MC33368 for motor control with power factor correction.

Referring to the simplified boost converter schematic diagram shown in Figure 3–6c and the critical conduction control mode current waveform shown in Figure 3–7, the operation of the converter can be described as follows. When the power

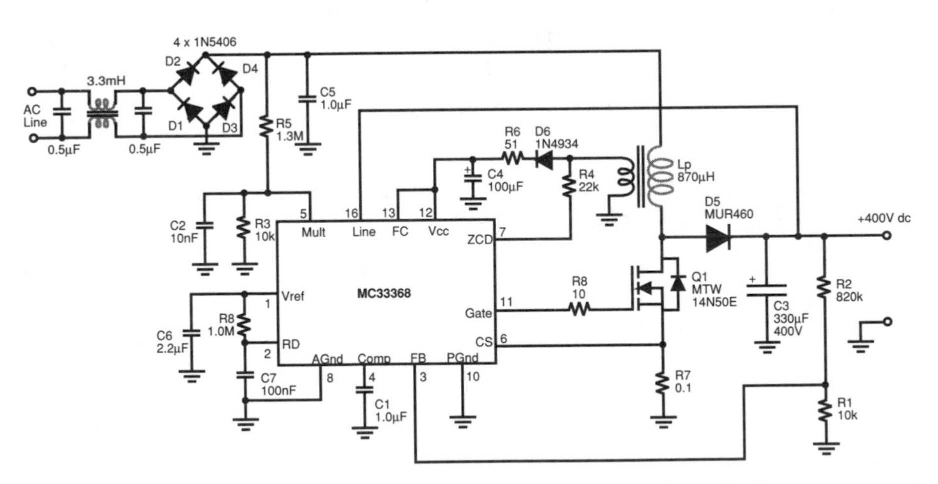

FIGURE 3–9 180 W universal input power factor controller schematic diagram.

switch turns on, one end of the inductor is tied to the ground, reverse biasing the diode and allowing the inductor to charge up. During this time the current in the inductor, which is the current of the AC line, increases linearly until the power switch is turned off. When the power switch is turned off, the voltage on the drain swings up to the output voltage (plus a diode drop), allowing the inductor current to flow through the output diode and charging up the capacitor.

Functional Blocks

During this period the inductor current is a linear ramp with a negative slope. By switching the power switch at a rate much faster than the input signal frequency and modulating the power switch off-time (with fixed on-time) relative to the input voltage amplitude, the inductor current waveform will track the input AC voltage waveform (see Figure 3–7). A description of each of the functional blocks of the controller follows.

Error Amplifier The error amplifier is a transconductance type, which means that it has high output impedance with controlled voltage-to-current gain. The noninverting input is internally biased at 5 V. The output voltage of the power factor converter typically is divided down by means of resistor divider and monitored by the inverting input. The error amplifier output is internally connected to the multiplier and pinned out for external loop compensation. Typically, the bandwidth is set well below 20 Hz so that the amplifier's output voltage is relatively constant over a given AC line cycle. In this way, the error amplifier monitors the average output voltage of the converter over several line cycles. This is another factor distinguishing PF converter from a typical switching power supply, which has a voltage feedback loop much faster.

Overvoltage Comparator Overvoltage comparison, one of several controller safety features, is incorporated to eliminate the possibility of runaway output voltage. This condition, which can occur during initial startup, sudden load removal, or output arcing, is the result of the low bandwidth that must be used in the error-amplifier control loop. The overvoltage comparator monitors the peak output voltage of the converter and, when exceeded, immediately turns off the switch.

Multiplier The multiplier is the critical element that enables this device to control the power factor. A single-quadrant, two-input multiplier monitors the AC haversines with respect to the ground. The multiplier output controls the current-sense-comparator threshold as the AC voltage traverses sinusoidally from zero to peak line, thus making the peak switching current to track the AC input voltage, and the preconverter load appears to be resistive.

Zero Current Detector The MC33368 operates as a critical-conduction-mode controller, which means that the next on time of the power switch is initiated when the inductor current reaches zero. This is sensed indirectly by monitoring when the auxiliary winding voltage falls below 1.2 V. The zero current detector sets the RS latch, thus initiating the power switch conduction time, which then is terminated when the peak inductor current reaches the threshold level established by the multiplier output.

The critical-conduction mode of operation has two significant benefits. First, since the power switch can not turn on until the inductor current reaches zero, the output rectifier's reverse recovery time becomes less critical, allowing the use of an inexpensive rectifier. Second, since there is no dead time between cycles, the AC line current is continuous, limiting the peak switch to twice the average input current.

Current Sense Comparator and RS Latch The current sense comparator input monitors the power switch current, which is converted to the needed voltage by inserting ground-referenced sense resistor R7 in series with the source of the power switch. Under normal operating conditions, the peak switch current is controlled by the threshold voltage of pin 6, where

$$I_{pk} = \frac{V_{th(Pin6)}}{R7}$$

When the preconverter is running at an extremely low line, inductor winding is shorted; and if output voltage sensing is lost, the power switch current can run out of control. Under these conditions, the current sense comparator threshold will be internally clamped to ±1.5 V and the maximum-peak switch current will be given by following expression:

$$I_{pk(max)} = \frac{1.5V}{R7}$$

The current-sense-comparator and RS-latch configurations used ensure that only a single pulse appears at the drive output during a given cycle. The current sense input to drive output propagation delay is typically 200 nsec.

Timer A watchdog timer function provides a means to automatically start or restart the preconverter if the drive output has been off for more than 385 sec after the inductor current reaches zero. The timer function eliminates the need for an external oscillator.

Output The MC33368 controller IC contains a totem-pole CMOS output driver specifically designed to drive the power MOSFETs. The gate output is capable of up to ±1.5 A peak current with a typical rise and fall time of 50 nsec with a 1.0 nF load.

Additional Features

All the functional blocks just described are essential to ensure a basic power factor converter operation. Nonetheless, the MC33368 controller offers a lot of additional advanced safety and performance enhancing features. Some of these follow.

Undervoltage Lockout The undervoltage-lockout (UVLO) circuit suppresses the gate output if the supply voltage, V_{cc}, drops below 8.5 V typically.

Quickstart During initial startup, when the compensation capacitor C1 is discharged, the quickstart circuit precharges the C1, allowing immediate drive output switching.

Restart Delay A restart delay pin is provided to allow hiccup-mode fault protection in case of a short circuit and prevent the converter from repeatedly trying to restart after the input line voltage has been removed.

Frequency Clamp In the AC line zero crossing, the output switching frequency clamp limits the minimum off time, determined by the values of R10 and C7. This allows discontinuous conduction operation, thus minimizing generated EMI and improving the power factor in this operating region.

Conclusion

The term *power quality* is being heard more frequently in recent years because of its impact on the users of electric power. The power factor correction brings benefits to a power distribution network by reducing rms current and increasing harmonic current content. It has been shown that implementing a modern, high-performance, cost-efficient active power factor correction often can help reduce the total system cost and increase the efficiency of AC power use.

References

Brown, Marty. *Power Supply Cook Book*. Boston, MA: Butterworth-Heinemann, 1994.

Cardinale, Vince. “Techniques for Improving Power Factor.” *Powertechnics Magazine* (April 1990).

Carter, Danis. “Power Factor Correction for Medical Power Supplies.” *EDN Magazine*, Europe (May 1998).

Mammano, Bob, and Bob Niedorf. “Improving Input Power Factor—A New Active Controller Simplifies the Task.” Unitrode Corp., Merrimack, N.H.

“MC33368 High Voltage GreenLine™ Power Factor Controller.” Data sheet, Motorola, Inc., 1997.

Sum, Kit. “Power Factor Correction for Single-Phase Input Power Supplies.” *PCIM Magazine* (December 1989).

Tenti, P., and G. Spiazzi. “Harmonic Limiting Standards and Power Factor Correction Techniques.” EPE Conference tutorial, Seville, Spain, September 1995.

CHAPTER 4

Designing High-Efficiency DSP-Based Motor Controls for Consumer Goods

AENGUS MURRAY

Analog Devices Inc., Motion Control Group

Electric motors are the major components in electric appliances such as refrigerators, washing machines, and clothes dryers. The energy consumed by the electric motor is a very significant portion of the total energy consumed by the machine. Controlling the speed of the appliance motor can both directly and indirectly reduce the total energy consumption of the appliance. The world's major domestic appliance manufacturers now are adding energy efficient features to improve their competitive position in the market. They also are motivated by the need to meet regulations on energy efficiency and water usage being introduced in Europe, Japan, and the United States of America in the next few years.

In many major appliances, advanced three-phase variable-speed drive systems provide the performance improvements needed to meet these new energy consumption targets. Digital Signal Processor-based (DSP) motor control systems offer the control bandwidth required to make possible the development of advanced motor drive systems for domestic appliance applications.

This chapter outlines some of the technical challenges involved in the design of fractional-horsepower drives for domestic appliances such as washing machines and refrigerators. In one application, an advanced back-EMF (electromagnetic force) sensing algorithm provides very efficient operation of a brushless permanent magnet motor in a refrigerator compressor. In a washing machine, field-oriented control of a three-phase induction motor increases the drum speed range, allowing for much more efficient spinning action.

Reduction of Energy Consumption in Domestic Appliances

Refrigeration Systems

The domestic refrigerator is a significant consumer of electricity because it is powered continuously throughout the year. It is estimated that, even for a small European country, a 30% reduction in power consumption by refrigerators could save the construction of a complete power plant along with a saving in fuel oil imports. This is even more important in the newly developing countries like India and China, where the electrical infrastructure is in need of significant investment.

A reduction in a refrigerator's power consumption may be achieved both by improving its ability to contain cold and by making its compressor unit more energy efficient. Thermal losses can be reduced by increasing the thickness of the wall insulation and improving door seals. However, this would require a significant investment in cabinet retooling, along with a reduction in the internal storage space. To solve the second half of the equation, appliance manufacturers have spent the last few years looking at ways to improve the refrigerator's cooling efficiency.

The standard compressor uses a single-phase induction motor connected directly to the AC line running at a fixed speed of 3,000 or 3,600 rpm. This means that the compressor runs almost continuously for rapid cooling but with a very low duty cycle in normal operation. An overall improvement in compressor efficiency can be achieved by reducing the speed of the compressor to match the cooling to that required for normal refrigeration operation. This reduction in the compressor cooling also improves the food storage quality by reducing the temperature variations within the cabinet. The high-speed operation is reserved for rapid cooling when the refrigerator is loaded with food or for fast freezing. A modern energy-efficient compressor has an electronic controller capable of running the compressor motor at its most efficient operating point of say 2,100 rpm and also at its maximum cooling point of say 3,600 rpm.

Washing Machines

Energy is directly consumed in the laundering process in the agitation of the clothes during washing and in the extraction of water during spinning. However, a very significant amount of energy is consumed in heating water for washing and heating air for drying the clothes. Appliance manufacturers have recently introduced energy efficient washing machines that require less water in washing and extract more water during the spinning process. Such a machine can dramatically cut the energy required to heat water for a wash and remove it from the clothing during drying.

European washers typically are horizontal-axis machines rather than the vertical-axis type generally used in North America. The drum in the horizontal-axis washing machine is only partially filled. The machine agitates the clothes by slowly turning the drum and letting the clothes fall into the washing water. This washes clothes more effectively and uses less water in the process. The efficiency of the clothes drying process is improved by increasing the final spin speed to extract more water. In the first stage of the spin cycle, the clothes are spun at a medium speed while the water is drained from the drum. The final spin, at a drum speed of up to 1,000 rpm, extracts much more of the remaining water than in a conventional vertical-axis machine. In these washing machines, an electronically controlled motor drives the drum through a belt drive system.

DSP Motor Control in Domestic Refrigeration Applications

System Requirements

Energy-efficient compressors require the motor speed to be controlled in the range 1,200–4,000 rpm. In fractional horse power applications, the motor of choice with the highest efficiency is an electronically controlled three-phase permanent magnet motor. Therefore, this is the compressor control system of choice for highly efficient domestic refrigeration systems.

In domestic refrigeration systems the compressor and motor are hermetically sealed within the same metal enclosure. The environment within the chamber is particularly harsh and does not allow the use of hall sensors typically used in other low-cost permanent magnet drives. A sensorless mode of operation, in which the motor acts as its own commutation sensor, therefore is essential. The target for this application is to provide a drive for a 200 W compressor motor with no sensors, of minimum size and cost, and meeting all the regulatory requirements for electromagnetic compatibility and safety.

Motor Control Strategy

To run the permanent magnet motor efficiently, it is important to synchronize the frequency of the applied voltage the position of the permanent magnet rotor. A very effective control scheme is to run the motor in a six-step commutation mode with only two windings active at any one time. In this case, the back-EMF on the unconnected winding is a direct indication of the rotor position. The rotor position is estimated by matching a set of back-EMF waveform samples to the correct segment of the stored waveform profile. This technique averages the data from a large number of samples giving a high degree of noise immunity. The control system, outlined in Figure 4–1, has inner position control loop that adjusts the angle θ_s of the applied stator field to keep the rotor in synchrony. The integrator input tracks the motor velocity when the rotor position error is forced to 0. The outer velocity loop adjusts the applied stator voltage magnitude to maintain the required velocity. The controller is capable of accelerating the compressor to its target speed within a few seconds and can regulate speed to within 1% of its target. The smooth running of the compressor also reduces audible noise. The lower operating speed helps minimize the temperature cycles in the cabinet and improves the food storage quality.

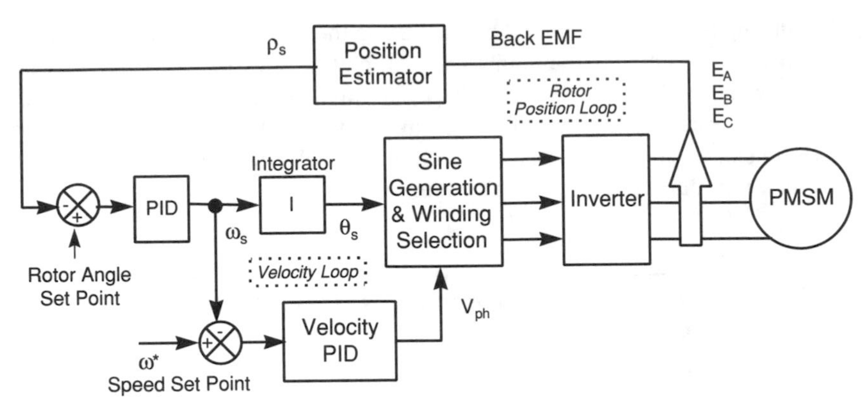

FIGURE 4–1 Sensorless control system.

Motor Control Hardware

The essential hardware in a variable-speed AC drive system consists of an input rectifier, a three-phase power inverter, and the motor control circuits. The input rectifier converts the input AC line voltage to DC voltage. The power inverter converts the DC voltage to three-phase AC voltages to drive the AC motor. The motor control processor calculates the required motor winding voltage magnitude and frequency to operate the motor at the desired speed.

A pulse width modulation (PWM) circuit controls the on- and off-duty cycle of the power inverter switches to vary the magnitude of the motor voltages. An analog-to-digital converter (ADC) allows the processor to sample motor feedback signals such as inverter bus voltage and current. In this sensorless control application, the motor-winding back-EMF signals are sampled to calculate to drive the motor at its most efficient point of operation. The voltage signal conditioning consists of resistive attenuators and passive filters. A simple transistor amplifier is used to capture the motor winding current by sensing the DC bus current. The controller uses this information to limit the motor starting current and to shut down the compressor in overload conditions.

The complete drive system, described in Figure 4–2, includes the electromagnetic interference (EMI) filter, the input rectifier, control power supply, motor control IC, signal conditioning circuits, power inverter, and gate drive circuits. A single chip DSP motor control IC, such as the ADMC330, integrates a high-speed DSP core with a multichannel A/D converter, a three-phase PWM controller, and communications ports. The DSP computing engine allows the processing of the many back-EMF data samples used to estimate the rotor position. The highly optimized motor control peripherals minimize the processor overhead in reading back-EMF samples and generating PWM signals for the power converter.

The DSP-based motor IC is the heart of the system. On power-up, the program performs initialization and diagnostic functions before starting the motor. The motor is started in open loop until the back-EMF reaches a minimum level, before

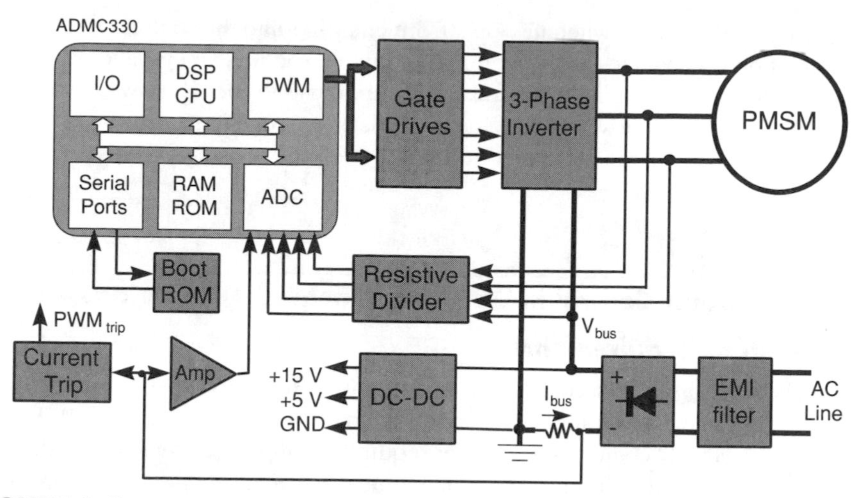

FIGURE 4–2 Permanent magnet synchronous motor (PMSM) control drive.

switching to running mode. Then, during every PWM cycle, the DSP uses the A/D converter to sample the motor back-EMF, the motor current and the bus voltage. The internal multiplexer selects the appropriate back-EMF signals to be converted. The software's control law calculates a new rotor position estimate and calculates the PWM duty cycle required, applying the required voltage to the motor. At particular values of estimated rotor position angle, the algorithm selects a new set of active motor windings by writing to the PWM segment selection register. The DSP algorithm also performs diagnostic functions, monitoring DC bus voltage, the motor current, and speed. In the case of overload conditions, the drive will be shut down and a restart attempted after a short time delay.

The drive power stage consists of a full three-phase MOSFET power inverter bridge and three integrated gate drive amplifiers. The rectifier common is connected to the control IC ground, and so the PWM outputs are connected directly to the gate drive inputs. The back-EMF signal conditioning consists of three matched high-voltage resistive dividers and a passive RC filter. The current amplifier circuit is synchronized to the PMW sampling frequency in such a way that it can determine the motor winding current from the DC bus current. The other elements of the drive solution are the addition of the control power supply and the EMC components to meet all the regulatory requirements. The very compact power supply design derives the +15 V and +5 V supplies from the 30 0V supply using a two-stage buck converter, thus avoiding the use of a bulky mains transformer.

A prototype system has demonstrated that it is possible for the drive electronics to be mounted on a single control card. The major challenges were in minimization of the control board size and manufacturing costs. The minimum size constraint on the board meant that the DSP motor control IC was placed within 2 in. of a MOSFET power inverter switching currents greater than 1 A from a 300 V bus.

To prevent any inverter switching noise from coupling into the control circuits, special attention was paid to the power circuit's layout, routing, and grounding. All the high-current-carrying component and tracks are close to the AC power and motor connectors. The final drive product met the customer cost targets and resulted in a 30% reduction in energy consumption by the compressor over fixed-speed single-phase motor operation.

DSP Motor Control in Washing Machine Applications

System Requirements

The drum in the horizontal axis washing machine is driven at speeds between 60 and 1,000 rpm. The motor, however, must run at speeds in the range 700–15,000 rpm. The universal "commutator"' motor requires a simple electronic controller and is widely used in European washing machines. However, universal motors have well-known problems of brush wear, low duty cycles, and limitations on the high-speed range. Three-phase AC induction motors provide advantages over universal motors through the elimination of brushes and a wider speed range. Thanks to recent advances in power electronics and digital controllers, three-phase variable-speed drives are being introduced into both European and North American washing machines.

To properly control a three-phase AC induction motor over a wide speed range, both motor current and motor speed information is required. Valuable information about the washing load can be inferred from the speed ripple and load torque of the washing machine motor. Speed ripple, for example, can be used to estimate the load unbalance before starting the spin cycle, which improves the mechanical reliability of the machine. The washing drive described here is for a 500 W AC induction motor with a speed range from 600 to 15,000 rpm. The challenge in this application was to match all the motor torque and speed specifications while meeting the cost goals of a domestic appliance application.

AC Induction Motor Control Strategy

The control of an AC induction motor (ACIM) is potentially much simpler than that required for a permanent magnet AC motor. The ACIM can be driven in open loop by a three-phase inverter, giving adequate speed control performance for many simple pump and fan applications. However, when a wide speed range and high dynamic performance is required, a field-oriented control scheme is necessary. In this case, the flux and torque currents are controlled independently to give a performance similar to that from a permanent magnet synchronous motor. In the low speed range of operation, the flux is kept constant and torque is directly proportional to the torque current. In the high-speed range, when the motor voltages are limited by the DC bus voltage, the flux is reduced to allow operation at higher speeds.

A direct stator field oriented control algorithm is described in Figure 4–3. The key motor variables are the flux and torque producing components of the motor cur-

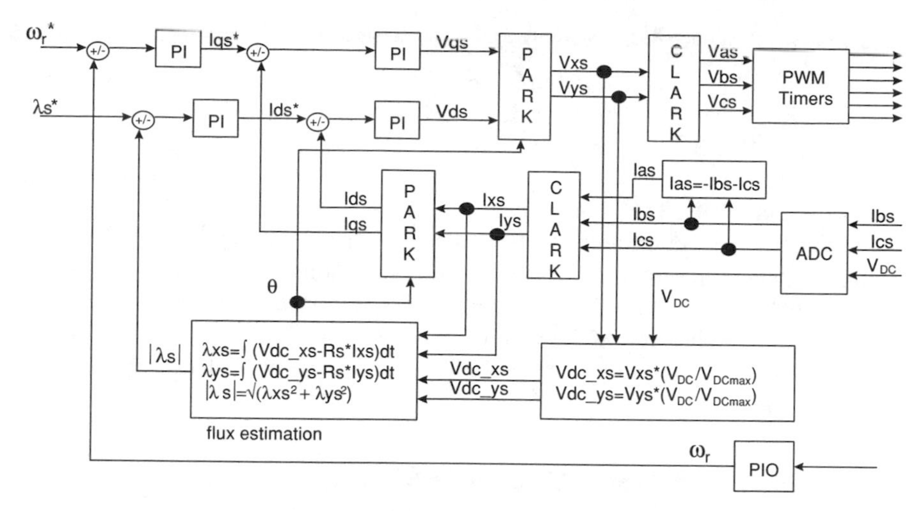

FIGURE 4–3 Direct stator field-oriented control scheme.

rents. The choice of reference frame is the key element that distinguishes the various vector control approaches from one another. In this scheme, a reference frame synchronized to the rotating stator flux is selected because of the availability stator current and DC bus voltage information (Xu and Novotny, 1991). A number of other field-oriented schemes require position information or stator flux measurements and are less suitable for this application, where controlled operation close to zero speed is not required. The Park and Clark reference frame transformation functions calculate the effect of the stator currents and voltages in a reference frame synchronized to the rotating stator field. This transforms the stator winding currents into two quasi-DC currents, representing the torque-producing (Iqs) and flux-producing (Ids) components of the stator current.

The stator flux angle is an essential input for the reference frame transformations. The stator flux is calculated in the fixed reference frame by integrating the stator winding voltages. In this system the stator voltage demands to the inverter are known, so the applied stator voltages can be calculated from the voltage demands and the DC bus voltage measurement. The flux estimation block uses stator current to compensate for the winding resistance drop. The output of this block is the stator flux magnitude and the stator flux angle.

Four closed control loops are used in this application. Two inner current loops calculate the direct and quadrature stator voltages required to force the desired torque and flux currents. The Park and Clark functions transform these voltages into three AC stator voltage demands in the fixed reference frame. The outer loops are the speed and flux control loops. The flux demand is set to a rated flux for below base-speed operation and is reduced inversely with speed for above base-speed operation in the "field weakening mode." Finally, the torque loop is the same as in any classical motion control system.

AC Induction Motor Control Hardware

The DSP-based AC induction motor system has hardware similar to the permanent magnet drive described previously. In this case, the motor is rated at over 500 W and so IGBTs are the power devices best suited. The feedback signals include the motor currents, the bus voltage, and a pulse train from a digital tachometer (see Figure 4–4). The motor-winding currents are derived from sensing resistors in the power inverter circuit. The DSP motor controller calculates velocity by timing the pulse train frequency from the digital tachometer. The DSP motor control IC communicates with the front panel washing machine control over an isolated serial link. This allows speed profile information to be downloaded to the controller and motor speed and torque information to be uploaded to the washing machine controller.

AC Induction Motor Control Software

One challenge in the development of the control software was to run four simultaneous control loops where the variables have a very wide dynamic range. A solution, which very much improved performance, was to use floating point variables for all the PI control loops. This extended the processing time somewhat but was not found to be a significant burden when using a 25 MIPS DSP core. The processor easily can handle the multiple interrupt sources from the A/D converter, the digital I/O block, the communications ports, and the timer. A number of useful device features of the device, such as the autobuffered serial port and the single context switch, made the task possible without significant overhead in pushing or popping a stack. Finally, the code development was somewhat simplified by the availability of motor control library functions in the internal DSP ROM.

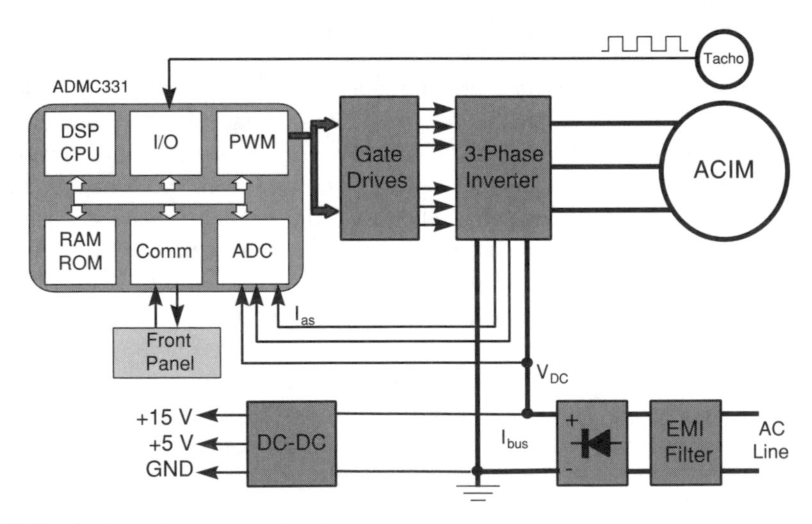

FIGURE 4–4 ACIM control hardware.

References

Xu, X., and D. W. Novotny. "Implementation of Direct Stator Flux Control on a Versatile DSP-Based System." IEEE Transactions on Industrial Applications, July-August 1991, Vol. 27, No. 4, pp 694–700.

Part II
Designing for Recyclability

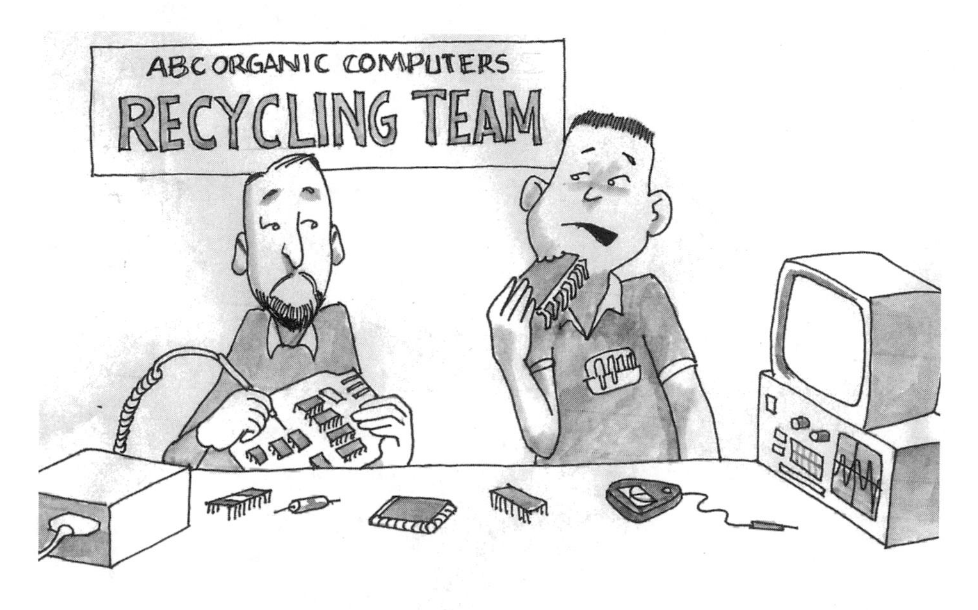

Remember, it's okay to eat any of the boards we can't fix, but don't forget to disconnect the power supply before you do!

CHAPTER **5**

Design for Disassembly, Reuse, and Recycling

PITIPONG VEERAKAMOLMAL AND SURENDRA GUPTA
Laboratory for Responsible Manufacturing, Northeastern University, Boston

Introduction

New electronic products usually are compact and equipped with the latest technology. They are replacing outdated ones at an astronomical rate. Ironically, a large number of outdated products are in excellent condition. Rapid product development coupled with a consumer appetite for latest models of products have caused consumers to discard outdated products even though they are still operational. This in turn leads to an increase in the quality of used and outdated products scrapped. Products made with reusable components, retrieved from discarded electronic products, not only can be cheaper but better. For example, electronic chips recovered from outdated computers can be "harvested" from boards at a fraction of their original production cost. These reclaimed ICs may well prove more reliable than new chips (if care is taken to protect them from thermal and static damage during removal) because they have survived an extended "burn-in" period during their service life.

Reuse and recycling of electronic products have been driven not only by the return on capital concept but also by the return to nature concept. Environmental awareness and recycling regulations have put pressure on manufacturers and consumers, forcing them to produce and dispose of products in an environmentally friendly manner. In many parts of the world, and especially in Europe, the regulations are becoming more stringent and manufacturers are required to recycle their products at the end of their useful lives. If the current trends continue, there is great promise for environmentally friendly companies who quickly meet the impending regulations to gain a competitive advantage in the marketplace.

To benefit from this new-found environmentalism, electronic manufacturers have to explore possible alternatives for designing environmentally benign products. This chapter provides an overview of the current techniques for design for disassembly, reuse, and recycling. First we introduce the "design for" concept and review the significance of environmentally benign design approaches. We also explore a variety of "design for" concepts that can guide product designers toward a specific design goal. Next, we investigate some product design guidelines and outline the steps required for the development of the design for disassembly, reuse, and recycling. Tools to evaluate product designs are described in the fourth section. The fifth section of this chapter provides case examples from major electronic product manufacturers in the United States and abroad.

The "Design for" Concept

During the past decade, interest has started to generate in designing products that not only satisfy functional specifications but also are easy to assemble and disassemble. More recent practices call for the inclusion of a host of other desired attributes. This concept, called *design for*, covers a wide range of design specialties; for example, "design for assembly" (DfA) and "design for manufacturing" (DfM). Lately, efforts have been made to incorporate environmental considerations into the "design for" concept. This is known as the *design for environment* (DfE), or *green design*, denoting environmental friendly engineering practices.

Since the design of a product has the highest influence throughout its life cycle, that is the first priority toward the greening of products (Graedel and Allenby, 1995). "Do it right the first time" is the phrase to describe the objective of green (life-cycle) design (Boothroyd and Alting, 1992). Green design has to capture the essence in every step of the product's life cycle to assess its impact on the environment (Figure 5–1). Traditionally, the design department used to pass the final product design to the manufacturing department with no regard to the difficulty in manufacturing. That practice, which became known as *over-the-wall engineering* (as if the designer throws the final draft over the wall to manufacturing), does not work in today's economic and regulatory environment. Today, *concurrent design* and *sustainable development* are the underlining keys to improve the interaction between the two domains. Concurrent design is a process that involves simultaneous and interactive team participation across various functions in a corporation. Sustainable development helps ensure that corporate plans are prepared and monitored continuously to achieve predefined short- and long-term goals. Such a structured cooperation also is required for DfE.

An all-encompassing term, *design for X* (DfX), is used to represent the multiple disciplines of design objectives. DfX, as referred to by Billatos and Nevrekar (1994); Hundal (1994); Marco, Eubanks, and Ishii (1994), and Graedel and Allenby (1995), for the multiplicity of "design for" concepts, includes factors such as disassembly, environment, quality, recycling, reliability, retirement (Ishii, Eubanks, and Marco, 1994), testability (Keoleian and Menerey, 1994), and usability. Some of the factors (and objectives) of design for X are presented in Table 5–1.

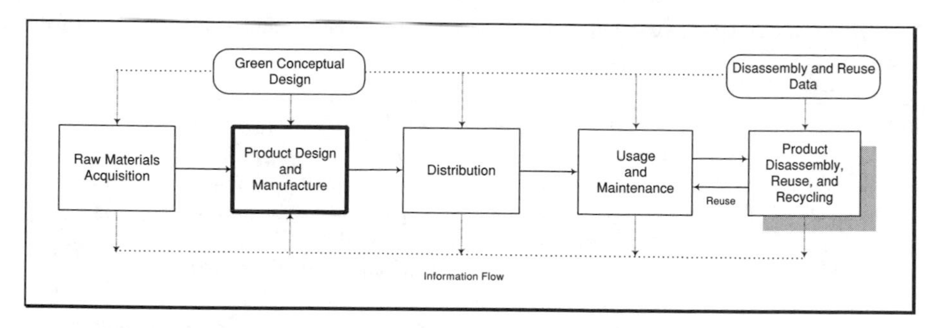

FIGURE 5–1 Product life cycle.

TABLE 5–1 DfX Design Practices

THE (X) FACTOR	OBJECTIVES
Assembly (A)	To enhance assembly tasks, including ease of assembly, error-free assembly, and use of common components in assembly
Compliance (C)	To consider the regulatory compliance required for manufacturing and field use, including such topics as electromagnetic emission and power consumption
Disassembly (D)	To consider designing for ease of disassembly: disassembly can be done for various reasons, such as maintenance, recycling, and remanufacturing; similarly, reuse and recycling cannot be carried out before products are disassembled
Environment (E)	To design a product that has minimal impact on the environment; life-cycle assessment (LCA) often is used to measure the impact on the environment
Logistics (L)	To address the management and movement of products and materials in the production networks
Manufacturing (M)	To integrate the design of the product to manufacturing processes and factory layout; DfM also can be described as the design of a product and the production process
Orderability (O)	To design products to facilitate the ordering process (from the customer's perspective), while taking manufacturing and distribution into account; DfO applications include assemble to order, make to order, and engineer to order
Product retirement (PR)	To accommodate the end-of-life product management that includes collection channels, component and material recovery options, disposal methods, as well as providing useful information to product retirement agencies
Quality (Q)	To enhance the consistency of a product's quality by establishing essential inspection points and allowing the ease of quality control (QC)
Recycling (R^1)	To design a product that is easy to recycle, using a minimum of different materials and individual components and providing an end-of-life material identification scheme

Table continued on next page.

TABLE 5–1 DfX Design Practices *(continued)*

The (X) Factor	Objectives
Reliability (R^2)	To design products that are reliable to operate, even under difficult operating conditions
Safety and liability prevention (SL)	To design a product to forestall misuse so as to prevent unreasonable and costly legal action; as well as adhere to industrial and safety standards and practice operational safety
Serviceability (S)	To focus on ease of initial installation as well as repairs and maintenance by consumers or service centers
Testability (T)	To design products that are easy to test, both in the factory and in the field

Green Design, Concurrent Design, and Sustainable Development

Green design initiatives were developed to address the environmental concerns of product life-cycle and production processes. Until recently, many companies were afraid that incorporation of green design would be enormously expensive, because their products and production facilities layout would have to be overhauled. The current consensus, however, is that, in many cases, green design not only can add to profits in the long run but also help avoid future regulatory problems.

Concurrent design is a modern engineering practice of congregating design principles from various business functions to enhance the integrity of the design process. Concurrent design leads to a better, greener product. It is based on the simultaneous design of product features and manufacturing processes. For example, for DfE, AT&T formed a "green product realization" design team that included representatives from several departments, such as product line management, marketing, research, design, product engineering, environmental health, and safety engineering (Keoleian and Menerey, 1994).

Sustainable development seeks strategic means to keep up with the endless waves of change without compromising future capacity. As far as our environment is concerned, sustainable development is a dynamic state that harmonizes economic activities with ecological processes (Keoleian and Menerey, 1994). By preplanning the product's retirement, design engineers can make appropriate iterative improvements to the design. Simultaneous planning of product design and product retirement logistics is known as *design for product retirement* (DfPR; Ishii et al., 1994).

Design for Disassembly, Reuse, and Recycling

Conceptually, design for disassembly, reuse, and recycling (DfDRR) is intended for end-of-life product management. The theme suggests that reusing and recycling products are important steps to slow down the rate at which our landfills are used up. Furthermore, when a product is sent to a landfill, not only are the precious components and materials wasted, but also, over the long haul, toxic substances in the product can leak out and contaminate underground soil and water. At the present rate of landfill depletion, it would be better to invest our efforts in disassembly than do nothing at all.

New developments in the component and material recovery systems, which integrate disassembly, retrieval, and recycling processes so that the consolidated system can function economically, have a potential to succeed by turning trash into treasure (Veerakamolmal and Gupta, 1998). Both reuse and recycling are desirable, since both lead to the reincarnation of resources. However, a contrast between reuse and recycling arises when we distinguish their benefits from the monetary point of view. Isaacs and Gupta (1997) orchestrated the comparison of a disassembler's profit from reuse and a shredder's profit from recycling. Designers may gain insight by comparing the different scenarios that reflect the current practices of reuse and recycling.

Navin-Chandra (1991) suggested the use of green indicators to evaluate the environmental compatibility of a component and compare various design decisions about feature selection and material choice. A product designer may replace a particular feature with a more desirable one and analyze the trade-offs. The optimal green indicator value shows the most preferred design parameter. He noted that, if expensive materials or components were used for DfDRR, then one has to ensure that they would be economically feasible to remove and reuse.

Product Design Guidelines

Due to a different lifetime expectancy of each component, coupled with a variability in product specifications, the end-of-life disassembly, reuse, and recycling have to account for individual product design characteristics. For instance, in mechanical products that are built with many moving parts, the components are known to have higher failure rates and need frequent replacements. On the contrary, modern electronic components tend to have longer life expectancies and can be recovered repeatedly for reuse. Here are a few practical guidelines for the design for disassembly, reuse, and recycling (Brennan, Gupta, and Taleb, 1994).

Modular Product Structure Consolidation of component modules can greatly simplify the tasks of disassembly by allowing easy identification of the various components. In this way, a small, up-front design effort can greatly reduce unnecessary disassembly steps. Additionally, modular structure can help reduce the costs of assembly, maintenance, and end-of-life recovery. In one very revealing study, Ishii et al. (1994) explored design for product retirement and material life-cycle methodologies and successfully applied a technique called *clumping* to the design of a coffeemaker.

Design of Functional Units Design of electronic components should incorporate a companywide universal data interface standard (such as the universal serial bus standard used in the computer industry) and consolidate functional units to enable the simplicity in reuse. For example, the Intel Pentium II microprocessor, which integrates a sizable cache memory unit to its processing unit, comes in a single enclosed protective casing. In the long run, this benefits the recovery (for reuse) or the replacement of the processor module. Another good example is the Cyrix Media GX microprocessor, which has a built-in display adapter and a digital-to-analog sound converting unit in a single chip. This dramatically reduces the size of the computer's main circuit board and the cost of additional display and sound cards.

Material Selection The number of material varieties in a product influences reuse and recycling efficiency. A product built with fewer components and materials greatly reduces the required logistics of sorting and processing. In addition, labeling of parts for the type of materials (for ease of identification) helps in the separation process and, thus, preserves the materials' purity. Plastic parts should be marked using standard marking schemes, such as ISO 11469, ISO 1043, or the U.S. recycling marking standards for plastics. Often, it is possible to mold material identification codes directly into the parts.

Minimize Waste and Harmful Contaminating Materials Designers should refrain from using toxic substances whenever possible. Fragile or hazardous materials should be easily identified to prevent any harm to disassembly operators. Alternative materials that are environmentally benign and easy to recycle should be considered. Warning labels attached to the product, or the component, can be helpful in identifying harmful substances during disassembly and recycling. Similarly, materials that are corrosive and may contaminate other materials during the recycling process should be documented.

Ease of Separation Products designed for ease of disassembly, reuse, and recycling require minimal effort to take apart. Some important factors that may influence the ease of separation are the need for specific separation tools or fixtures and the orientation of the components' layout during disassembly. Designers concerned with disassembly should avoid types of fasteners (e.g., screws, glues, and welds) that may undermine disassembly efforts. Fasteners made with a clip, snap fit, or Velcro are easier to separate and require less energy to take apart. Fasteners that require special tools to remove can increase the setup time or impede the recovery process all together.

These guidelines can help identify the basic requirements for green product design. In practice, however, each company may be motivated to individually create the resource for migrating to the new paradigm. Each company always must take into account product-specific characteristics. For example, while snap-fitted components used in the design of a refrigerator can be easily taken apart with a special separation tool, Hewlett-Packard and AT&T found it cumbersome to take apart snap-fitted components in their computer workstations. Furthermore, the migration process can be complex and may require different amounts of developmental time for different product platforms. However, the experience gained from a particular disassembly operation can be helpful in the designing of disassembly shops for other products. Table 5–2 outlines the steps required for the designing of green products (Steinhilper, 1994).

TABLE 5–2 Steps for Designing Green Products

Step 1. Thoroughly analyze the product platform and required end-of-life tasks
Analyze and structure product platform
Analyze disassembly, reuse, and recycling tasks
Analyze material and information flow
Establish action plans
Point out potential improvements

Step 2. Determine the degree of disassembly, reusability, and recyclability of products and components
Develop disassembly, reuse, and recycling criteria
Evaluate the materials for disassembly, reuse, and recycling potential
Evaluate various designs for disassembly, reuse, and recycling
Document the possible ways to reuse and recycle subassemblies and materials
Document potential improvements
Carry out the required improvements

Step 3. Plan return logistics and information flows between production and end-of-life processing
Organize the return of products from consumers by selecting between the existing and alternative distribution and collection channels
Develop the technologies and equipment for the return logistics
Develop an information system for the return flows to provide feedback to designers
Generate a plan for internal and external material and information flows
Transfer knowledge from CIM (computer integrated manufacturing) to CIR (computer integrated recycling)

Step 4. Develop and design reliable and visionary solutions for disassembly, reuse, and recycling
Plan technical and time capabilities
Determine suitable disassembly, reuse, and recycling processes
Determine suitable disposal processes
Perform make or buy decisions for the recycling and disposal processes
Evaluate economic benefits
Establish future technical, economical, ecological, and environmentally friendly goals for recycling and disposal
Integrate production, usage, and end-of-life processing

Step 5. Prepare comprehensive guidelines for future green product design
Prepare product structure guidelines
Prepare material selection guidelines
Prepare fixture and joining technique guidelines
Recommend an appropriate configuration for the product platform
Prepare green manufacturing process guidelines
Prepare economic evaluation guidelines
Establish clear guidelines for an environmentally friendly design
Document important design measures
Establish the curriculum to train product designers the techniques of green design and manufacturing

Tools for Design Evaluation

This section outlines a series of evaluation tools recently developed to assist or evaluate various aspects of DfX (Table 5–3). At Stanford University, Ishii et al. (1994) used a methodology to design a product for retirement using hierarchical semantic network that consists of components and subassemblies. LINKER is a product representation scheme to model the semantic network and solve the disassembly problem by pointing out a list of necessary network links to disassemble.

From the Robotics Institute at Carnegie-Mellon University, Navin-Chandra (1994) developed an evaluation methodology for design for disassembly (DfD). He developed software, called *ReStar*, that optimizes the component recovery plan by taking into account various attributes of the product, such as the type of fasteners used and the accessibility to components and subassemblies (i.e., tool/hand access).

Isaacs and Gupta (1997) of the Laboratory for Responsible Manufacturing at Northeastern University have suggested an evaluation methodology that enables an automobile designer to measure disassembly and recycling potential for different automobile designs. With respect to the designs, the method uses goal programming to analyze the trade-off between the profit aspiration levels of the disassembler and the shredder.

Johnson and Wang (1995) used a disassembly tree in planning for product disassembly and material recovery opportunities. The technique, which tries to suggest selective disassembly of a product by performing a profit/loss analysis, considering various combinations of components, is featured in a software package called *EDIT*.

A group of researchers from the University of Iowa studied the design of products that can be easily disassembled for maintenance. Software, called *Design Evaluation for Personnel, Training, and Human Factors* (DEPTH), was developed to search for all geometrically feasible disassembly sequences that can be performed by a technician to identify the optimal operation time and cost (Vujosevic et al., 1995).

Subramani and Dewhurst (1991) investigated procedures to assess service difficulties and the associated costs at the product design stage. A computer program was written to model the product's structure and store it in the form of a disassembly diagram. A metric for serviceability was used to assess an overall rating of the product's design in comparison to its expected lifetime servicing costs.

The very first industrial application for green product design was introduced by AT&T. The elements of green design in electronics were carefully studied with the objective to revolutionize green production, usage, and end-of-life reclamation. The DfE assessment technique introduced is called the environmentally responsible product matrix, or ERPM (Graedel and Allenby, 1995). The matrix consists of five attributes for environmental concern: materials choice, energy use, solid residue, liquid residue, and gaseous residue. Another dimension of the matrix lists five stages of a product's life cycle: premanufacturing, manufacturing, packaging and transportation, consumer use, and refurbishing, recycling, or disposal. A product design expert has to identify the environmental effects on the array of design options that are evaluated across the life cycle. The matrix elements are assigned a numeric determinant ranging from 0 (highest impact on the environment) to 4 (lowest impact). Once an

TABLE 5–3 DfX Evaluation Tools

Title (Software)	Objective	Approach	Modeling Technique
Design for Product Retirement and Material Life Cycle (LINKER)	Design for product retirement (DfPR); addresses the methodology that evaluates a clump and its compatibility	Disassembly cost analysis (DCA) level of material compatibility	Hierarchical semantic network of components and subassemblies (nodes) and the relationships (links) represent actual connections
ReStar: A Design Tool for Environmental Recovery Analysis (ReStar)	Automated evaluation and automation in design; product design indicator; handles various types of fasteners, subassemblies, tool/hand access	Five decision points for tracking costs and revenues; looks at product recovery, not material recovery	Multiobjective version of A* (special branch-and-bound) optimization algorithm to solve traveling salesman problem of disassembly path combinations
A Decision Tool to Assess the Impact of Automobile Design on Disposal Strategies (Goal Programming)	Evaluate different product designs and maximize profit for both disassembler and shredder	Disassembler and shredder profit aspiration levels; investigates the optimal quantity of materials removed by disassembler prior to shredding	1. Multicriteria decision making: goal programming (GP) 2. Cost/benefit evaluation
Planning Product Disassembly for Material Recovery Opportunities (EDIT)	Disassembly of product; Recovery of specific material or groups and specific components or parts	Profit/loss margin (PLM): 1. Selective disassembly 2. Disassemble entire or majority of product to optimize PLM	Disassembly tree (DT) consists of part, subassembly, disassembly operations; free nodes; disposal cluster, material cluster
Simulation, Animation, and Analysis of Design Disassembly for Maintainability Analysis (DEPTH)	Develop procedure for disassembly sequence; time and cost prediction to evaluate whether the disassembly sequence can be performed within defined limits	Analysis criteria: 1. Time prediction 2. Cost prediction 3. Human factor analysis	Modeling and identification of all geometrically feasible disassembly sequences; human factor analysis using simulation and animation modeling

Table continued on next page.

TABLE 5–3 DfX Evaluation Tools (*continued*)

TITLE (SOFTWARE)	OBJECTIVE	APPROACH	MODELING TECHNIQUE
Automatic Generation of Product Disassembly Sequence (DAD)	Assessment of service and maintenance difficulties in product design	Optimal sequences for product disassembly	1. Rational model 2. Disassembly diagram (DAD) 3. Brunch and bound optimization algorithm
AT&T's Environmentally Responsible Product Matrix (ERPM)	Determine DfE value, called *environmentally responsible product rating*	Requires a product design expert to evaluate degree of environmental impact; in environmental impact evaluation scheme, 0 is the highest and 4 is the lowest	A 5×5 matrix of attributes; rating is the sum of the matrix elements (since there are 25 matrix elements, a maximum product rating is 100)
Apple Product Environmental Specification Tool (APES)	Knowledge-based approach to managing a range of specific environmental objectives	Environmental design criteria: ecopolicies, ecogoals, ecodetails, ecotest, and ecodeclare	Relational database linked to the Apple product environmental goals (APEG) database system

evaluation has been finalized for each matrix element, the aggregate environmentally responsible product rating is computed (a maximum product rating is 100 because altogether there are 25 matrix elements).

Apple Computer presents another interesting industrial application for DfX. The company increasingly has emphasized the greening of products in addition to optimal operational performances. Pioneered by the Environmental Technologies and Strategies (ETS) group, Apple Computer designed the Apple product environmental specification (APES) tool to manage a range of specific environmental objectives. The goal of APES is to provide design engineers with environmentally specific design data; that is, ecopolicies, ecogoals, ecodetails, ecotests, and ecodeclare. APES is programmed in Filemaker, a popular relational database software package, and linked to the Apple product environmental goals (APEG) database system (Matzke, Chew, and Wu, 1998).

Cases

Major electronic manufacturing companies have taken proactive steps toward the greening of electronic products. This has encouraged future product designers to emphasize on reducing parts, rationalizing materials, and reusing components. Companies from both the United States and abroad wishing to compete in the global market must adopt the dictates of the emerging market—one of which is led by environmentalism. This section provides several interesting case examples of design for disassembly, reuse, and recycling in the electronics industry.

Xerox launched its green manufacturing program with the objective of reducing costs by reusing its photocopy components (Bylinsky, 1995). Some of the major improvements that resulted in a total cost savings of $200 million a year are

- Improved layout design of potentially reusable parts in the machines to make them easily accessible.
- Using snap-fitted fixtures in place of screws.
- Using standardized components across the entire product platform.

Hewlett-Packard (HP) designed a new chassis and housing concept for its computer workstation product line in response to the shorter life cycles for computer products, faster development and production times, and steadily decreasing market prices. The new concept, HP-PAC, was intended to accommodate quick assembly and disassembly. To make recycling easier, product enclosures needed to be disassembled at least as quickly as they were originally assembled. To achieve this goal, HP employed a new method that uses the geometrical forms of a products' components (i.e., disk, speaker, power supply, CPU board, and fan) to fit them together in a jigsaw fashion within a chassis. HP's designers soon realized that the raw material used to build the structural layout had to meet several critical requirements. These include the ability to withhold large tolerances, to be nonconductive (to hold and protect electronic components), and to be able to hold components without fasteners (snap fits were not used because they can damage electronic circuit boards and other components during disassembly). Expanded polypropylene (EPP) was chosen for the chassis since it has all the suitable qualifications and is 100% recyclable. The HP-PAC workstation showed a dramatic 90% reduction in disassembly time. The result also reflected a substantial reduction in the number of mechanical parts, screw joints, assembly time, transport packaging, and housing development costs (Mahn et al., 1994).

IBM, one of the largest computer manufacturers, established component recovery facilities to disassemble and recover reusable components. At the Reutilization Center in Endicott, New York, IBM laid out two disassembly lines—a stationary disassembly line for larger computer machines and a conveyor-driven disassembly line for personal and notebook computers. The center works closely with IBM's Engineering Center for Environmentally Conscious Products (ECECP) in Raleigh, North Carolina, to improve future computer designs. Endicott's process includes customer shipment, receipt and inventory verification, process preparation, disassembly, sorting, and component recovery. Not only was IBM able to achieve DfE in its future products design, during 1994 to 1997, the reutilization facility had processed over 70 million pounds of equipment. In addition to the environmental benefits, the reclamation effort saved IBM over $50 million through internal product reuse. The operation realized another $10 million worth of income through industry standard component sales and another $5 million through the sale of recycled commodities (Grenchus, Keene, and Nobs, 1997).

Sony also incorporated the DfFE principle into its product development process. At the Sony Disassembly Evaluation Workshop in Stuttgart, Germany, products are taken apart to assess the reuse and recycling qualities of electronic parts. The product categories include television, compact stereo system, VCR, portable telephone, plus notebook and desktop computer. During disassembly, every step is clearly documented and recorded on video. At the end of the process, every component is carefully weighted and registered, with the resulting data placed in a software spreadsheet for analysis. The results are shared with the design engineer to help improve future designs (Ridder and Scheidt, 1998).

In addition to the efforts by private companies, industrial organizations have targeted various studies at the possibility of designing an automated system to extract information on products in the form of an electronic identification system. The identification system would include information such as physical structure, bill of materials, components, and fixtures. The system can be beneficial to procurement agencies or product designers as an evaluation and design modification tool.

Two product identification systems have been developed in the United States. An identification representation was developed at the National Institute of Standards and Technology, called the *product data exchange standard* (PDES). The future use of PDES is for organizations to transfer complex product information electronically. The aim is to use advanced information technology to read the PDES data file and evaluate aspects of separation, recycling, or hazardous contents (Navin-Chandra, 1991). Another form of intelligent identification system has been designed to enhance the potential of reuse and recycling at the end of the electronic products' lives. "Green Port" is an electronic memory installed within each product. Future recyclers will be able to access information provided by the product's manufacturer, the service technicians (who will record repairs and part replacements), and the sensors that monitor the equipment's operating conditions (e.g., humidity and temperature). This system would be of great benefit to disassembly planners for quality control and the estimation of components' reusable life (Dillon, 1994).

Conclusions

A perfect phrase to describe how today's businesses synchronize both ends of a product's life cycle is *making ends meet*; that is, the design of products on one end and the end-of-life reclamation on the other. Companies in the field of computers and consumer electronics, home appliances, and automobile manufacturing are tapping into the trend of selling green products for commercial as well as environmental reasons.

To entice consumers with the most up-to-date technology, companies are trying harder than ever to design products that accommodate end-of-life upgrade. This, in turn, offers consumers an array of choices whether to buy or to lease a product, while they also consider trading in an old product for a new one or upgrading an existing product with refurbished, state-of-the-art components.

One may conclude that the phenomenon helps move products off the shelves more quickly, allowing comsumers with limited budget to gain access to refurbished, higher-end products at an earlier phase of the market cycle. On the other hand, this directly benefits the environment by offseting the level of detrimental effects due to the depletion of natural resources and the disposal of products.

References

Billatos, S. B., Nevrekar, V. V., 1994, "Challenges and Practical Solutions to Designing for the Environment," Proceedings of the 1994 ASME National Design Engineering Conference, DE-Vol. 67, 49–64.

Boothroyd, G., and L. Alting. "Design for Assembly and Disassembly." *Annals of the CIRP* 41, no. 2 (1992), pp. 625–636.

Brennan, L., S. M. Gupta, and K. Taleb, K., 1994, "Operations Planning Issues in an Assembly/Disassenbly Environment." *International Journal of Operations and Production Management* 14, no. 9 (1994), pp. 57–67.

Bylinsky, G. "Manufacturing for Reuse." *Fortune* (February 6, 1995), pp. 102–112.

Dillon, P. S. "Salvageability by Design." *IEEE Spectrum* (August 1994), pp. 18–21.

Gatenby, D. A., and G. Foo. "Design for X (DFX): Key to Competitive, Profitable Product." *AT&T Technical Journal* 69, no. 3 (1990), pp. 2–13.

Graedel, T. E., and B. R. Allenby. *Industrial Ecology.* Englewood Cliffs, NJ: Prentice-Hall, 1995.

Grenchus, E., R. Keene, and C. Nobs. "Demanufacturing of Information Technology Equipment." Proceedings of the 1997 IEEE International Symposium on Electronics and the Environment, May 5–7, 1997, San Francisco, pp. 157–160.

Hundal, M. S. "DFE: Current Status and Challenges for the Future." Proceedings of the 1994 ASME National Design Engineering Conference, 1994, DE-vol. 67, pp. 89–98.

Isaacs, J. A., and S. M. Gupta. "A Decision Tool to Assess the Impact of Automobile Design on Disposal Strategies." *Journal of Industrial Ecology* 1, no. 4 (1997), pp. 19–33.

Ishii, K., C. F. Eubanks, and P. D. Marco. "Design for Product Retirement and Material Life-Cycle." *Materials and Design* 15, no. 4 (1994), pp. 225–233.

Johnson, M. R., and M. H. Wang. "Planning Product Disassembly for Material Recovery Opportunities." *International Journal of Production Research* 33, no. 11 (1995), pp. 3119–3142.

Keoleian, G. A., and D. Menerey. "Sustainable Development by Design: Review of Life Cycle Design and Related Approaches." *Journal of the Air and Waste Management Association* 44, no. 5 (1994), pp. 645–668.

Mahn, J., J. Haberle, S. Kopp, and T. Schwegler. "HP-PAC: A New Chassis and Housing Concept for Electronic Equipment." *Hewlett-Packard Journal* (August 1994), pp. 23–28.

Marco, P. D., C. F. Eubanks, and K. Ishii. "Compatibility Analysis of Product Design for Recyclability and Reuse." *Computers in Engineering* 1 (1994), pp. 105–112.

Matzke, J. S., C. Chew, and T. S. Wu. "A Simple Tool to Facilitate Design for the Environment at Apple Computer." Proceedings of the IEEE International Symposium on Electronics and the Environment, May 4–6, 1998, Oak Brook, IL, pp. 202–206.

Navin-Chandra, D. "Design for Environmentability." Proceedings of the 1991 ASME Design Technical Conference, DE-vol. 31, pp. 119–125.

Navin-Chandra, D. "The Recovery Problem in Product Design." *Journal of Engineering Design* 5, no. 1 (1994), pp. 65–86.

Ridder, C., and L. G. Scheidt. "Practical Experiences in the Sony Disassembly Evaluation Workshop." Proceedings of the IEEE International Symposium on Electronics and the Environment, May 4–6, 1998, Oak Brook, IL, pp. 94–98.

Steinhilper, R. "Design for Recycling and Remanufacturing of Mechatronic and Electronic Products: Challenges, Solutions and Practical Examples from the European Viewpoint." Proceedings of the 1994 ASME National Design Engineering Conference, DE-vol. 67, pp. 65–67.

Subramani, A. K., and P. Dewhurst. "Automatic Generation of Product Disassembly Sequence." *Annals of the CIRP* 40, no. 1 (1991), pp. 115–118.

Veerakamolmal, P., and S. M. Gupta. "Design of an Integrated Component Recovery System." Proceedings of the IEEE International Symposium on Electronics and the Environment, May 4–6, 1998, Oak Brook, IL, pp. 264–269.

Vujosevic, R., T. Raskar, N. V. Yetukuri, M. C. Jothishankar, and S. H. Juang. "Simulation, Animation, and Analysis of Design Assembly for Maintainability Analysis." *International Journal of Production Research* 33, no. 11 (1995), pp. 2999–3022.

CHAPTER 6

Defining Electronics Recycling

CRAIG BOSWELL
HOBI International, Dallas

The ability of design engineers to effectively design more recyclable products is enhanced by an understanding of the recycling process. The basics of recycling are simple. The effectiveness of the recycling process is affected by the ability to collect the product to be recycled, extract or liberate the target materials, and return such materials for use. These basic concepts apply as well to the recycling of electronics products as to the recycling of aluminum cans. An understanding of the implementation of these basic concepts as they apply to electronics products can bring design for recyclability (DfR) in to focus.

An analysis of the basics of the electronics recycling process begins with an understanding of the materials being recovered. The list of materials is as varied as the bill of materials list for an electronic product. The primary materials targeted by the recycler are high-valued materials such as precious metals, aluminum, and copper. However, the recycler also must be concerned with recovery of all hazardous materials and attempts to profitably recover lower-value materials such as ferrous metals and plastics.

The second important aspect of the recycling process is minimizing costs. The costs involved in the process are twofold. The first is the cost to liberate the recyclable materials. The second cost is in the logistics and transportation required for collecting the products. Thoroughly developed DfR plans will address both costs involved in material liberation along with logistics and collection issues.

Recycling Technologies

Two primary technologies have emerged in the electronics recycling process. The first is manual disassembly and the second is destructive disassembly or "grinding." An understanding of these two technologies is important for proper implementation of DfR concepts in product design. The primary technology being used is manual disassembly, which incorporates hand tools and methodologies similar to product assembly. This process, however, is not synonymous with reverse assembly. Labor costs in the disassembly process often can be minimized through the use of techniques such as shearing assemblies apart. Product design will dictate when time-saving steps such as these can and cannot be implemented. A designer incorporating design for assembly concepts will address some DfR concerns, but there are a number of distinctions between design for recycling and design for assembly or reparability. DfR focuses attention on unique items such as material recyclability and separation techniques.

A number of recyclers now use the alternative "destructive" disassembly method. This process incorporates "grinding" or "shearing" as a means to reduce the size of the products, followed by any number of material separation techniques. The process is similar to the shredding process used for recycling automobiles. Once the product has been shredded, magnetic separation is used to reclaim ferrous materials. Gravity separation, among other techniques, then can be used to separate other metal, plastics, paper, and glass. The advantage of this destructive disassembly technique is that it minimizes labor costs. The disadvantage is that it tends to yield more contaminated materials and eliminates the potential for reuse of subassemblies, which can enhance total reclamation value.

The recycling technology being employed, manual disassembly or destructive disassembly, defines the applicability of many DfR principles to a given design. DfR concepts that focus on reduction of disassembly time will have little applicability to a product that ultimately is shredded. Determining what technology will be used to recycle a product is a critical step in the DfR process. This is a simplistic step if the manufacturer has a plan for end-of-life disposition. The designer simply has to be aware of the technology being used by the manufacturer's captive recycling operations. When this information is not available, two metrics generated in the DfR analysis of a product, estimated disassembly time and recyclable material value, can be used as a predictor. If disassembly times are significant and recyclable material value is small, the chance a product will be recycled using a shredding technology is greatly increased. This is especially true for products with little reuse potential, such as mobile communications devices, which often are of little or no value for reuse due to rapid product obsolescence.

Materials Considerations

DfR considerations can be broken down in to two broad categories:

1. Material considerations.
2. Disassembly considerations.

An understanding of material considerations will require analysis of not only the raw materials used in the product but also how these materials are assembled into the final product. The materials portion of the analysis centers on the relative recyclability and toxicity of the materials. The portion of the analysis centering on assembly techniques focuses on barriers that can be created during assembly to the liberation of clean, recyclable materials.

The relative *recyclability of materials* can be broadly defined as the ability and desirability of reprocessing the material. This definition reflects the two characteristics of the material that enhance or limit the recyclability. The first characteristic is the ability to reprocess the material such that its physical characteristics closely reflect the characteristics of virgin material. The second characteristic is the desirability of using recycled material as measured in its cost versus virgin material.

During material-recyclability analysis the product should be evaluated for potential closed-loop recycling options and the potential for reuse of entire parts and subassemblies. *Closed-loop recycling* is defined here as the process of reintroducing the recovered raw materials into the manufacturing stream for that specific product. *Reuse* is defined here as the recovery of partial or complete assemblies for remanufacture in new products. A significant competitive advantage can be gained from products with well-developed reuse programs through raw material and assembly cost avoidance. As an example, large copiers returned from customer lease are sent through a recovery program not only for the recovery of plastics to be reground and mixed with virgin material but also for the recovery of entire assemblies, such as motors and housings. A recovery program such as this often includes high-value integrated circuits such as ASIC devices.

The steps to developing a successful reuse program such as this include analyzing the potential for testing and verification of recovered assemblies. A logistical system also must be developed for recovery of postconsumption product. Additionally, the designer must develop the disassembly procedures necessary to recover usable parts and subassemblies. A final consideration in a plan to incorporate recovered or recycled material in a particular design is gauging its potential impact on the consumer's perception of the product.

The majority of material recovered from products for recycling follows an open-loop recycling path. That is, the material is returned to raw material and can be used in the manufacture of other products, often not even resembling the product from which the material was recovered. Table 6–1 provides a list of the commonly recycled materials found in most information technology products, roughly ordered by their relative value to the recycler.

A product's relative recyclability ultimately is enhanced or restrained by the inclusion of materials that are inherently recyclable and have a significant value on the recycled material market. Although recycled material markets have been developed for a broad range of materials, as seen in Table 6–1, material selection decisions still can make recycling less attractive or impossible. For example, polyethylene terephthalate (PET) is an extensively recycled form of plastic at the municipal level. Yet PET is a relatively low-value plastic and therefore seldom recovered when the logistics of recovery add even small costs to the process.

In addition to the inherent material attributes, the recyclability of a material can be significantly decreased by how it is incorporated into the product during

TABLE 6–1 Commonly Recycled Material Types (in descending order of reclaimed value)

ELEMENTS	COMPOUNDS	COMPONENTS
Platinum	ABS plastic	Integrated circuits
Gold	ABS-FR plastic	Motors
Palladium	Stainless steel	Power supplies
Silver	PVC	Displays
Nickel	Polyethylene	Lead acid batteries
Copper	Steel	NiCad batteries
Zinc	Cardboard	
Aluminum	Glass	
Mercury		

assembly. For example, captive steel inserts in aluminum chassises require an additional processing step for separation, reducing the recovered value and, therefore, the recyclability. Labels added on the surface of plastics can have the same effect. The label material is a contaminant in the plastic recycling operation and can degrade the properties of the recycled material. Removal of labels from plastic parts often is cost prohibitive, making recovery of the plastic no longer economically viable. As a result, otherwise recyclable parts may be sent to incineration or even landfill.

Finally, a review of the toxicity of materials used in the product is an essential step in determining a product's environmental impact at the end of its life. The inclusion of hazardous heavy metals, such as lead in solder and cadmium in portable storage devices, often is a necessity of electronic product design. At end of life, these hazardous materials will have to be recovered and processed, unless they are eliminated through product design improvements. There are methodologies for the safe recovery of these heavy metals; however, the recycler must be able to identify, segregate, and aggregate these materials for the recovery process.

The potential release of hazardous materials in the recovery process includes toxins released in post-disassembly processing. The post-disassembly processing of plastics with brominated and chlorinated fire retardants represents such a concern. These fire retardant materials have the potential to produce dioxins if the plastic is incinerated for energy generation at the end of life. The use of these additives can prevent the recycler from considering energy conversation as an alternative to disposal of plastics in landfills.

Disassembly Considerations

The logistical issues involved in recovering electronic products at the end of life are significant. The goal of this process is to liberate recoverable materials at a minimum cost. In manual disassembly, the cost is measured by disassembly time, which is proportional to the labor cost of disassembly. The minimum disassembly time can be defined as the time to disassemble the product to the appropriate level of disassembly using the optimum disassembly methodology. In many cases, the determination of the optimum disassembly methodology can be an arduous task. The recycler is subject to learning curve effects similar to those experiences in the assembly process, which can be seen as inefficiency in the disassembly process. The potential for these types of inefficiency is significantly affected by product design. Figure 6–1 provides an example of this learning curve effect. Product design considerations such as the visibility and ease of access to fasteners can significantly reduce the learning curve, eliminating some of these inefficiencies from the process.

The optimum disassembly time is affected by a variety of product characteristics, including the number of fasteners that must be removed, the number of materials used within the design, and the time necessary to separate dissimilar materials. The optimum disassembly time is not necessarily equivalent to the time to completely disassemble the product such that all dissimilar materials are separated; for example, removing adhesives, coatings, and labels. The electronics recycler's goal is to disassemble to the point of maximum return. This point can be determined through the use of a net revenue curve, like the one shown in Figure 6–2.

The y-axis of the net revenue curve represents the liberated material value from product disassembly less the cost to disassemble. The x-axis is the time to disassemble. The economic goal of the recycling process is to operate at the most positive point in the net revenue curve. In some cases, the recycler is unable to operate at the peak of this curve due to the need to recover parts bearing hazardous materials, such as mercury relays. In these cases, the recycler must disassemble to the point at which these materials can be recovered and processed in an appropriate fashion. Product design establishes the parameters for the net revenue curve by determining the purity, recyclability, and rate of recovery of materials within the design.

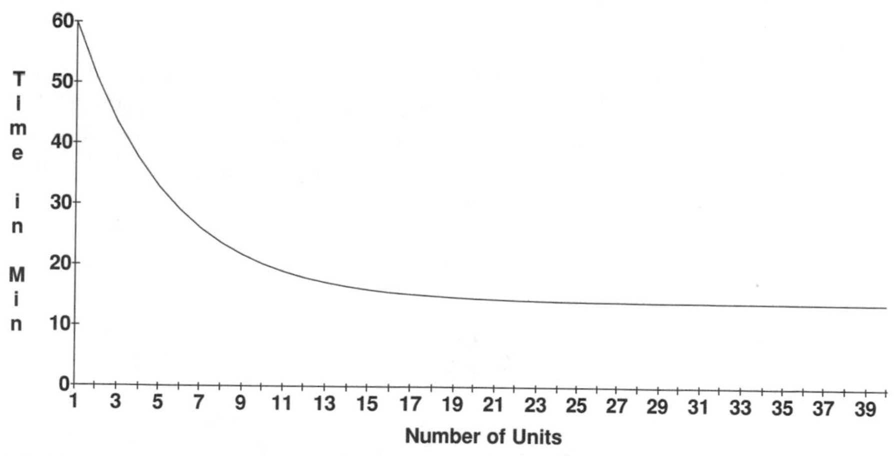

FIGURE 6–1 Disassembly learning curve.

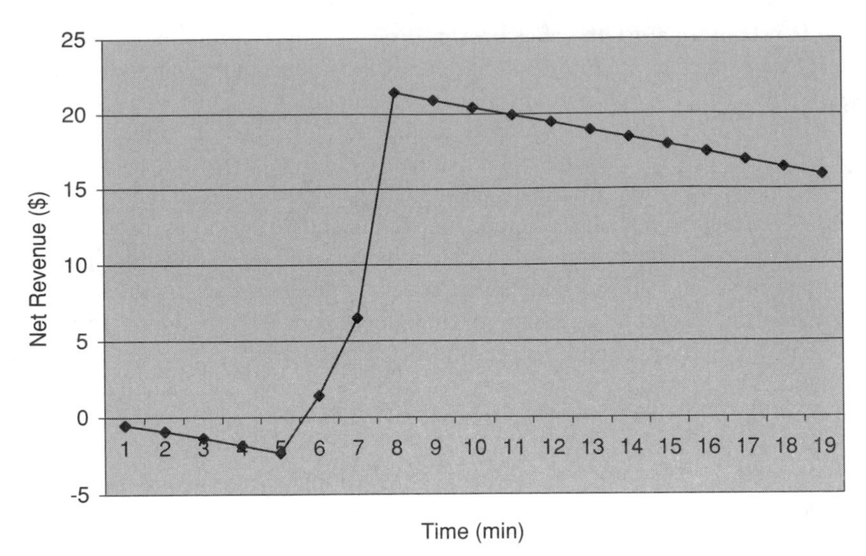

FIGURE 6–2 Net revenue curve.

Design for Recycling Specifics

The goal of DfR analysis is to highlight characteristics of a product that affect its recyclability. The output of the DfR analysis is an understanding of the product's recyclability and a list of potential product improvements. Designers wishing to improve the recyclability of their products can work within three broad categories: increasing the value or recyclability of the liberated material, decreasing the time to liberate the material, and reducing or eliminating hazardous materials.

Recovered Material Value

DfR concepts directed at improving recovered material value encompass both improving the quality of the recovered material and highlighting the potential for choosing more recyclable materials. For the most part, any contaminate added to a material could decrease the value recovered in recycling. Items that require particular attention are those involving the joining of dissimilar materials, including dissimilar plastics and metals. In general, dissimilar materials should be joined with fasteners or clips whenever possible to ensure they can be separated easily. Adhesives and welds should be avoided.

The relative recyclability of materials is affected substantially by market considerations. However, some materials, such as foam and rubber, seldom are recovered in a recyclable form and the weight of these materials should be kept to a minimum. This includes the use of these types of products in product packaging. In most cases, packaging material is not designed into the recovery system, and the best designs keep these materials at a minimum.

Disassembly Time Reduction

Thorough DfR analysis includes an analysis of the time (labor cost) necessary to liberate materials in the demanufacturing or recycling process. The time to liberate materials is affected by a variety of design variables; for example, the number and variation of fasteners, the modularity of the design, and the ease of access to fasteners. Variation in these and other design attributes can have a significant impact on disassembly time.

As an illustration, a simple list of potential design changes can be made for fastener technology. This list would include an overall reduction in fasteners. Consistency in fastener usage (for example, all Phillips-head screws) is very important. In addition, the selection of fastener types can play a significant role in disassembly time. Phillips-head screws are preferred over hex head because they are less likely to strip with high power tools, and clips are preferred over welds.

Recycling is significantly enhanced by design improvements that enhance the accessibility of parts. Therefore, modularity in design can be either a benefit or a hindrance to recycling. Modular designs that create easier part access and make optimum disassembly steps more obvious are a benefit. Modular designs that create a greater number of parts and a greater variation in materials are a hindrance (one large aluminum chassis typically is easier to recover than six small modular frames). It is important to stress that any DfR improvements implemented to reduce manual disassembly time are of little value if the most probable end-of-life processing technology for the product will be destructive disassembly. In destructive disassembly, the two most important product attributes are the variation of materials contained in the product (which should be kept at a minimum) and the relative separability of these materials.

Hazardous Material Elimination

Regardless of the recycling technology chosen for a product, the elimination of hazardous materials results in substantial reduction in potential end-of-life environmental impact. These improvements involve the identification of alternative materials or technologies for changes in product material. Often these improvements extend beyond a specific design. They can involve the development of completely new processes. Examples of these types of changes would be the development of lead-free solder or the elimination of cadmium from portable storage devices. These changes require a DfR program that incorporates research and development, extending beyond incremental improvements to current designs. The payback for these improvements can be quite significant as measured in reduction of product environmental liability.

Quantifying DfR Results

An often-overlooked aspect of a DfR program is defining a methodology to quantify results and allow comparative analysis between competing designs. A quantitative assessment of design improvements targeted at either decreasing disassembly time or increasing liberated material value can be gained by an analysis of the net revenue curve. Figure 6–2 provides an example of this type of curve. DfR improvements that decrease disassembly time increase the peak magnitude of the net revenue curve by shifting the peak to the left (increasing the net revenue generated in the process). DfR improvements, which increase the value of the liberated materials, do not shift the peak of the curve but increase its magnitude by increasing the revenue generated in the disassembly process. Obviously, this type of measurement can be employed only when the design has matured enough to allow disassembly times and recycled content to be estimated. In early design stages, such as the conceptual design phase, more qualitative techniques can be employed. These qualitative techniques often employ a figure of merit or grading system. Criteria such as proposed contained material variations, relative material toxicity, weight, and size can all be a part of the grading system. These qualitative approaches are best employed for comparing various design proposals. Applying these DfR concepts as early in the design process as feasible can be the key to a successful program. Design changes that would not be cost effective to implement in later design stages can be implemented at a much lower cost in early phases of design.

References

Allenby, B., and T. Graedel. *Industrial Ecology.* Englewood Cliffs, NJ: Prentice-Hall, 1995.

Boswell, C. “The Economic Impact of Design for Disassembly on the Electronics Recycling Process.” Proceedings of the Fourth International Congress on Environmentally Conscious Design and Manufacturing, July 23-25, 1996, ECM Press, Albuquerque, NM, 1996.

Boswell, C. “A Feedback Strategy for a Closed Loop End-of-Life Process.” International Conference on Clean Electronics Products and Technology, Institution of Electrical Engineers, Washington, DC, 1995.

Ching, Stephen K., J. Ray Kirby, and O. Dewey Pitts. “Plastics Recycling Issues for the Computer Industry: Progress and Challenges.” IEEE International Symposium on Electronics and the Environment, Dallas, TX, 1996.

CHAPTER 7

Sensor-Based Data Recording for Recycling: A Low-Cost Technology for Embedded Product Self-Identification and Status Reporting

Markus Klausner and Wolfgang M. Grimm
Robert Bosch GmbH, Stuttgart, Germany

Arpad Horvath
Carnegie Mellon University, Pittsburgh

Introduction

Traditionally, consumers have been disposing of used products at the end of their lives. Product takeback imposes the responsibility for a postconsumer stage on manufacturers by requiring them to collect and recycle their products when they reach the end of their lives. Legislation is a major driving force behind product takeback, typically with the goals of allocating waste management costs to producers, reducing the volume of waste generated, and increasing the use of recycled materials (OECD, 1996).

It has been common industrial practice to recycle end-of-life products for their materials. Most design-for-environment guidelines aim at improving products in terms of their recyclability. However, materials recycling might be unattractive in terms of its economic efficiency. Materials often constitute a very small fraction of the product value (e.g., the materials of an average power tool are worth $3, whereas the manufacturing cost is $50). Further, only a fraction of the materials can be reclaimed, and the quality of reclaimed materials may be inferior to virgin materials. The revenues from reclaimed raw materials alone are unlikely to cover collection and disassembly costs. Hence, materials recycling may result in a financial loss, imposing additional costs on manufacturers. Alternative methods for higher levels of product recovery, such as reuse of parts or components from end-of-life products and remanufacturing, are desirable from both the private and social perspectives since they reclaim a higher fraction of the value embedded in a product. If, for example, an electric motor with a rated lifetime of 1,000 hours was used for only 50 hours during the first use stage, why not reuse the motor?

Unfortunately, no information on the remaining lifetime and the quality of a used motor is available or can be obtained easily. Inferior quality of used components, uncertainty about the remaining lifetime, and the rapid obsolescence of reused components frequently are cited arguments against the reuse of components. Some components, such as electric motors, power supplies, and other basic product subsystems, are less subject to obsolescence and innovation, as their technology is comparably stable. This leads us to the problem of assessing the remaining lifetime. While similar strategies can be developed for each type of component, this study focuses on assessment methods that enable reliable, cost-effective reuse of electric motors. Even though we focus on electric motors, most of the work presented in the chapter readily can be generalized for any electronic or mechanical component. We briefly discuss this issue in the last section.

Tests have been developed to assess the reuse potential of certain components. For example, Xerox Corporation developed a test using enveloped vibration energy measurements to discriminate between good and bad used motors to assess the reuse potential of AC induction motors of copiers (Reyes et al. 1995). Here, we describe electronic data logging as a superior alternative to testing. Electronic data logging is the recording of data indicating the degradation of components during the use stage of a product by an electronic device integrated in the product.

Implementation of Product-Integrated Electronic Data Logging—The EDL Concept

Only few concepts have been proposed for storing data for product recovery using a product-integrated electronic device. An approach outlined by Scheidt and Zong (1994) is based on a so-called identification unit that stores static and dynamic "green data," which are accessed via a "green port." At this writing, no prototype based on this concept has been implemented (T. Seidowski, personal communication, 1998). Independent from this approach, we at Bosch have developed and implemented an integrated electronic data log (EDL) that stores data obtained from sensors indicating the degradation of electronic and electromechanical components (Grimm et al., 1998; Klausner et al. 1998a, 1998b). The result of these efforts is an EDL for electric motors, a product-integrated device used to measure, compute, and store parameters correlated with the degradation of an electric motor aiming at the reuse of electric motors and other components of electromechanical end-of-life products.

Our two main design objectives for an EDL prototype for electric motors were

- *Minimization of extra cost attributed to the EDL*, since each product using an electric motor has to be equipped with the EDL, which results in higher initial manufacturing cost.
- *Small size*, as the EDL would be implemented in highly integrated products without modifying the housing and the geometric dimensions.

Product-Integrated EDL Hardware

The EDL prototype that follows, shown in Figure 7–1, meets both design objectives and consists of the following components:

- A circuit board including a microcontroller and EEPROM memory.
- Sensors for the measurement of temperature and current.
- A wireless interface to transmit data from the EDL to an electronic reader; in the first prototype, this was realized with a low-current LED.
- A power supply that provides the DC voltage to supply the microcontroller and sensors. The power supply is not required for a wide range of battery-powered products like cordless power tools, where the DC voltage from batteries can be used.

One of the first approaches to integrating the EDL into a small consumer product and testing its functionality is shown in Figure 7–1. This figure depicts how the EDL could be located inside the housing of a right-angle grinder, one of the most densely packed power tools, without modifying the original design. We did not experience problems when implementing EDLs in various kinds of power tools where space was very limited. The power supply of the EDL is connected to the terminals of

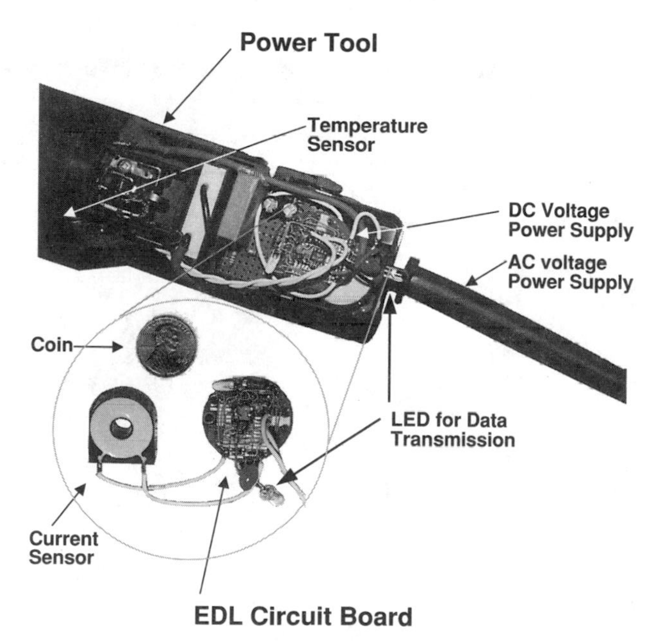

FIGURE 7–1 The first EDL prototype, consisting of circuit board with microcontroller and data memory, current sensor, temperature sensor (not shown), and power supply. For a large-scale application, custom ICs could be developed. For size comparison, a U.S. penny is shown.

the motor. A capacitance ensures that the EDL can safely finish writing data when the motor is switched off.

EDL functionality includes

- Counting the number of starts and stops of the motor.
- Storing the runtime in each individual use cycle as well as the accumulated runtime.
- Recording and compiling sensor information, such as the motor temperature and the power consumption in each individual use cycle.
- Classifying and evaluating the recorded data.
- Computing and storing peak and average values of all parameters of interest.

To achieve a large recording capacity with a much smaller, and thus less-expensive, data memory (preferably the microcontroller's internal EEPROM), the measured parameters are assigned to classes instead of recording a chain of data sets for each use cycle. This approach reduces the data memory size needed to record 50 parameters for 10,000 use cycles from 488 KB to less than 1 KB. Figure 7–2 illustrates this approach, using a total of 29 classes (9 for the temperature, 8 for the current, and 12 for the runtime data). The number of classes and their boundaries are application specific. This approach embeds the disadvantage of losing the correlation between the parameters measured (e.g., current and temperature shown in Fig-

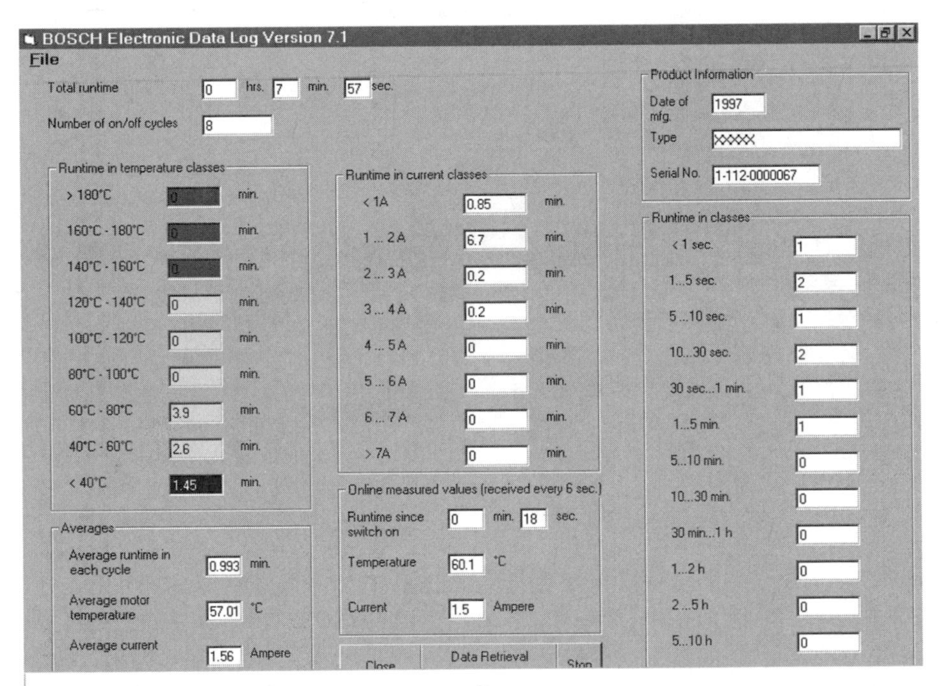

FIGURE 7–2 Screencopy of a software prototype for data visualization (Source: Klausner, 1998b).

ure 7–2). However, this problem can be overcome by combining uncorrelated EDL data with data from laboratory experiments. Software then can estimate the correlation. The first implemented EDL prototypes can record data for an accumulated runtime of approximately 2,300+ hours.

Three bytes in the EDL memory store a unique product identification, like a serial number, that can be used to link the set of dynamic data in the EDL to external static information on the product (discussed next).

EDL Interface and Electronic Reader

Data stored in the EDL is transmitted to a reader using a low-cost, low-current LED, which is located at an easily accessible part of the product's housing. Every time the on/off switch of the product is pressed, the data set stored in the EDL is sent via the LED at a rate of 9,600 baud, indicated by a short flashing of the LED. The data transmitted via the LED is received by a reading device connected to the RS 232 port of a computer. It consists of an array of photo diodes and an electronic device to amplify and convert the transmitted data, plus the necessary RS-232 interface circuitry. The LED also can be utilized for other purposes; for example, to indicate that a service inspection is due since the brushes are worn out.

We investigated other means for transmitting the data stored in the EDL, such as infrared transmission and high frequency (Grimm et al., 1998), and concluded that the LED has the lowest cost of all options. Possible shortcomings associated with the LED option are discussed in Grimm et al. (1998).

Software for Data Visualization and Interpretation

Software was developed to visualize, store, and analyze the data retrieved from the EDL. Data such as total runtime, individual runtime in each use cycle, the associated motor temperature and current, and peak and average values of those variables are visualized on the screen (Figure 7–2). A classification algorithm allows us to discriminate between reusable and non-reusable used motors based on the recorded data.

Some EDL Design Considerations

An EDL design has to be robust, similar to the black box in an aircraft. Therefore, the EDL to a great extent should be independent from failure or damage to the product in which it is implemented. Consider the previously described EDL prototype. To retrieve the EDL data, the product must be connected to a power supply, and both the switch and the LED must be functioning. Therefore, a better but unfortunately more expensive design would use radio frequency for data transmission. The EDL would communicate to the reader via an antenna, and the reader would provide energy to read the EDL data. This design would be similar to contactless smartcards. EDL data retrieval would be independent from the connection of the product to a power supply and a functioning switch. While this option is clearly preferable for product recovery from a technological viewpoint, it is more expensive than the LED-based solution.

Another design aspect is the validation of the data recorded by the EDL. They have to be checked for plausbility, and failures of sensors must be detected. Tampering with EDL data must be prevented by using a design that makes alteration of collected data by the user or a third party almost impossible.

Standardization

The interface for data retrieval and the data format have not yet been standardized (Grimm et al., 1998). If the EDL data were accessible to recyclers and an EDL design could be customized such that it could be used by different manufacturers and for different products, unit costs could be significantly lowered. This would require an EDL design that can be adjusted to different applications. It also implies a stand-alone EDL instead of the integration of EDL functionality in existing controls.

If used components are reused, the transfer of EDL data associated with reused components from a previous product's EDL to the EDL of the current product employing the used component may become an interesting issue. This would require a standardization of the data format. In this context, it seems interesting to discuss the degree of centralization of EDL data gathering. One could think of a design with one EDL per product on the one extreme and a design with individual EDLs on the component level on the other. This is particularly relevant for MEMS-based EDLs (discussed later) as they would be applied in a decentralized manner.

An industrywide standardized EDL for electronic products is the focus of one project proposal in the context of the European CARE Vision project.

An Information System for Product Recovery

End-of-life costs can be reduced and the reclamation of value from end-of-life products improved if the dynamic data obtained from the EDL are combined with external data relevant for product recovery (e.g., demand for used components and remanufactured products) and further static data on the product (e.g., materials composition, disassembly sequence). Static data is created at the design and manufacturing stages, while external data elements reflect the current market environment. The information system for product recovery (ISPR) integrates these static and dynamic data and automates the classification of returned end-of-life products (Klausner et al., 1998a). For example, the ISPR would check whether there is demand for a remanufactured model of a returned end-of-life product, using the external data linked to the product via the unique product identification stored in the EDL (Klausner, 1998). In a next stage, the ISPR would identify reusable parts, components, and subassemblies based on the evaluation of the data stored in the EDL. If remanufacturing is not possible (since there is either no demand or the product technically is not remanufacturable), materials recycling (which might involve the reclamation of some parts) would be recommended and supported by a generated disassembly sequence optimizing revenues from reclaimed materials.

Economic Efficiency of the EDL in a Reuse Scenario

Manufacturing Cost Savings

The cost target for the EDL ought to be determined by the economic efficiency of reusing components from end-of-life products. The EDL is economically attractive only if the additional manufacturing costs attributed to EDL implementation are offset by cost savings from reuse. Therefore, we developed an economic model addressing this problem for the EDL for electric motors (Klausner et al., 1998b).

Since all motors of a product line have to be equipped with an EDL, the initial manufacturing cost will increase due to the additional cost of the EDL and its integration into the product. Unfortunately, only a fraction of the motors equipped with the EDL is likely to be returned, and only a portion of the returned motors actually can be reused. A manufacturer therefore is faced with the question of whether the additional cost of the EDL is justified by the savings resulting from the reuse of a fraction of the motors equipped with the EDL. To answer this, we compare the net present value (NPV) of the total cost of equipping all motors with an EDL and reusing a fraction of them (cost C_{reuse}) to the NPV of the total cost of newly manufactured motors not equipped with an EDL (cost C_{new}). Taking into account the costs of screening and reclaiming used motors, we compare the difference between the two NPVs of C_{new} and C_{reuse} over two motor life cycles (Klausner et al., 1998b).

We denote the mathematical product of the fraction of motors returned and the fraction of returned motors reusable as the recovery rate. Figure 7–3 shows the

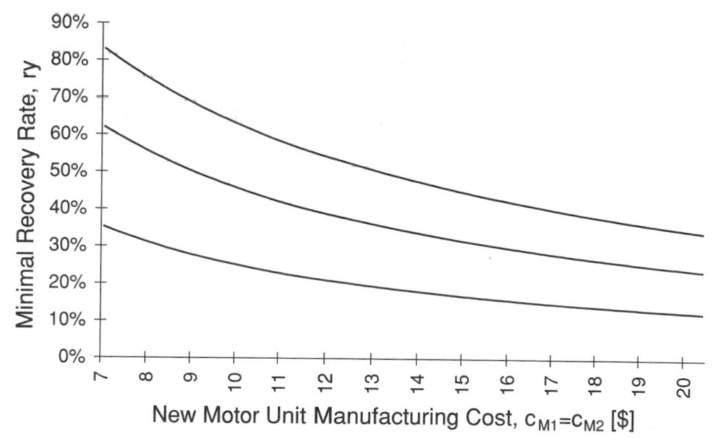

FIGURE 7–3 Recovery rate that must be exceeded for profitable motor reuse based on EDLs as a function of motor cost for different costs of the EDL (Source: Klausner et al, 1998b).

minimal recovery rate required to offset additional manufacturing cost by cost savings from reuse as a function of motor cost. For example, if motor manufacturing cost (without the EDL) is \$15 and the EDL cost is \$2, a recovery rate of 32% would be needed to justify the additional cost of the EDL (Figure 7–3). If 50% of all returned motors are reusable, 64% of the motors manufactured would have to be returned.

Accounting for Misclassifications

Ideally, the classification software correctly classifies all motors as reusable or non-reusable. In actuality, however, misclassifications are unavoidable (Figure 7–4). As a result, a fraction of motors classified as reusable might fail in the second life cycle (false positives, FP) and a fraction of motors rejected for reuse might turn out to be reusable (false negatives, FN). Misclassifications result in additional costs, which we integrated in our economic analysis (Klausner et al., 1998b).

The cost of an FN, c_{FN}, is the cost of substituting a newly manufactured motor for a motor falsely rejected for reuse. Estimating the cost of an FP, c_{FP}, is more difficult. A motor originally classified as reusable, which fails later when placed back in a product, may lead to serious consequences including negative impact on the image of a manufacturer and loss of future contracts. As a result, quantifying c_{FP} is subjective and difficult to justify. The most conservative estimate for c_{FP} may be the warranty cost for a defective motor. However, a manufacturer concerned about quality may use an extremely high cost estimate, taking into account that the indirect effects of motor failure might be prohibitively expensive.

Estimating the fractions of TP, FP, FN, and TN is very difficult. The yield is equivalent to the sum of the fractions of TP and FP and known. Since, however, the relation between TP and FP generally is unknown, the best solution is the application of good engineering judgment. Repair statistics are bad estimators for the fractions of FP, since the eventual fate of a product equipped with a defective motor can hardly be predicted. The product may be disposed of, stored, and so forth, so that a manufacturer has no complete information on the actual number of failures during the entire use stage of a product.

		Actual Motor Behavior	
		Will Not Fail	Will Fail
Motor Classified as	Reusable	True positive (TP)	False positive (FP) **Cost c_{FN}**
	Non-reusable	False Negative (FN) Cost c_{FP}	True Negative (TN)

FIGURE 7–4 Classification of used motors including misclassifications.

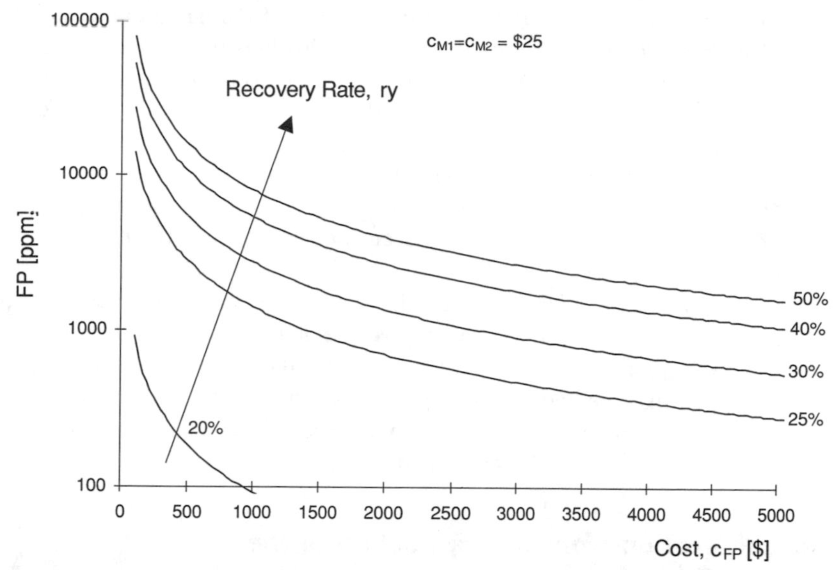

FIGURE 7–5 Maximum number of false positives (FP) that must not be exceeded depending on both the cost of an FP and the recovery rate (Source: Klausner et al, 1998b).

Figure 7–5 depicts the maximum number of FP (in parts per million) that must not be exceeded to obtain a profit from motor reuse. It is based on the ED depending on both the cost assigned to an FP and the recovery rate for a motor manufacturing cost of $25 and an EDL cost of $2. The analytical approach behind Figure 7–5 is described in (Klausner, 1998; Klausner et al., 1998b). Figure 7–5 represents a guide to determine the required classification accuracy of the software processing the EDL data. At a recovery rate of 30%, less than 2,726 ppm FP would be acceptable if a cost of $1,000 is assigned to each FP (Figure 7–4). If we assigned a cost of only $100 to an FP, then a maximum of less than 27,263 misclassifications would be acceptable, given that all other conditions remain unchanged.

Further Application Scenarios

In addition to being an enabler for high levels of product recovery, the EDL might be used in the following scenarios (Grimm et al., 1998):

- *Leasing based on use intensity.* Instead of lessees paying for the time they are leasing a product, the EDL would enable the lessor to charge a fee based on equivalent operating hours (EOH; Klausner, 1998). This would not only imply a fairer pricing mechanism but also counteract the incentive to abuse leased products. Applications include power tools, construction machinery, and rental cars.

- *Quality management and market research.* The EDL helps to monitor customer behavior, thereby providing valuable insights for product design.
- *Service and maintenance or warranty claim assessment.* Misuse or overuse could be easily identified. Causes leading to failure modes would become transparent.
- *Use intensity-based warranty periods.* Instead of offering a warranty period of fixed length from the date of purchase, the warranty could apply to the first *n* number of EOH, rewarding customers who use their product less intensively.
- *Pricing of used products.* As the EDL allows one to reconstruct the entire use history of products and detect possible abuse, pricing of used products becomes more transparent and less risky for the buyer. Traditional pricing indicators like age and odometer readings cannot provide this information, thus implying higher risks for the buyer. These risks result in a lower price than achievable with EDL-equipped products.

Considerations for the Application of the EDL to Other Products

The main motivation underlying the EDL is to substantially increase product end-of-life value. It accomplishes this by providing information on product use that is essential for product recovery and would be unavailable otherwise. Products that typically qualify for EDL implementation include electromechanical systems and electronics. The degradation of most electromechanical systems is strongly correlated with use intensity. Therefore, an EDL for an electromechanical product would be similar to the EDL for electric motors, recording a set of application-specific parameters strongly correlated with degradation and wear. In contrast, intensive use does generally not degrade electronics and yet implementing an EDL to improve electronics recovery still might make sense.

Extreme environmental conditions (e.g., high temperature and humidity) and improper product handling (e.g., product fell on the ground, product was exposed to high stress or strain) could prevent product or subassembly reuse. Therefore, one might be interested in recording parameters that exceed certain critical thresholds (e.g., temperatures that lead to critical temperature-induced stresses). Microelectromechanical systems (MEMS) offer opportunities for low-cost recording of such parameters. Another major advantage of MEMS is their small size, allowing them to be implemented in all kinds of electronics. For example, microengineered pressure sensors could record whether circuit boards were excessively bent, such as during disassembly. As appealing as EDLs appear, they should only be implemented for product recovery if they are superior to tests or visual inspections in terms of economics and information availability. In addition to their use for product recovery, EDLs could enhance the analysis of product failures as outlined already.

References

Grimm, W. M., H. Horber, M. Klausner, and W.-H. Rech. "Product-Integrated Electronic Data Log as an Enabler for Reuse, Repair, Quality Management, and Market Research." Proceedings CARE Innovation '98, The Second International Symposium, Vienna, 1998.

Klausner, M. "Design and Analysis of Product Takeback Systems." Unpublished Ph.D. thesis, Carnegie Mellon University, Pittsburgh, 1998.

Klausner, M., W. M. Grimm, C. Hendrickson, and A. Horvath. "Sensor-Based Data Recording of Use Conditions for Product Takeback." Proceedings of the IEEE International Symposium on Electronics and the Environment, Chicago, 1998a, pp. 138–143.

Klausner, M., W. Grimm, and C. Hendrickson. "Reuse of Electric Motors of Consumer Products: Design and Analysis of an Electronic Data Log." *Journal of Industrial Ecology* 2, No. 2 (1998b), pp. 89–102.

OECD. "Extended Producer Responsibility in the OECD Area, Phase 1 Report," Working Paper No. 66. Paris: OECD, 1996.

Reyes, W., M. Moore, C. R. M. Bartholomew, R. Currence, and R. Siegel. "Reliability Assessment of Used Parts: An Enabler for Asset Recovery." Proceedings of the IEEE International Symposium on Electronics and the Environment, Orlando, FL, 1995, pp. 89–94.

Scheidt, L.-G., and S. Zong. "An Approach to Achieve Reusability of Electronic Modules." Proceedings of the IEEE International Symposium on Electronics and the Environment, San Francisco, 1994, pp. 331–336.

Part III

Green Design Automation Tools

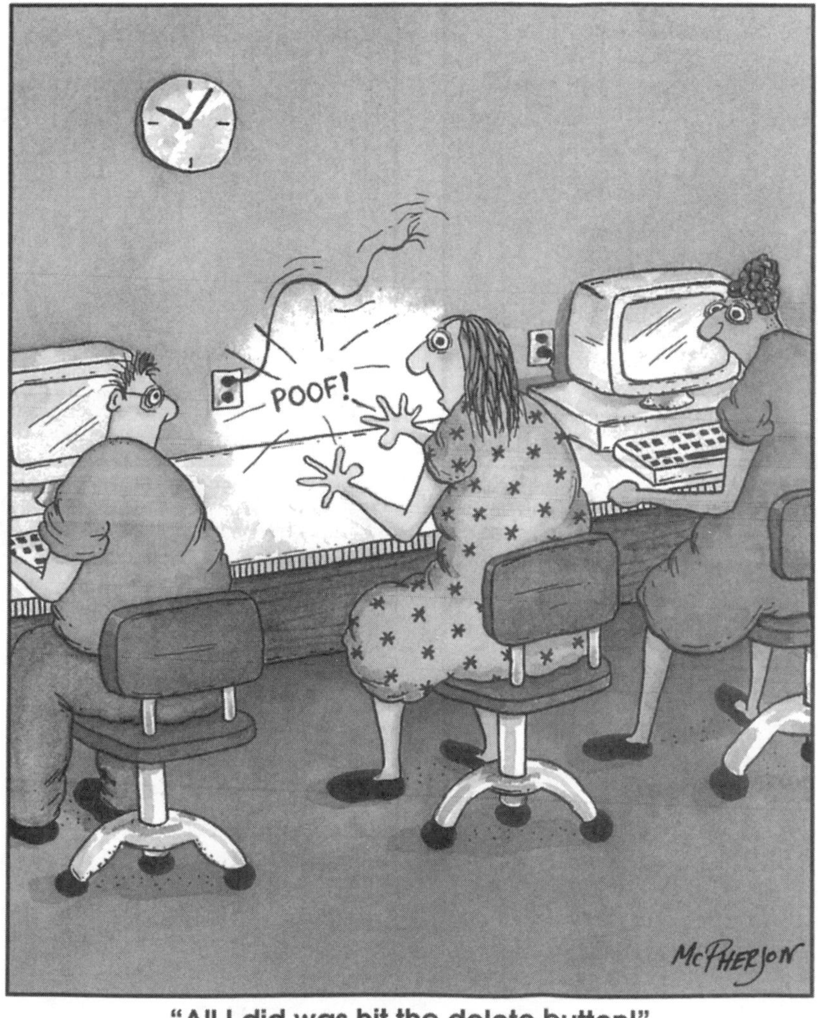

"All I did was hit the delete button!"

CHAPTER **8**

A Survey of DfE Software

JOAN WILLIAMS
Federal Reserve Bank

The proliferation of automated tools for environmental design is truly on an S-curve. Environmental regulations from above as well as education on green design and a demand from below have fueled the need for some way to identify, measure, and especially incorporate environmental impact into product design. Life cycle assessment (LCA) provided the fundamental methodology used to evaluate the materials selection, production, distribution, use, and disposal costs associated with a product during its complete life cycle. Now, design-for-environment (DfE) proponents have rapidly applied this approach to systematic design practices, both automated and manual, which minimize these costs at the time of design. Currently, the proliferation of such design practices is coming to the steepest part of the S-curve, where the groundwork for some standardization has been made but much room is left for further innovation.

This survey will take on the characteristics of a "snapshot" analysis, where a rapidly developing market makes it difficult to create a listing that is either comprehensive or absolute and a snapshot of the landscape is pragmatic. The quantity of products being developed using both DfE and LCA, and the speed of evolution of existing products, impedes the job of describing a comprehensive collection of commercially available products. Ranking the available tools and discussing them in superlative terms is unreliable for the purpose of this text, since models are continually refined and, of course, the best tool is the one that best meets the requirements of a particular design.

Many resources for locating the right software tools are becoming available. In this chapter, the "still frame" analysis will concentrate on the evolution of these products parallel to the evolution of the DfE movement and identification of resources that will lead any product designer to the appropriate software tools.

DfE Software Classification

Contemporary DfE activities roughly fall in a spectrum between identification of environmental impact and total product design according to environmental design metrics (Table 8–1). On one end of the spectrum lies the identification of environmental costs, usually categorized as LCA. In their purest forms, LCA tools are particularly useful for facilitating and documenting compliance with environmental regulations. As the consideration of life cycle stages and environmental concerns become less qualitative and more quantitative, tools are categorized as DfE; that is, they influence environmental impact at the design phase.

It is difficult to place different types of environmental software, over 2,000 currently marketed, into tidy categories. The EPA and the Research Triangle Institute (RTI) established general categories to organize a broad range of environmental software in its 1995 "Incorporating Environmental Costs and Considerations into Deci-

TABLE 8–1 Design for Environment (Where is DfE today?)

Phase	Metrics	Application	Product Designer's View	Examples
0—Problem Recognition	None	Select products and processes—typically those with high visibility	Guidelines	Meeting regulations or compliance
				Qualitative or subjective approaches
1—Problem Articulation	Few	Generic product categories and technology families	Available as a consulting activity	Design-for-Environment Energy/Mass Balance LCA
2—Metric Formulation	Concise	Selected specific products	Available during the design process (but not part of general design methodology)	Design for Manufacturability/Assembly Design-to-Cost Design-for-Reliability
3—Product Impact	Mature	Every applicable product	Integrated into the design process/ methodology	Design-for-Test Performance (electrical, thermal)

Source: Pitts, 1997.

sion-Making: Review of Available Tools and Software" (Table 8–2). The publication was critical and timely for this emerging market. It not only provided badly needed organization but also offered assessments and recommendations for selected vendors in each product category. In this classification system, DfE tools could be located in several of the project-focused (as opposed to managerial) product categories, where the key function of the software is design and where a systematic, ecoefficient approach to metrics, design practices, and analysis methods is taken (Fiksel, 1996).

Digital Equipment Corporation and the MIT Program on Technology, Business and Environment classify DfE tools according to three primary attributes. First, a tool's applicability to product development stages will indicate whether a tool may be used for simply establishing project goals or actually developing detailed designs. Second, its degree of applicability to product life-cycle stages determines how appropriately life-cycle stages are applied to a product's design and how many

TABLE 8–2 EPA/RTI Classification of Environmental Software Systems (1995)

	Name	Description
Class 1	Cost Estimating Software Systems	Products designed for cost estimation. Usually used by project managers to estimate conceptual and/or detailed project costs
Class 2	Scheduling and Cost Control/Analysis Software Systems	Products designed to automate project scheduling, monitoring, cost control and performance measurement. Used by project managers to maintain project schedules and budgets according to plan
Class 3	Risk Assessment and Contingency Analysis Software Systems	Products designed to assess risk (not necessarily project related)
Class 4	Environmental Management and Regulatory Compliance Software Systems	Products designed to track waste and waste management costs, primarily to comply with environmental regulations
Class 5	Remediation Project-related Software Systems	Products designed to address different areas of remediation projects, including cost estimation and scheduling, RI/FS planning and risk analysis, and cost tracking
Class 6	Financial Analysis Software Systems and Tools	Products designed to provide information and methods for the financial analysis of projects (usually applied to pollution prevention projects)
Class 7	Environmental LCC and Impact Analysis Software Systems and Tools	Products that identify, estimate and/or analyze environmental costs for specific projects, areas, or as generic tools
Class 8	Waste Reduction Software Systems and Tools	Products designed to provide general or project/facility-specific guidance on methods to effectively manage wastes or environmental costs

Source: Sharma, Elwood, and Weitz, 1995.

life-cycle stages the tool supports. Finally, a tool's degree of decision support accounts for the type of data output generated. Inventory tools generate raw data, impact tools aggregate the data, and improvement tools generate design alternatives that minimize environmental impact (Roll and Ehrenfeld, 1997). Using this system can help designers organize available tools and choose the ones most suitable for their specific projects.

Product Evolution and Diversity

In the early 1990s, European companies began to experiment with LCA at the design level through checklists and guidelines. They also applied matrices by plotting some blend of LCA life-cycle stages (materials acquisition, manufacturing and testing, use/reuse/maintenance, and disassembly/waste management) against an applicable list of environmental concerns. Checklists, guidelines, and matrices were an improvement over LCA tools in product development, since LCA tools normally require a significant amount of data and knowledge of processes. Also, LCA tools typically are time consuming, and inherently, design must be completed quickly to speed products to market. For DfE principles to become widely adopted, designers needed a way to implement them quickly.

Above all, LCA tools produced qualitative assessments, and designers needed a quantitative assessment to compare impact and choose design alternatives. Results produced by LCA tools usually were a subjective assignment of a value on a 1–4 scale, oftentimes weighted, to a particular environmental impact concern. These were beneficial for internal assessments but were not standardized or comparable for external review. This standardization problem was, and still is, associated with checklists, matrices, and DfE software products that employ different metrics, methodologies, data requirements, levels of customization, and specific hardware requirements.

However, this lack of standardization has a positive tilt. The number of unique tools on the market address the diverse needs of designers and project managers. Also, both ready-made, often-customizable, applications and tailored applications offered by consultants bring continually evolving applied DfE principles to the mainstream. In this section, we briefly explore two commercially available DfE software tools, each with a contrasting approach to DfE but a common goal to make embracing DfE principles practical in the corporate environment.

In 1997, a consortium of Alcatel Alsthom, IBM, Legrand, Schneider Electric, ADEME (French Environment Agency), Thomson Multimedia, and the ECOBILAN group (Ecobalance, Inc.) released EIME (Environmental Information and Management Explorer). The tool, aimed at designers and development staff, was an attempt to capitalize on ECOBILAN's LCA experience while creating a way for corporations to standardize their strategy for integrating DfE principles.

The tool relies on flexible interfaces, generic environmental data, and a focus on reduction of mass and energy (materials acquisition, manufacture, and use life-cycle stages). Its database contains the most common materials and parts used in electronic design, as well as process and transportation modules. Company-specific requirements can be added, and designers using the tool receive a warning when they attempt to use materials that have been prohibited by company policy or legislation (Figure 8–1). This feature improves standardization and regulatory compliance, but it also saves valuable time by avoiding potential errors. The application also facilitates recyclability by maintaining a "To Do" list throughout the product's design. For example, the system will let a designer know when a recyclable component should be marked as such later in the design process.

DfE 1.0 provides a different incentive for companies to incorporate DfE principles: the bottom line. The tool performs a cost and environmental assessment coanalysis of future products, concentrating on disassembly at the end of the product's life. The tool, jointly produced by U.S.-based Boothroyd and Dewhurst, Inc. (BDI), and the TNO Institute of the Netherlands, was awarded *Industry Week*'s 1996 Technologies of the Year Award. It results from BDI's background as a pioneer in

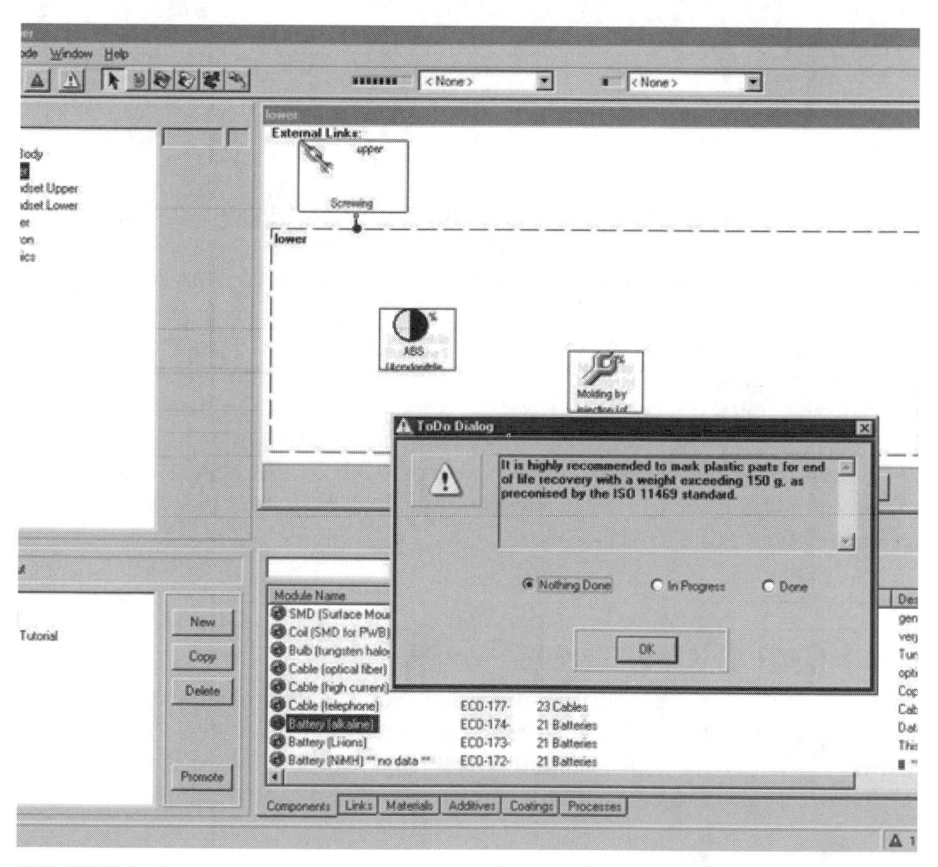

FIGURE 8–1 DfE software can be used to alert a designer to materials selection problems.

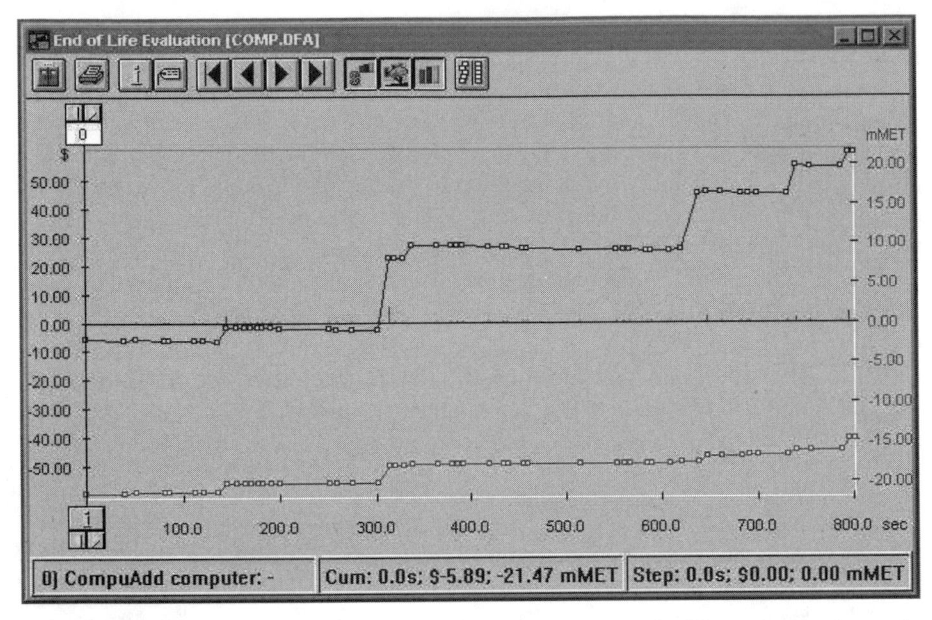

FIGURE 8–2 DfE software can be used to perform analyses for life-cycle planning and design.

DfA (design-for-assembly) applications, and TNO's proprietary MET (materials, energy, toxicity) points value assessment metric for quickly determining environmental impact. The application uses the metric to analyze and maximize a product's end-of-life recovery potential and resulting cost benefits. The financial return curve, a juxtaposition to the environmental impact curve on DfE 1.0's graphical interface, shows the company's potential profit or loss as each component in the planned product is disassembled (Figure 8–2). Essentially, the tool determines the point at which it becomes uneconomical to continue disassembling a part or product.

Compared to the EIME software product, this type of simulation tool, with its focus on the disposal and reassembly life-cycle stages, proves how varied the life-forms of DfE software tools can be.

Software Resources and Guides

EM Magazine, a publication of Air and Waste Management, published (July 1997 issue) and updated (October 1998 issue) a comprehensive environmental software products buyers' guide including over 900 offerings. Software and vendors for the following functions are included ("Environmental Software Problems," 1998):

Air
Ground water
Hazardous and toxic materials

Land use
Occupational safety and health
Soil and geology
Surface water
Transportation
Waste disposal and treatment
Waste water
General environmental
Calculations and equations
Control and remediation
Cost and finance
Design
Graphics
Modeling
Physical and chemical data
Pollution prevention
Risk assessment
Audits and compliance
Data management
Facility operation
Geographic information systems
Inventory
Monitoring
Permit tracking
Regulations
Research
Emergency response and planning
Hazards and operability studies
Labels and manifests
MSOSs
Public right to know
Releases and spills
Reporting
Site assessment
Training

In addition, the EPA's "Incorporating Environmental Costs and Considerations into Decision-Making: Review of Available Tools and Software" is available both on-line (http://www.epa.gov/opptintr/acctg/rev) and in print from the EPA.

Acknowledgments

My special thanks to Brian Glazebrook, Lisa McCafferty, and Greg Pitts for their invaluable help in preparing this chapter.

References

"Environmental Design Tools." In *Product Development and the Environment*, ed. Paul Burall, pp. 115–130. Hampshire, England: Gower Publishing, 1996.

"Environmental Software Products." *EM Magazine* (October 1998), p. 83.

Fiksel, Joseph. "Conceptual Principles of DfE." In *Design for Environment: Creating Eco-Efficient Products and Processes*, ed. Joseph Fiksel, p. 55. New York: McGraw-Hill, 1996.

Gilligan, John (Boothroyd and Dewhurst, Inc.). At mailto:info@dfma.com or http://www.dfma.com.

Glazebrook, Brian (Ecobalance USA; ECOBIAL Group). At brian_glazebrook @radian.com.

Mizuki, Coleen, Cynthia Murphy, and Peter Sandborn. "Implementation of DfE in the Electronics Industry Using Simple Metrics for Cost, Quality and Environmental Merit." Microelectronics and Computer Technology Corporation (MCC), MCC-ENV-019-98, 1998.

"New DfE Software Addresses Economic, Ecological Aspects of Product Recycling." *Business and the Environment* 7, no. 12 (December 1996), p. 11

"New Software for DfE and Analysis of Product Lifecycles." *Product Stewardship Advisor* 1, no. 1 (May 1997), p. 12.

Pitts, Greg. "DfE and Takeback of Electronic Products in the U.S." Microelectronics and Computer Technology Corp. (MCC), presentation to End of Life Electronics Products—Takeback Conference, London, November 25–26, 1997.

Roll, Monica (Digital Equipment Corp.), and John Ehrenfeld (Massachusetts Institute of Technology Program on Technology, Business and Environment). "Implementing Design for Environment: A Primer," pp. 15–16. Digital Equipment Corp., Maynard, MA, March 1997.

Sharma, Aarti, Holly Elwood, and Keith Weitz. "Incorporating Environmental Costs and Considerations into Decision-Making: Review of Available Tools and Software." U.S. Environmental Protection Agency, RTI Project Number 5774-3, September 1995.

CHAPTER 9

Design for Environment: A Printed Circuit Board Assembly Example

SUDARSHAN SIDDHAYE AND PAUL SHENG
University of California, Berkeley

Introduction

Integration of factors concerning environmental impact during manufacture, use, and disposition of the product is an emerging issue in design of electronics. The drivers for this in electronics include certification standards such as ISO 14000 and British standard 7750; ecolabeling programs such as Energy Star, Blue Angel, and TCO; increasing internalization of waste mitigation and disposal costs into the product cost; and an increasing need for environmental accountability in global supply networks. One important aspect of product design for environment (DfE) in electronics is the consideration of the environmental impact during the manufacturing stage. In particular, a significant contributor to life-cycle environmental impacts is the fabrication and assembly stages of a printed circuit board. Process models can be used as an analytical tool to develop environmental performance indicators for products. These process models, while modeling the manufacturing waste streams, also implicitly model the product parameters and can be used conveniently for product design optimization.

This part of the chapter will introduce the techniques based on process modeling and product optimization that can be applied to printed circuit board assembly design to minimize the environmental impact. Although the focus of this part is on PCB assemblies, after studying these techniques, one easily can apply the principles to other product optimization problems.

We first talk briefly about the process models for PC board fabrication. A waste-stream weighting scheme, which is extremely useful for comparing two or more dissimilar waste streams, then is introduced. After that we discuss an optimization algorithm that will seek a balance between the various board design parameters, such as board area, number of layers, and number of boards on a panel, to come up with the physical board design with the minimal manufacturing waste per board. The results of a case study will be presented to give the reader an idea of how the technique can be implemented. Last we qualitatively discuss specific issues such as how to incorporate various design constraints, how to extend this analysis to packaging and the semiconductor manufacturing level, and how this piece of analysis fits into the overall life-cycle analysis of a product.

Process Modeling

Manufacturing a printed circuit board assembly consists of three parts: (1) semiconductor manufacture, (2) electronic packaging manufacture, and (3) bare-board fabrication and component assembly. Despite a tremendous flexibility in process selection in semiconductor manufacturing, there is somewhat limited room for product optimization to achieve better environmental results. In electronic packaging, one can choose from a wide array of packages. However, in most cases, the functional requirements very quickly narrow the choice to a few types.

For bare-board fabrication, about 7% of the material used actually goes into the product and the remaining 93% is emitted as process waste (Allen, 1997). Hence, minimizing the process waste is the most logical way to minimize the environmental impact of a circuit board. The process steps include laminate core fabrication, resist coating, exposure, development, copper etch, resist strip, oxide treatment, lamination, drilling, desmear and copper plating, and solder masking, as shown in Figure 9–1.

We can model the thermochemical and thermomechanical behavior of various process steps involved in fabrication to predict the waste streams. As an example, the waste streams from the etching operation can be modeled in terms of the board parameters as

$$m_{Cu} = \rho_{Cu}(1 - K_{Cu})\,A_{core}\,t_{Cu} \quad (9\text{–}1)$$

$$m_{etc} = m_{Cu}\,(M_{CuCl2}/M_{Cu}) \quad (9\text{–}2)$$

$$m_{Cu2Cl2} = m_{Cu}\,(M_{Cu2Cl2}/M_{Cu}) \quad (9\text{–}3)$$

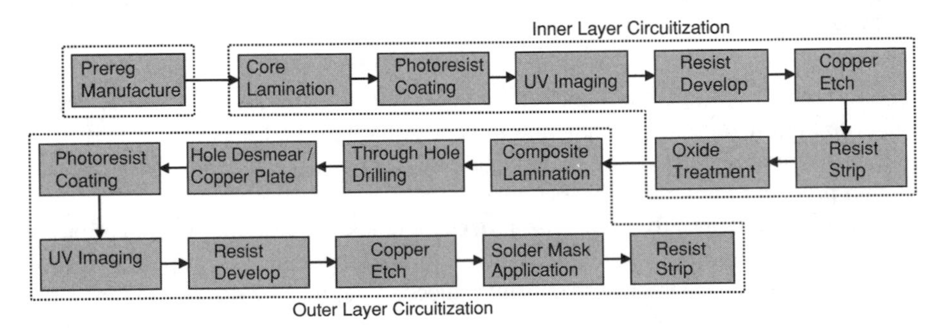

FIGURE 9–1 Process steps in PCB fabrication.

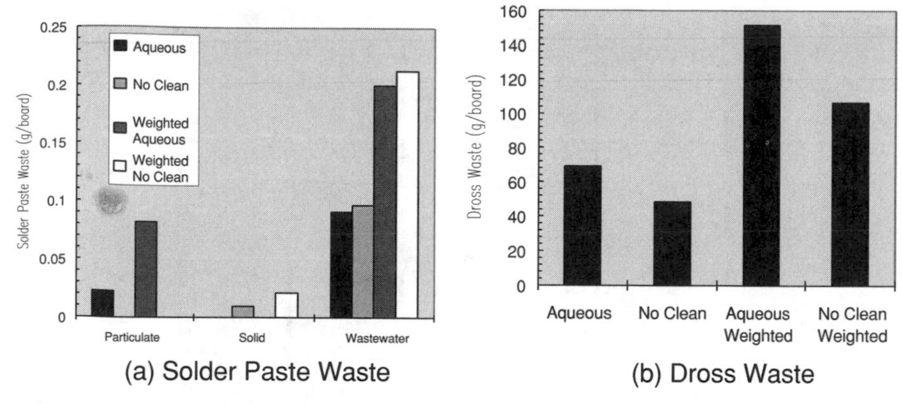

FIGURE 9–2 Process model estimates for reflow and wave solder processes.

where m represents the mass, M represents the molecular weight, A represents the area, t represents the thickness, and K represents the fraction of copper retained on the board after etching, for a particular layer. Similar models can be formulated for component assembly operations such as stenciling, component placement, reflow, wave solder, and board cleaning. A complete set of models can be found in Siddhaye and Sheng (1997) and Worhach and Sheng (1997). These models must be validated using the actual waste-stream data collected at the fabrication site. Figure 9–2 shows the model estimates for reflow and wave soldering processes.

Health Hazard Assessment

It is crucial to be able to compare the raw mass of these waste streams. This can be achieved using some kind of health hazard assessment method like the health hazard scoring system described in Srinivasan, Wu, and Sheng (1995). This system computes a scalar weighting factor called the *health hazard score* (HHS). This number is calculated for a particular waste stream using its health hazard potential data (carcinogenicity, reactivity, flammability, dermal irritability, inhalation toxicity, oral toxicity, and eye irritation), its phase (solid, solid particulate, liquid, vapor, or aerosol), and the safety practices on site. This number essentially brings two dissimilar waste streams to the same level of hazard for the purpose of mutual comparison.

The categorical hazard score, H, is determined based on the information from various sources such as the American Conference of Governmental and Industrial Hygienists (ACGIH) threshold limit value (TLV) data and the Registry of Toxic Effects of Chemical Substances (RTECS) database.

To introduce phase effects with chemical hazard subscores, a phase matrix, P, can be constructed to partition the hazard share for each factor among the different physical phases using the Kepner-Tregoe method, where each coefficient is assigned a fractional value from 0 to 1.

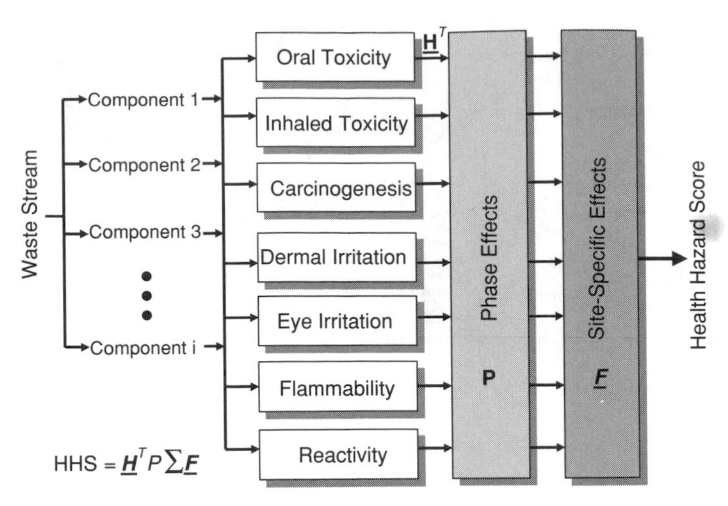

FIGURE 9–3 Health hazard scoring method.

The final factor to consider is site modeling. Since each site in which manufacturing occurs is different in terms of facilities design, equipment, and work practices, these site-specific factors have a significant influence on waste-stream environmental impact. However, these factors are largely qualitative in nature (e.g., wearing protective garments, continuous monitoring of the process). A major challenge, therefore, is to reduce qualitative site information into a quantitative form, which can be evaluated along with chemical hazards and phase.

One approach is to construct a set of pairwise evaluations comparing toxicity (oral and inhaled), carcinogenesis, irritation (dermal and eye), reactivity, and flammability using the analytic hierarchy process (AHP), a method that ranks pairwise comparisons between various factors. Successive comparisons set up a matrix. Initially, a subjective set of priorities is elicited from the user regarding the different factors (such as toxicity, reactivity, flammability). These priorities then are placed into an AHP matrix.

The schematic of the HHS method is shown in Figure 9–3. Examples of categorical hazard scores are shown in Table 9–1. An example phase matrix is shown in Table 9–2, and an example AHP matrix is shown in Table 9–3.

TABLE 9–1 Score, H_i, for "Reactivity"

Score	Reacts with
9	Metals, oxidizing agents, acids, bases, moist air, water, etc.
8	Metals and moist air
7	Metals
6	Air (moist)
4–5	Oxidizing agents
1–3	Acids or bases
0	No known substance (inert)

TABLE 9–2 An Example Phase Matrix

	PHASE				
HAZARD	SOLID	LIQUID	AEROSOL	VAPOR	SOLID PARTICLES
Oral toxicity	0.3	0.4	0	0	0.3
Inhalation toxicity	0	0	0.5	0.3	0.2
Eye irritation	0	0	0.4	0.4	0.2
Dermal irritation	0.2	0.5	0	0	0.3
Carcinogenicity	0	0.3	0.3	0.3	0.1
Reactivity	0	0.5	0.2	0.2	0.1
Flammability	0.1	0.6	0.1	0.1	0.1

Based on this matrix, a 1-×-7 fate and transport column, vector $\boldsymbol{F}$, can be calculated. A rank value is determined through the following equation:

$$R_1 = \left(\sum_{j=1}^{k} X_{ij} \right)^{1/k} \tag{4}$$

where X_{ij} are the elements of the k-×-k prioritization matrix, $\mathbf{X}$. Here, $k = 7$, the number of effects of interest. The elements of $\boldsymbol{F}$ then are determined by a simple normalization:

$$F^{(i)} = R_i / \sum_{i=1}^{k} R_i, \; i = 1, \ldots k \tag{5}$$

For the matrix in Table 9–3, the $\boldsymbol{F}$ vector is

$$\boldsymbol{F} = [0.01\ 0.05\ 0.07\ 0.43\ 0.03\ 0.21\ 0.20]^T \tag{9–6}$$

The environmental impact index, or health hazard score for the ith waste stream and the jth phase (HHS_{ij}) can be calculated as shown in eq. (7), where $\boldsymbol{H}_i$ is the 1-×-7 vector of the raw score $[O, I, E, \ldots, F]$ for the ith waste stream, $\boldsymbol{P}_{ij}^{'}$ is the

TABLE 9–3 Example AHP Matrix for Site-Specific Prioritization

$$X = \begin{array}{c} \\ O \\ I \\ E \\ D \\ C \\ R \\ F \end{array} \begin{array}{ccccccc} O & I & E & D & C & R & F \\ \end{array}$$

	O	I	E	D	C	R	F
O	1	1/5	1/10	1/30	1/2	1/20	1/20
I	5	1	1	1/10	2	1/5	1/5
E	10	1	1	1/6	2	1/4	1/3
D	30	10	6	1	15	2	3
C	2	1/2	1/2	1/15	1	1/5	1/8
R	20	5	4	1/2	5	1	1
F	20	5	3	1/3	8	1	1

transpose of the jth column of the phase matrix for the ith waste stream. $\boldsymbol{H}_i\boldsymbol{P}_{ij}$ is a 1-×-7 vector equal to the element-by-element product of $\boldsymbol{P}_{ij}$ and $\boldsymbol{H}_i$:

$$\text{HHS}_{ij} = \boldsymbol{H}_i\boldsymbol{P}_{ij} \bullet \boldsymbol{F} \qquad (9\text{–}7)$$

Once derived, an overall HHS index can be written for chemical species with multiphase pathways in terms of the mass fractions of the different phases as

$$\text{HHS}_i = \sum_j \text{HHS}_{ij} M_j / \sum_j M_j \qquad (9\text{–}8)$$

Board Optimization

Deciding the Variables of the Problem

Once equipped with a set of process models and hazard assessments, we can analyze a particular board design. Keeping the functionality of the board untouched, we can change its physical design and observe the change in the waste-stream generation impact. First, we intuitively decide which factors will have the most significant impact on the waste stream. In circuit boards, we observe from the process models that the number of layers, number of boards tiled on a single panel, and the board area are the key design parameters. We cannot vary the number of pins or components at this point because that will hamper the functionality of the board and our focus is not on devices on the board.

Deriving Interparameter Relationships

Changing certain design parameters affects other design parameters. For example, changing the dimensions of the board requires recomputing the copper fraction for every layer. Hence, we need to derive relationships between various parameters. These relationships serve as the equality constraints of the optimization problem. In our board example, we need to derive three formulas:

1. *Copper fraction of the signal layers.* Balakrishnan and Pecht (1995) derived a relationship for the average length of a copper trace on a board as

$$L_{\text{avg}} = (A+1)\frac{\sqrt{A_r}}{6(n-1)\sqrt{A_s}}\left[1 + \sqrt{2A_s/N_l(A_s^2+1)}\right] \qquad (9\text{–}9)$$

where A_s is the aspect ratio, A_r is the routable area of the board, N_l is the total number of component pins, and n is the average net size. From this, we can write the copper fraction as

$$K_{\text{cu-board}} = (L_{\text{avg}}\, N_{\text{int}}\, t_{\text{trace}}) / A_b \qquad (9\text{–}10)$$

where

$$N_{\text{int}} = N_l(n-1)/n$$

2. *Number of boards per panel.* Boards can be arranged on a rectangular panel in two possible orientations, as shown in Figure 9–4. If we denote the length and breadth of the board and panel by L_b, W_b, L_p, and W_p, respectively, then the number of boards for the two orientations will be as follows.

Orientation 1: If $G_L > W_b$, then

$$N_b = \text{Int}\,(L_p/W_b)\ \text{Int}\,(W_p/L_b) + \text{Int}\,(L_p/L_b) \tag{9–11}$$

otherwise

$$N_b = \text{Int}(L_p/\,W_b)\ \text{Int}(W_p/L_b)$$

Orientation 2: If $G_w > W_b$, then

$$N_b = \text{Int}\,(L_p/\,L_b)\ \text{Int}\,(W_p/W_b) + \text{Int}\,(W_p/L_b) \tag{9–12}$$

otherwise

$$N_b = \text{Int}\,(L_p/\,L_b)\ \text{Int}\,(W_p/W_b)$$

We must calculate the number of boards per panel using these formulas and choose the orientation that gives the maximum number of boards per panel. This way, more material will go into the product and less into the manufacturing waste.

3. *Total number of signal layers.* The number of signal layers can be estimated given the routable board area, A_r, and the number of "reference components," N_{ref}, using the density approach described in Balakrishnan and Pecht (1995). The number of reference components is equivalent to the number of components when all components are weighted with reference to a 14-pin DIP component as one unit. The categorical functional dependence is given in Table 9–4.

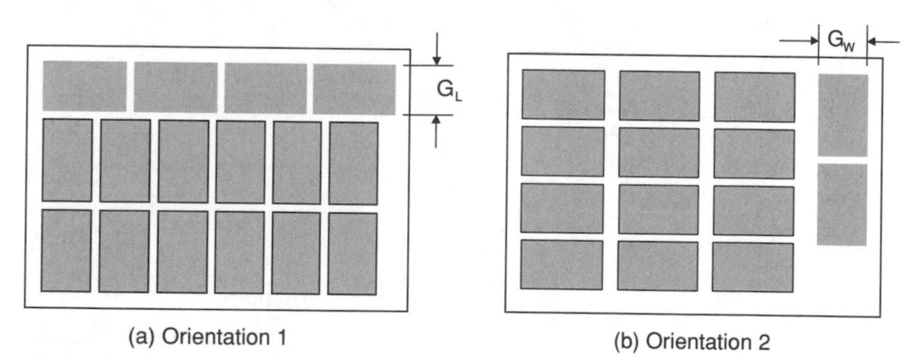

FIGURE 9–4 Two panel layouts.

TABLE 9–4 Signal Layer Estimation

A_r/N_{ref} (SQ. IN/14-PIN DIP)	$N_{s\text{-layers}}$
Above 1.0	2
0.8–1.0	2
0.6–0.8	4
0.42–0.6	6
0.35–0.42	8
0.2–0.35	10
0.0–0.2	10+

Optimization

Once we derive the process models and the preceding relationships, we can follow a procedure like the one depicted in Figure 9–5 to optimize the board design parameters. The results of such an optimization are shown in Figure 9–6. The plot shows the weighted mass of the waste streams on per board basis as a function of the board dimensions. From this plot, we can choose the dimensions of the board corresponding to the minimum waste.

We also can observe the effect of relaxing a constraint or imposing an additional constraint on the optimization problem. These constraints easily can be imposed or removed during the waste-stream calculation from process models.

Several useful conclusions can be drawn from these plots:

- The minimum waste does not necessarily occur for the smallest or thinnest (i.e., fewest layers) board size.
- A large variation (more than 100% in the plots shown) in the amount of waste per board occurs as we vary the dimensions and the number of layers of the board. Hence, the scope for waste minimization through design optimization is tremendous.
- The choice of panels also makes a difference in waste generation. Hence, whenever a variety of panels is available, we must calculate which to choose.

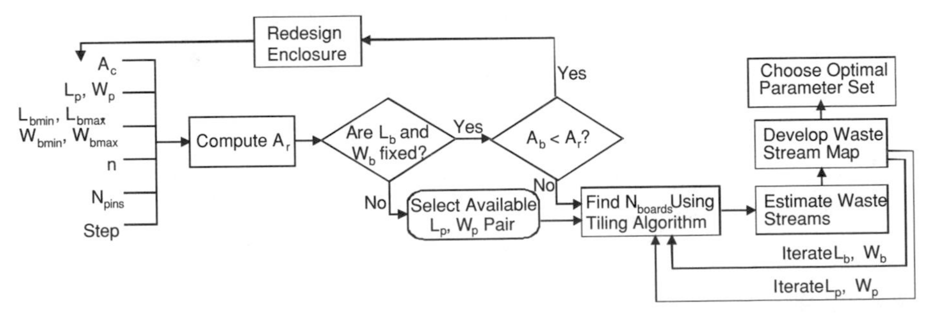

FIGURE 9–5 Board design optimization procedure.

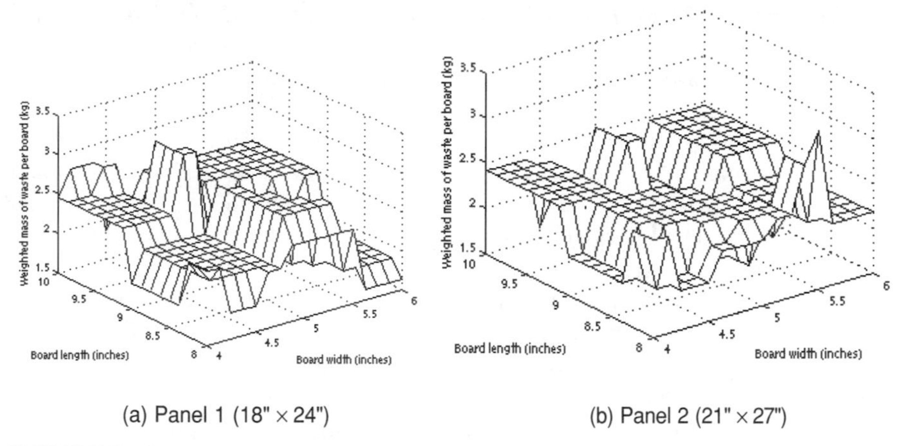

(a) Panel 1 (18" × 24") (b) Panel 2 (21" × 27")

FIGURE 9–6 Waste mass as a function of board dimensions for two different panel sizes.

Extending the Scope of Analysis

A bare board is only one component of an overall printed circuit board assembly. Hence, it is important to perform a similar optimization analysis on every component of the assembly. Also, design variation in one component sometimes necessitates the design variation in another. For example, making the board smaller may allow the use of flip-chip ball grid array components, which may not be as environmentally benign as quad flat packages because of the potential worker exposure hazard in the solder-bumping process. Therefore, the optimization procedure eventually can be extended to incorporate selection of component packaging. Electronic packaging presents discrete choices of package types. We can formulate the process models for each package type as a function of a functional parameter, such as the pin count. For semiconductor or die manufacturing, environmental issues largely are a function of waste mitigation at the manufacturing process; currently, limited opportunity is available to effect environmental decisions through design changes. However, a change in technology brings about major changes in process steps, chemicals used, and process mechanics and a resulting significant change in process waste. Therefore, process models for semiconductor manufacturing must predict the waste per die as a function of the yield (which is a function of die size and wafer size) and the technology used.

So far, we have examined mainly design optimization of a product for minimum process waste. One aspect neglected in this analysis was the amount of material going into the product itself and its eventual fate. Although manufacturing wastes represent the dominant life-cycle impact for printed circuit boards, we cannot neglect the environmental impacts of use and disposition phases of the life cycle for other components of a circuit board or computer. Life-cycle analysis (LCA) examines a product from the time its raw material is mined to the time when the product is disposed back into the environment. So LCA looks at material and energy flows in mining, material refinement, manufacturing, use, consumption, and disposal (which includes recycling, reuse, remanufacturing, incineration, deposit in a landfill, etc.) associated with a particular product. While LCA conceptually is straightforward, to implement such analyses requires a great deal of data that often are unavailable or of low quality. LCA is extremely data intensive, and while results can be found for some comparisons, often the data are so poor that little can be learned from them. Furthermore, few have agreed on how the multiple health and environmental impacts of a product's life cycle can be compared to those of another product, making between-product comparisons difficult.

LCA is an attempt, ultimately, to draw a quantitative connection between the existence of a product (its manufacture, use, and disposition) and environmental impact. DfE is an attempt to incorporate this information (i.e., connections, analyses) to minimize environmental impacts of design decisions.

One can say that, just as more traditional engineering models help designers predict the performance of their design (in terms of speed, weight, energy consumption, and other more standard measures of performance), LCA is a model that predicts for designers the environmental performance of their designs.

References

Allen, David. "Life Cycle Assessment and Design for the Environment." Tutorial Notes, IEEE Symposium on Electronics and the Environment, San Francisco, CA, May 1997.

Balakrishnan S., and M. Pecht. *Placement and Routing of Electronic Modules*, pp. 59–96. New York: Marcel Dekker, 1993.

Siddhaye, S., and P. Sheng. "Integration of Environmental Factors for Process Modeling of Printed Circuit Board Fabrication," Proceedings of the IEEE International Symposium on Electronics and the Environment, San Francisco, May 1997, pp. 226–233.

Srinivasan M., T. Wu, and P. Sheng. "Development of a Scoring Index for the Evaluation of Environmental Factors in Machining Processes: Part I, Formulation." *Transactions of NAMRI* 23 (1995), pp. 115–121.

Worhach, P., and P. Sheng. "Integration of Environmental Factors for Process Modeling of Printed Circuit Board Assembly." Proceedings of the IEEE International Symposium on Electronics and the Environment, San Francisco, May 1997, pp. 218–225.

CHAPTER **10**

Toward Integrated Product Life-Cycle Design Tools

BRIAN GLAZEBROOK
Ecobalance Inc.

Introduction

A number of different approaches to design for environment (DfE) have emerged as market pressures and regulations drive businesses to consider environmental issues *during instead of after* product development. They cover the spectrum from life-cycle assessment (LCA) to guidelines for designing for disassembly. LCA itself is a rigorous standardized methodology (ISO 14040) that has been used by industries to examine product options or investment decisions relevant to a company's product line. Conducting a full LCA is very difficult for those unfamiliar with the method, such as design teams charged with the development of complex products (e.g., electronic devices or cars). Similar to LCA, the other approaches to DfE address specific concerns but are not all encompassing. Most companies require a more integrated DfE tool, which provides life-cycle data and addresses regulatory and consumer concerns.

Approaches to Design for Environment

Design for environment can be defined as "a system approach to design that incorporates environmental, health and safety concerns over the full product life cycle" (Glazebrook, 1996). In other words, DfE bridges the gap between product development and environmental management, where up until recently environmental concerns have focused on the impact of specific sites rather than an entire product. Prior to the development of software tools tailored specifically for DfE, companies applied a variety of different methodologies to address the product environmental impacts, including

- Design guidelines (e.g., checklists and matrices).
- Design for disassembly (DfD).
- Life-cycle assessment (LCA).

Design guidelines that consist of qualitative methodologies developed to address product-related environmental issues driven by customer demands (e.g., recycled content in products), market constraints (e.g., ecolabels), and regulatory constraints (e.g., removal of cadmium). These design tools normally are developed or outlined by the in-house EH&S staff (based on its understanding of relevant environmental issues) and put into use by the company's designers. Generally, these qualitative tools can be divided into either checklists or matrices. A checklist is used to outline materials banned or restricted from use in a product, describe internal requirements for recycled material content, or highlight regulations relevant to the design process. Matrices are broad, qualitative decision tools used by design teams to assess the perceived impact of a product's life-cycle stages on input and output such as raw material consumption, energy consumption, and emissions. The design team uses this information to determine where in the product life cycle it should focus its efforts on reducing the impact.

The advantage of the guideline methodology is that it is developed in-house and directly reflects the interests and goals of the company. Setting guidelines also is a practical and quick method for making design changes. This can be useful in a rapidly changing design environment.

An example of the use of this methodology is IBM's product environmental profile (PEP) document. A PEP is required for all new or modified products carrying the IBM logo, and its contents vary depending on the type of product. The information that a PEP contains can run the range from a simple list of potentially harmful substances to a more-detailed list that includes information on energy, consumables, and standards compliance. The focus of the document is to allow development engineers to target the reduction of hazardous materials use or improve the environmental benefits during product use, without having to conduct a complicated life-cycle assessment of the product.

The weakness of this methodology lies in the generally short-term focus of the guidelines; that is, they are formulated to address current environmental concerns or regulatory issues but do not always address the comprehensive, multimedia environmental impact of a product. Additionally, the qualitative nature of these tools makes the process very subjective. Checklists focus on environmental concerns, such as recycled content or banned materials, that are driven by policy, consumer demand, or marketing concerns, which are not necessarily supported by concrete environmental data. Matrices reflect the subjective weighting of types of impact by staff members who may not have the expertise to accurately gauge the impact of a product, either at a particular life-cycle stage or on a particular emission.

Design for Disassembly

Design for disassembly (DfD) targets the end-of-life impact of a product's design. The focus is to improve the design of a product so that it can be disassembled with the least environmental impact and cost. The methodology addresses manufacturing issues such as the number of fasteners in a product, the time to disassemble a product, and the recyclability or energy content of product materials.

Since the methodology requires an understanding not only of design but also of the end-of-life issues relative to materials and subassemblies, DfD can be a complicated methodology for product designers. A number of software tools are available that assist them in determining the optimum design for disassembly, without requiring the tools to be aware of all of the environmental issues. Some tools allow a user to assess the impact on the environment of stopping disassembly at various points in the process, which can be useful in determining the point at which the benefit of disassembly diminishes.

The advantage of the design for disassembly approach is that it addresses concrete design issues (number of fasteners, the type of material used) that directly affect the end-of-life of a product. Basing the methodology on quantitative data permits a clear determination of the trade-offs between different product designs. DfD also is practical, in that disassembly effects can be directly translated into economic impact.

However, the narrow focus of the design for disassembly methodology in fact can be a disadvantage. With its narrow focus on the end of a product's life, it ignores other life-cycle stages (such as product manufacturing or use) that may have a more profound effect on the environmental impact of a product. Additionally, designing a product for disassembly does not necessarily address legislative concerns that may affect how a product is designed.

Life-Cycle Assessment Methodology

Life-cycle assessment used as a DfE tool addresses particular questions:

- Should a specific material or process be restricted?
- What end-of-life processes should be promoted?
- Does a specific regulation (e.g., an ecolabel) make sense from an environmental point of view?

In comparison to a more qualitative approach, LCA methodology focuses on the quantification of potential forms of environmental impact. This is done by performing an analysis of material consumption and emissions from the materials acquisition, manufacturing, distribution, use, and end-of-life steps of the product life. An LCA is carried out in four phases, which have been standardized under ISO 14040: definition of the project goal and scope, compilation of an inventory of relevant system inputs and outputs (LCI; see Figure 10–1), impact assessment, and interpretation of results.

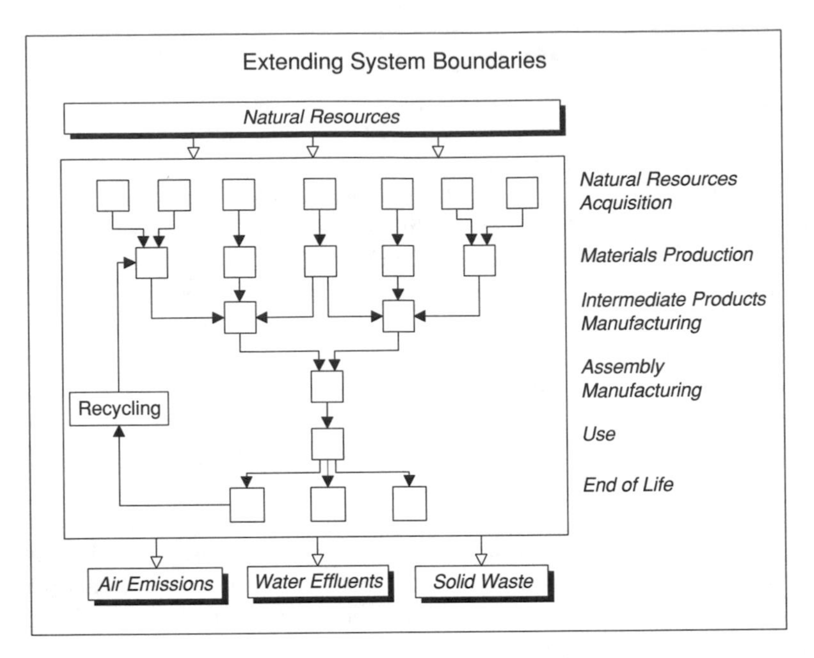

FIGURE 10–1 Life-cycle assessment boundaries.

Life-cycle assessment is a useful tool for some applications, because it can help detect the shifting of environmental burdens from one life-cycle stage to another (e.g., lower energy consumption during use is achieved at the cost of much higher manufacturing energy consumption) or from one media to another (e.g., lower air emissions at the cost of increased solid waste). Because the set of flows calculated during an LCA often is very large, subsets of the flows sometimes are consolidated or aggregated to facilitate interpretation, especially when two or more products or processes are being compared.

This consolidation or aggregation of flows has been given the (possibly misleading) name *life-cycle impact assessment* (LCIA). In fact, it is *not the actual impact* of the environmental flows in the inventory that are estimated using LCIA but a *series of impact indicators*. These indicators are generated by consolidating and aggregating the inventory flows using information about their relative potential strength of influence with respect to separate categories of potential environmental impact. The results within each LCIA impact category are useful for comparison of one product or process versus another but have little meaning in an absolute sense (i.e., relative to estimating the actual environmental impact of a product or process).

LCA provides the objective information needed for decision making and helps clarify environmental debates, where specifications and priorities often are implicit. However, because of the inherent limitations of its general methodology—data scope, system modeling, and data interpretation—LCA is not the best-suited tool for day-to-day design for environment. We can examine each of the LCA's three stages briefly to understand their shortcomings:

1. *LCA data scope*. All material input and output are taken into account by LCA methodology but not other information also of interest to design teams (e.g., environmental regulations that apply to a specific product or manufacturing process). Nor does it distinguish between what is in the product and what is emitted. Things like safety, noise, and power consumption also are not taken into account. For end-of-life issues, the LCA methodology does not include data on the ease of recycling or integrating reusable components.
2. *Systems modeling*. Because most manufacturers make complex products and outsource a significant share of the production, it can be difficult, time consuming, and expensive to collect the data to carry out a full LCA. Also, some systems modeling is difficulty due to the data uncertainty for product's end of life because it is nearly impossible to collect real data on end-of-life processing at the design stage. End-of-life effects also are difficult to anticipate for complex products with long lifetimes.
3. *Data interpretation*. Impact assessment methods are not standardized yet and are still subject to much debate and research. Indeed, emissions most often take place in chain reactions with synergistic or antagonistic effects that are not well known or documented. This explains why results of an LCA are difficult for designers and others who are not environmental experts to interpret.

Toward an Integrated Life-Cycle Design Tool

Each of these three DfE methodologies (Guidelines, DfD, and LCA) is designed with specific goals, with its particular advantages and disadvantages, but the whole process falls short of the loftier goal of being "a system approach to design that incorporates environmental, health and safety concerns over the full product life cycle." Each approach addresses discrete aspects—regulatory, end of life, life cycle—all of which can be incorporated into a broader, more robust life-cycle design tool that draws on the best traits from all three. Such a tool would provide that

- Life-cycle inventory data are enhanced by data relative to mechanical assembly and information on compliance with internal and external standards.
- The end of a product's life is dealt with through design-related indicators.
- Impact assessment results are condensed into either a single index or a series of simple indicators.

The index of indicators should be organized in a way that is easy to understand and allows designers to identify opportunities for product improvement. (Note that this is likely not compliant with the ISO 14042 standard for LCA, which requires that the presentation of final results be transparent and unambiguous. Therefore, extra care should be taken in presenting single indices as a result.)

A life-cycle design tool would require a comprehensive database that incorporates simplified LCI data in the form of aggregate life-cycle information for individual materials, components, and processes. An additional database would be necessary on the impact at the end of a product's life for different assembly methods. Finally, both these quantitative datasets would need to be supplemented with an extensive database covering regulatory and restricted materials, which could be tailored to a company's needs and interests.

It would be simplistic to say that melding the previous DfE methodologies would be sufficient to create a suitable life-cycle design tool. The volume of data required, as well as the nature of the different datasets, requires the incorporation of additional organizational elements into the tool. These elements not only will make the tool more flexible but also more adaptive to the specific corporate environment:

- *Separate roles for the designer and the environmental expert.* A product designer is not likely to be fully aware of all the forms of the environmental impact in certain material or design choices. Therefore, the environmental aspects of the tool should be disassociated from the design aspects. This would relieve the designer from maintaining a current life-cycle database, updating regulations, and keeping abreast of current material restrictions (see Figure 10–2).

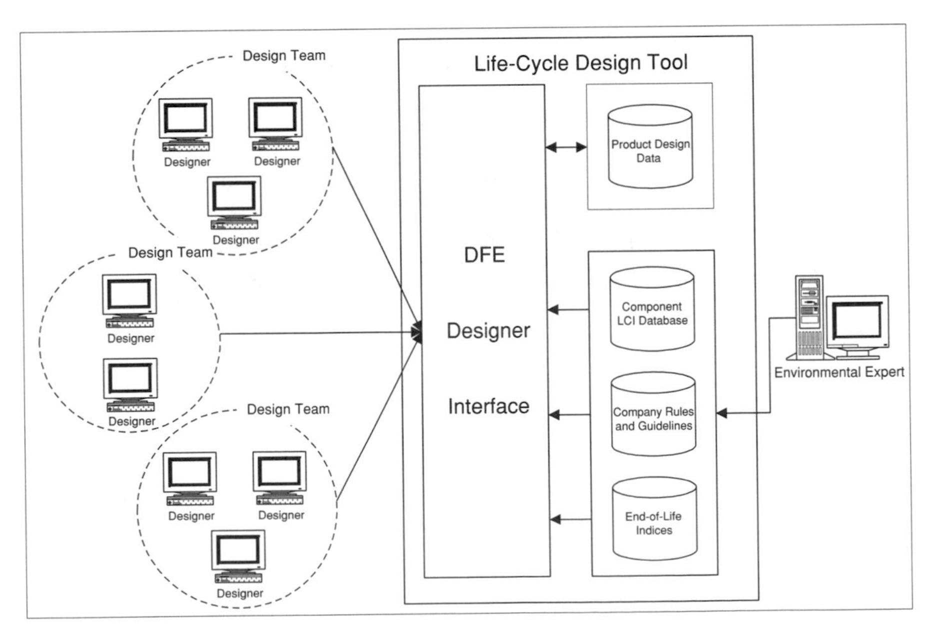

FIGURE 10–2 The designer's and expert's DfE roles.

- *Common database for all environmental data.* Most companies employ multiple designers to work on a specific product or product components. A centralized, common database for environmental information is important, so that all designers are working off of the same set of data. This would also ease the separation of the environmental and design roles, since it would only require the environmental "expert" to maintain one database.
- *Interactive design guidelines.* The benefit of incorporating guidelines into the design tool comes from the ability of a company to tailor its designs to consumer or market concerns. However the benefit of a single design tool is lost if many of the guidelines designers must use are provided in separate books or checklists. Therefore, the guidelines should be neatly integrated into the tool, so that once certain material or process choices are made, the appropriate guidelines are triggered.
- *Mechanism for updating guidelines.* While the guidelines should be interactive, they also should be easily updated. Since regulations, material restrictions and consumer demands change constantly, the DfE tool should be able to keep pace with these changes. This could be accomplished through an interface that would allow environmental experts to easily update or create guidelines.
- *Dialog between suppliers and the company.* The product development process is not a black box for many companies; designers rely on parts or materials produced by suppliers to manufacture a product. For the data relevant to the life-cycle impact of a product to be relevant to the product, and not merely generic substitute data, input from suppliers is key. This not only assures that data are accurate but keeps suppliers involved in the DfE process.
- *Simple update of the life-cycle inventory database.* Aside from the need for supplier specific information in the life-cycle inventory (LCI) data, the database should also contain the latest information on more generic processes or materials. Relying on outside consultants to provide this information can be costly, especially when some of the data are publicly available. A mechanism to allow updates or additions to the database is important to ensure the reliability of the life-cycle data.
- *Integration of tool with CAD/PDM.* Enterprise product data management (PDM) has become instrumental for many large and medium sized companies as a tool to consolidate the volumes of technical information they generate. The life-cycle design tool should provide the capacity to interact with a company's PDM, so that the DfE data is consolidated with CAD, supplier, cost, and other data. This would facilitate the integration of environmental concerns into the design process and allow a company to compare designs based on a number of different factors, including feasibility, cost, and environmental impact.
- *Simple customization by the user.* While companies are beginning to subscribe to the idea of DfE, many still are hesitant to implement a design tool that does not meet their direct concerns or integrate easily with their current

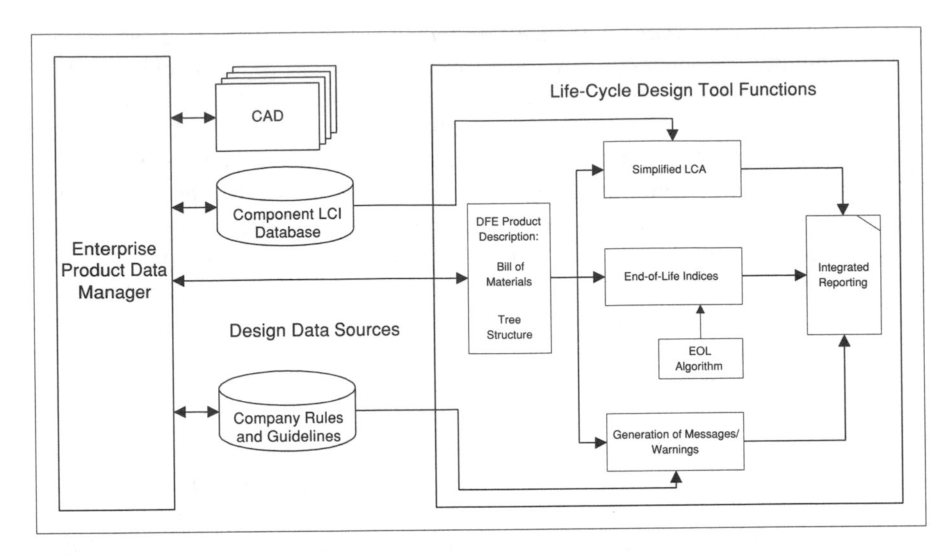

FIGURE 10–3 Integrated life-cycle design tool.

design process. A modular life-cycle design tool allows users to customize the tool to their specifications, which not only facilitates its use but also smoothes the integration of DfE into the design process.

Figure 10–3 presents a summary of how such an integrated life-cycle design tool is used for DfE within a company. The functions that the tool provides would encompass all the design for environment methodologies discussed, with adjustments so that all are provided in one tool. The advantage of the approach is that the design process becomes easier for the designer and the company, since the environmental data are incorporated into the overall design process.

References

Brinkley, A., and T. Mann (IBM Corporation). "Documenting Product Environmental Attributes." Paper presented at the IEEE International Symposium on Electronics and the Environment, San Francisco, May 5–7, 1997, pp. 52–57.

Fiksel, Joseph, ed. *Design for Environment*, New York: McGraw-Hill, 1996, pp. 3-5.

Miller, Ed. "PDM Moves to the Mainstream." *Mechanical Engineering* (October 1998), pp. 74–78.

Section II
Materials and Process Issues

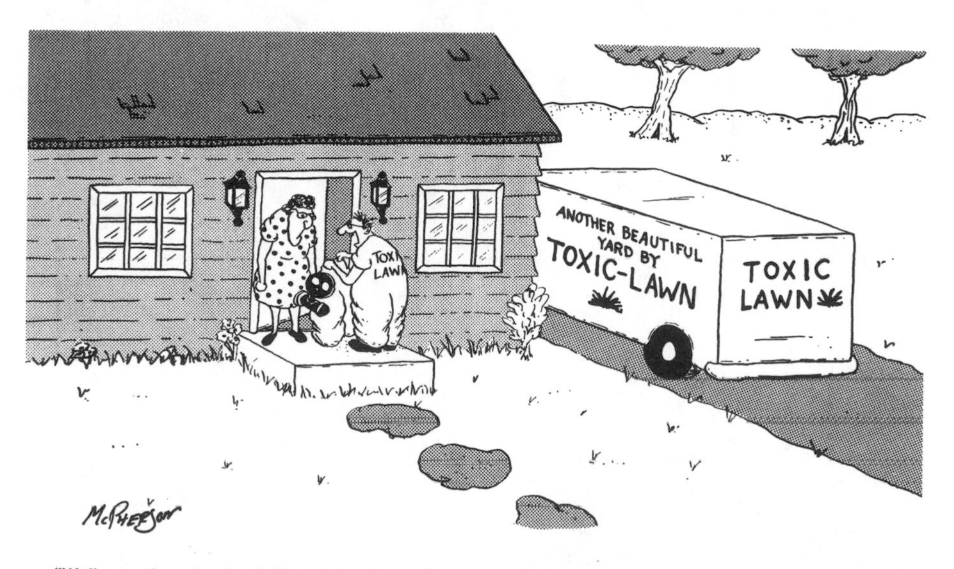

"Well, your lawn's all set, Mrs. Fertstein! Here are some hermetically sealed protective suits and some respirators in case someone actually needs to walk on the lawn this summer."

Introduction: Electronic Manufacturing Processes and the Environment

CHRISTOPHER RHODES

Introduction

Electrons don't weigh much, about 9×10^{-28} grams each. A piece of paper weighs about 4 grams. Both items can be used to store data, but it takes far more energy to create a piece of paper and move it 100 kilometers than to create and move the data-equivalent collection of electrons. In this respect, the electronic revolution made possible by telecommunications and computers already is a step in the environmentally friendly direction.

The electronics revolution holds tremendous potential for environmental benefits in all sorts of ways. Books can be printed on demand. This would be a vast improvement over the current process, where most books are overprinted, shipped, returned, and pulped because the publishers have to guesstimate demand and because it is much easier to overprint a run than reprint if you run out. With electronics, you print what you need, when you need it.

Electronics also can cut the environmental damage caused by travel. People can send their brains instead of their bodies to the office by telecommuting. This cuts congestion, pollution, gasoline consumption, and land development for newer, bigger roads.

Outside of commuting, teleconferencing and videoconferencing can cut business travel. Why fly a dozen people across the country to sit in a room and talk when those wonderful little electrons can carry everyone's words and images anywhere they need to be?

For that matter, why drive down to your library or ship a rare book from library to library to meet demands when the Internet allows everyone access to enormous data resources, including resources on how to design a better tomorrow? In these and dozens of other ways, electronics can and do facilitate a better standard of living with less environmental damage.

On the other hand, the electronics revolution has spawned its own problems. The equipment required to handle the electronic traffic—computers, modems, phones, monitors, printers—and the processes used to manufacture this equipment have created a new set of environmental effects.

While electronics manufacturing is significantly "greener" than many other types of manufacturing, it does present its own problems. Semiconductor manufacturing, for example, consumes enormous quantities of water. Almost all electronics use lead, although the amount used is very small compared to the lead used in lead-acid batteries in cars. Circuit board manufacturing requires a variety of hazardous materials.

The authors in this section tackle the challenges posed by electronics to help ensure that the environmental benefits of electronics use are not negated by the environmental effects of electronics manufacturing.

John Lott of DuPont, vice-chair of the IPC Environmental, Health and Safety (EHS) Committee, presents data on the environmental effects of printed wiring board (PWB) manufacturing. A 1993 life-cycle environmental assessment of a computer workstation found that PWBs accounted for the largest use of energy and water as well as the greatest amount of hazardous waste generated in manufacturing the workstation. Dr. Lott's paper assesses the environmental effects of certain PWB manufacturing processes.

One PWB manufacturing step that has received considerable attention in recent years is the process used to make PWB holes conductive. In manufacturing a PWB, holes are drilled through the nonconductive laminate. These holes will be used to conduct electricity from one side of the board to the other or to interior layers of the board, but first the holes must be made conductive. Traditionally, a process using formaldehyde makes these drilled holes conductive.

Another environmental concern of electronics manufacturing is the tin-lead solder widely used to solder electronic components onto the circuit board. Although this uses a relatively small amount of lead compared to other lead uses in the United States and the world, it still is an environmental challenge. William Trumble of Nortel looks into soldering processes that do not use lead.

By tackling these and other environmental challenges, the electronics industry hopes to make this not only a connected world but also a cleaner, better one.

Part IV
Materials Selection for Electronic Products

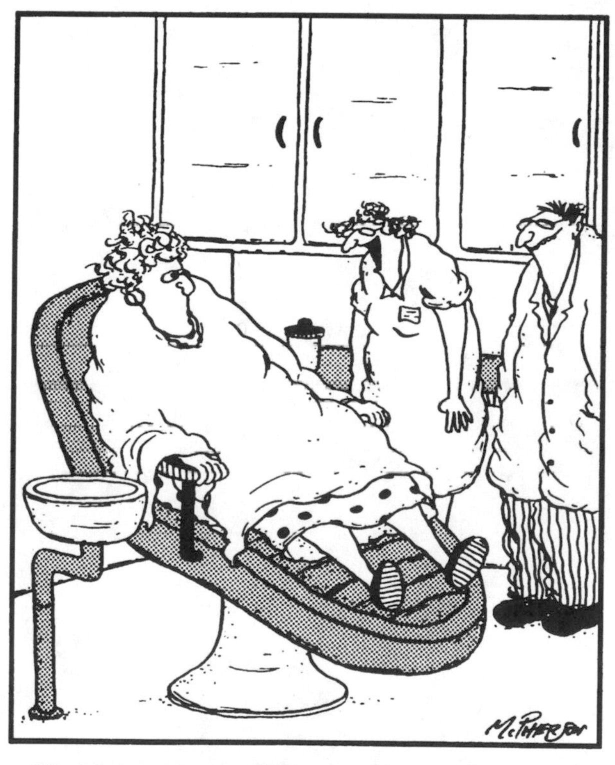

"Dr. Vernley prides himself on his commitment to 100 percent organic dentistry. Today he'll be using bamboo drill bits, a yucca extract painkiller, and adobe fillings."

CHAPTER 11

Selection of Plastics Using Cost, Structural, and Environmental Factors

WILLIAM TRUMBLE

Retired from Nortel Networks, Nepean, Canada

Introduction

Plastics, when used within their design envelope, are very environmentally and cost efficient. When used within the boundaries of their physical design properties, plastics are more effective than glass, ceramics, wood, or metal. They are a good electrical insulator, light weight, and some plastics can be molded into very large complex shapes that would require many parts and assembly operations for other materials.

Many references assist the designer in selecting the right material for an application. Some of the best sources for design information are the suppliers of the platters materials, *Modern Plastics Encyclopedia*, and the large reference manuals from the American Society of Materials. When embarking on a design project using plastic materials, contact the suppliers of the candidate materials and involve them in the project from the start. Suppliers like GE or Bayer have years of experience with their materials and can provide information on how to accomplish the design intent of the candidate plastic. Table 11–1 illustrates how a material was selected for an electronics enclosure used outdoors. This table would not be possible without the early participation of the supplier. Selecting the plastic whose properties for the design intent is the most cost-effective, environmentally friendly material selection.

Some Plastic Classes and Their General Features

To optimize cost and structural integrity, the classes of plastics must be broken down. Like other materials, plastics have a property window beyond which, if the plastic is used, the material will fail, causing product cost and environmental impact to rise. Before you select a material for a design, list the important performance factors

TABLE 11–1 Outdoor Terminal Materials Selection Matrix—Cover

Property	Method Used	Value Needed	Materials											
			Lexan 923	Lexan 923 Painted	Valox 357	Valox 365	Valox GF 42OSEO	Noryl 190	Noryl HS2000	S Cycolac V100	VC Geon 85856	S Cycolac V100	VC Geon 85856
Plastic type			PC	PC	PBT	PBT	PBT-Glass F	PPO	Min F PPO	ABS	PVC	ABS	PVC
Tensile strength break (psi)	ASTMD638	—	9000	9000	7000	6000	17000	6000	9500	700	6308	700	6308
Tensile modulas yield (psi)	ASTMD638	—	325000	324000	320000	300000	800000	325000	500000	340000	460000	340000	460000
Elongation %	ASTMD638		7	7	110	120	3	60	25	140	140	140	140
Notched izod impact (ft.lb/in.)	ASTMD638	23°F	12	12	10	12	1.2	7	3.5	3	17	3	17
		–40°F	1.8	1.8	0.8	0.8	0.8	3	1.5	1.2	0.7		
Unnotched izod (ft.lb/in.)		23°F			60	60	13						
		–40°F											
Gardner impact st. (ft.lb/in.)	ASTMD3029	73°F		Improved	32	29	N/A	17	21.1	20	10	20	10
		–40°F				8	3						

Property	Method Used	Value Needed	Materials										
			Lexan 923	Lexan 923 Painted	Valox 357	Valox 365	Valox GF 42OSEO	Noryl 190	Noryl HS2000	S Cycolac V100	VC Geon 85856	S Cycolac V100	VC Geon 85856
Chemical resistance to:	Bellcore												
Bug spray	TR-TSY		Fair	Fair	Good	Good	Good	Fair	Fair	Poor	Good	Poor	Good
Oil base Paint			Poor	Good	Very good	Very good	Very good	Good	Good	Poor	Excellent	Poor	Excellent
Water dispersion lubes	TR-TSY		Fair	Good	Very good	Very good	Very good	Good	Good	Poor	Good	Poor	Good
Ammonia	Household		Poor	Poor	Very good	Very good	Very good	Good	Good	Excellent	Excellent	Excellent	Excellent
Road salts			Good	Good	Excellent	Excellent	Excellent	Excellent	Excellent	Good	Excellent	Good	Excellent
Fertilizers			Good	Good	Excellent	Excellent	Excellent	Excellent	Excellent	Good	Excellent	Good	Excellent
Herbicides			Fair	Fair	Good	Good	Good	Good	Good	Poor	Good	Poor	Good
UV Stability*	BNR		Fair	Very good	Very good	Very good	Very good	Good	Good	Fair	Good	Fair	Good
DTUL 264 psi ©	ASTM648		132	N/A	99	121	204	88	110	95	71	95	71
Flammability (in.)	UL94	V-O	0.058	0.14	0.025	0.031	0.035	0.058	0.0621	0.059	0.0621	0.059	0.0621
CTE	ASTME831	10^5 mm/ mm°C	3.8	3.8	5.19	3.8	1.4	4	2.5	5.5	3.2	5.5	3.2
Cost ($US)	GE Est (Col)	Per lb.	1.96+ 4.00	1.96	1.94	1.96	2.06	1.74	1.87	1.60	1.43	1.60	1.43
Sp. Gr.			1.2	N/A	1.34	1.33	1.62	1.08	1.24	1.2	1.47	1.2	1.47

* on black or white pigmentation

Note: Cycolac, Noryl, Valox, and Lexan are trademark names for plastic products produced by General Electric Plastics. Geon is a trademark name by Geon.

for the design, reduce the factors to material properties, then decide on the quantitative limits of each property. When you complete this iteration, write it down in table form. In the table, write the designed properties use columns of candidate materials against the requirements. Do the table before you start the design and with the help of your plastic supplier. A sample table is included in this lesson. The primary classes of plastics are thermoset and thermoplastic polymers.

Thermoset Plastics

Some typical thermoset plastics are epoxies, phenolics, polyesters, polyimides, and rigid urethanes. These materials are formed by combining two or more components and applying sufficient heat to cure the material to a rigid mass. Most of the thermosets are rigid but not very strong, so most are reinforced with substances such as glass fibers, glass matrices, carbon black, other fibers, or other fillers. These fillers most often are selected for a specific design requirement, such as cost or radiation resistance.

Most of the thermosets, except the phenolic and melamine, are sensitive to moisture. Some electrical and mechanical properties will degrade with exposure to heat, air, moisture, or sunlight over time. Many of these issues are addressed and tests recommended in the Underwriters Laboratory documents 246A, 246B, long-term properties of polymers. Unlike in the past, many types of thermosets can be reclaimed but with cost and time. The problem with recycling thermosets is not the plastic but what is on or in the plastics.

A prime example of a plastic part that is hard to dispose of is FR-4, the most commonly used substrate material for printed circuit boards. A typical returned FR-4 circuit board consists mainly of epoxy, and filler (usually glass fiber and silicone sizing agents), and electronic components (ICs, resistors, capacitors, connectors, etc.), but there is a host of other materials found in greater or lessor quantities. These include things like copper pads and traces, residual solder, as well as ink, tapes, and labels. Often, boards are coated with solder mask compounds (often acrylic, sometimes epoxy) and treated with flame-retardant compounds such as polyaminides or brominated aromatics.

As with all material system recycling, the base material is tough to recycle. The attachments make recycling very expensive. All the thermosets are made of organic materials. This means that, given a high enough temperature, these materials will burn. To guard against burning, in printed circuit boards, the plastic usually is treated with a flame retardant. The most frequently used are brominated aromatic hydrocarbons, which give environmentalists fits. Despite all efforts at any cost, no one has found a flame retardant as effective as the brominated hydrocarbons—so far.

Thermosets have their place in the design of electrical components. This applies especially to the filled thermosets because of their low coefficient of thermal expansion and their ability to maintain a significant proportion of their mechanical and electrical properties over the thermal operating ranges of most electronic systems. With the proper type and amount of filler, the epoxies and silicones can be formulated to be very conductive thermally or electrically and maintain this conductivity for a long time.

Thermoplastic Plastics

The thermoplastics included in this class range from low-density polyethylene (in wrapping film) through nylon and polyester to liquid crystal polymer. These plastics are characterized by a loss of mechanical properties then softening with the application of heat. The thermoplastics are further divided into two classes: amorphous and crystalline. The amorphous plastics get softer with increasing temperature but do not transform into a liquid. Crystalline plastics soften with heat up to a certain temperature, then turn to a liquid. Typical amorphous plastics are polyvinyl chloride polystyrene and polycarbonate. Typical crystalline plastics are nylon, high-density polyethylene, and polyesters such as polyethylene butylene terephthalate (PBT).

The differences between these two materials become most apparent in injection molding. It is possible to exchange one amorphous or crystalline material with another, but you can't cross over. In addition to the homopolymer (one chemical entity) are a myriad of copolymers, alloys, and blends. The variety is so large it is bewildering to the average designer. The advice of a supplier helps.

A product made of thermoplastic plastics can be formed in many ways, including vacuum forming, extrusion, injection, molding, and stamping. Methods of assembly include ultrasonic welding, gluing, bolting, and snap fills. Methods of forming or assembling thermosets are more limited, but flexible enough to meet most design intents.

The mechanical properties of thermoplastic vary across a very wide spectrum. Low density polyethylene can have modulus lower than some rubbers while the liquid crystal polymers, such as Kevlar (trademark plastic of DuPont) or Xydar (trademark plastic of Hoechst Celanese), can be as tough as aluminum or brass alloys. This spectrum is the best reason to build a requirement property table.

Such a table can help you select the best material for the least environmental impact, often for little or no additional cost. It is important to understand that processing conditions contribute between 60 and 70% of the performance of a plastic part, especially on injection molded parts. Carefully monitor the mold, design, and process parameters to maximize the value of the part with a minimal cost. In this feature, the devil is in the details.

Critical properties of thermoplastic deteriorate with exposure to heat, air, moisture, and sunlight over time. Properties such as impact strength, tensile strength at breaking, elongation at breaking, and brittle temperature can deteriorate significantly within two years if the environmental metal stress is high enough. Underwriters Laboratory Bulletins UL746 A&B address these issues and suggest the appropriate tests.

Some plastics deteriorate significantly when in contact with some metals and exposure to air. The combination that occurs most frequently in electrical technology is polyethylene in contact with copper and its oxide to air or water (dissolved oxygen). Failure to be cognizant of this situation can lead to disastrous results (always check for consequences with metal-plastic contact).

In theory, the process for recycling thermoplastics is easy. You just grind up the parts, put the regrind into the process hopper, and start all over—provided the reground material is not contaminated. Contaminated plastic is death to the reground material and any virgin plastic with which it is processed.

When designing for recyclability, consider these thoughts:

- Contamination includes glues, paints, labels, type residues, and solvents spilled onto the plastic.
- A little contamination can cause a lot of damage. I've seen 1 pound of acrylic ruin 2,000 pounds of styrene, as well as contaminate the process machinery.
- When specifying postconsumer plastic in your product, make sure it is analyzed. Postconsumer plastic has the most varied pedigree of all.
- Always check the molders or other plastic part suppliers for the required discipline and housekeeping around the machine.
- A regrind of polycarbonate, nylon, and polyester must be dried to the specified moisture content just like the virgin material before reusing.
- Many of the plastics used in the electronics or electrical industry, such as ABS, polyethylene, and polycarbonate, are stable to normal thermal conditions if processing. A regrind percentage of 25% often is used. Be very careful when using a polyvinyl chloride regrind. It scorches and burns easily and the scorched material catalyzes further action in the process to cause more scorching.
- A program to use postconsumer plastic is fraught with danger. The composition of a bin of reground material can be widely varied as to the kinds of plastics in the container. The condition of any of these plastics can be contaminated with inks, adhesives, and the like, potentially increasing the recycling problem further because of the resulting contamination of the host plastic.
- Direct metallization of plastic (vacuum deposited) does not affect the mechanical properties of the plastic. This is because the metal is inert to the plastic and in reality contributes a very low volume contribution. A test performed by GE Plastics yielded plastic that looked ugly but was mechanically usable.
- To aid in the recycling of plastics, ISO standard 11469 specifies how each plastic should be identified. Here is an example for 20% glass filled polycarbonate: >PC-GF20<. This identifying code should be molded into each part or somehow associated with the product.
- The American Plastics Council has generated an excellent pamphlet for designing with plastics: "Designing for the Environment, A Design Guide for Information and Technology Equipment." Call Al Mateu at (202) 371–5319 to obtain a copy.

CHAPTER 12

Battery Selection and Application—Environmental Considerations

GEORGE L. YENDER
Yender Associates

This chapter addresses the environmental issues surrounding batteries for the product designer seeking a primary or backup power source for a product or product feature. Rather than concentrate on the details of battery design, we focus on the environmental issues unique to batteries, explore how they relate to environmental design principles, and summarize currently available application choices and alternatives. Recycling considerations are discussed and the segment concludes with a view of the future.

Environmental Issues Involving Batteries

Two fundamental environmental issues associated with batteries are volume and hazardous content. The volume of batteries introduced to the market is escalating rapidly as new product applications are released each year. Market demand for mobility and convenience has fueled this growth, leading to battery-powered cellular phones, camcorders, toothbrushes, and remote control products undreamed of as recently as ten years ago. A mass balance requires that whatever enters the use stream must leave it at some point, entering the waste stream as either energy or waste mass.

The second fundamental environmental issue with batteries is exacerbated by the first. Toxic heavy metals such as cadmium, lead, and mercury are used in batteries and eventually enter the waste stream, contaminating air, water, and soil if not properly managed. For example, until the early 1990s, mercury was used in alkaline manganese dioxide, zinc carbon, and mercuric oxide battery cells, which entered the waste stream in billions of units (Fishbein, 1997).

When spent batteries are not recycled, materials are irretrievably lost and, worse, may be contaminating the environment we depend on for life. To address these issues, it is important to understand the technology of batteries and to develop environmental principles to deal with the impact.

Battery Technology and Classification

Storage batteries are devices that convert chemical energy into electrical energy utilizing a positive electrode, negative electrode, an electrolyte and case, either sealed or unsealed. They typically are classified into primary batteries and rechargeable batteries. Battery packs are made up of individual battery cells, either in parallel or in series, with external leads or terminals for interconnection with the product.

Primary batteries are initially charged, installed in a product, and discharged throughout their life cycle. This continues until they reach a lower limit, where the remaining charge is insufficient and the battery must be replaced. Primary batteries often can be found in items such as flashlights, toys, portable audio products, hearing aids, and implanted medical devices.

Rechargeable batteries typically are rechargeable over many cycles, using an external source to restore a discharged battery to a higher state. They often are used in automobiles, emergency lighting, portable phones, hand tools, and power backup systems.

Other subclassifications of rechargeables include SLI (starting, lighting, and ignition) batteries; lead-acid and nickel cadmium rechargeable batteries are two of the most common examples. Yet another classification distinguishes between dry cell, wet cell, and gel cell batteries, which refer to the physical state of the electrolyte. Sealed and unsealed batteries refer to the design of the seal and usually are associated with venting of gasses or with the need to perform maintenance on liquid electrolyte.

Battery Application Design Principles

In addition to legally mandated requirements, the product designer is responsible for understanding the environmental impact of his or her design. A popular concept is that of sustainable development, environmental design, or product stewardship. Designers wishing to develop responsible design practices can be guided by the "Three Rs": reduce, reuse, recycle.

The hierarchy is intentional. First, the product designer should endeavor to specify the least amount of material necessary to achieve product function, cost, quality, and durability. By extension, the energy to create the materials, manufacture, distribute, and operate the product are all part of the goal to *reduce*, sometimes referred to as *life-cycle analysis*. A full analysis also considers energy required to recycle the product at its end of life. In most instances, the product designer has less control over the earlier elements of the life cycle but more direct control over the energy demand of the product during use and disposal.

The goal to *reuse* is met by designing a product so that it can be used many times over. Rechargeable batteries are an excellent example of reusability.

Recycle, the third principle of sustainable development, involves reclamation or extraction of material from an end-of-life product for reuse as raw material. Applied to batteries, it would be desirable to recycle the contents of all primary batteries instead of disposal in a landfill. Pilot programs to economically extract manganese, zinc, and cobalt in fact are being tested. Rechargeable batteries, too, eventually reach the limit of the recharge cycles they can sustain and enter the end-of-life phase. Lead acid batteries already are actively recycled (with varying degrees of environmental quality) in virtually all parts of the world. In the best processes, all components of the lead-acid battery are recycled, including the sulfuric acid electrolyte and plastic case ("Exide and the Environment," 1998). Nickel and cadmium are actively recycled in Europe, Japan, and the United States.

Battery Application Choices and Environmental Features

Based on environmental design principles and product features, the product designer has several battery types from which to choose. Colin Vincent provides a comprehensive discussion of available battery technologies (Vincent, 1996). The most common battery chemistries used in the marketplace today are tabulated in Table 12–1.

Laws and Regulations

A brief review of battery laws is necessary because product designers must engineer products for compliance. As noted, the two primary environmental impacts of batteries are volume and toxic content. Governments in most industrialized countries have enacted battery laws to address these impacts. Five separate requirements characterize the nature of these laws:

1. Restriction of heavy metal content (Ca < .025%, Hg < .025%, Pb < 0.4%, as percentages of battery weight).
2. Ease of battery removal.
3. Standardized marking.
4. Mandated collection and restricted disposal.
5. Submittal of battery management plans and periodic reporting.

While standard, cataloged battery cells typically comply with regulations, custom battery packs are the responsibility of the product designer, who must specify material content, marking, and removability. Because many of these laws undergo

TABLE 12–1 Summary of Environmental Criteria and Features for Battery Selection

Rechargeable Batteries				
Battery Type	**Typical Applications**	**Positive Features**	**Negative Features**	**Overall Environmental Features/Alternatives**
Lead Acid and Small Sealed Lead Acid (SSLA)	SLI Battery Back-up	Good for harsh application environments Easily rechargeable over hundreds of cycles Relatively high voltage Most mature collection and recycling technology	Low energy density Heavily regulated worldwide Narrow temperature range for efficient operation Heavy, bulky	Highly compatible with 3Rs Contains heavy metal Leaking batteries may spill sulfuric acid electrolyte Alternatives: none
Lithium-Ion (LiION)	Principal power source for laptop computers, consumer electronics, Electric Vehicles	High energy density Rechargeable over many hundreds of cycles No heavy metals, no toxic electrolytes Regulated for transportation	Costly Sensitive recharge controls reqd	Immature recycling/ reclamation technology Alternatives: NiMH
Nickel-Cadmium (NiCd)	Portable tools, consumer electronics, commercial principal power sources, commercial power back-up systems	Excellent re-chargeability Favorable energy density Excellent for high power drain applications 2nd most mature collection and recycling technology	Contains heavy metal (Cd) Heavily regulated worldwide Recharging must be carefully managed to avoid "memory" effects	Heavy metal content requires strict controls for disposal Recycling technology well advanced Alternatives: NiMH or LiION in some applications
Nickel Metal Hydride (NiMH)	Portable consumer products, laptop computers, Electric Vehicles	Excellent energy density Rechargeable for hundreds of cycles No toxic content Mature collection and recycling technology	Not recommended for high torque requirements (hand tools)	Favorable 3R performance Mature technology for reclamation of Nickel Alternative: LiION

Primary or Non-recharegable Batteries				
Battery Type	Typical Applications	Positive Features	Negative Features	Overall Environmental Features/Alternatives
Alkaline Manganese Dioxide	Consumer products: flashlights, torches, toys, portable audio products, air monitoring/smoke detectors	Low Cost No Hazardous material content Favorable performance under high drain conditions Easiest access for replacement worldwide	Not rechargeable (with some exceptions) Heavy metal content regulated worldwide Efficient operation over limited temp range	Incompatible with 3Rs Very limited reclamation technology Alternatives: rechargeable Alkaline or Zinc Carbon
Lithium Manganese Dioxide ($LiMnO_2$) or Lithium Polycarbon-monofluoride	Coin and cylindrical cell applications in consumer electronic products: cameras, pagers, remote controls	Direct replacement for mercuric oxide coin cells High energy density Long life No heavy metals but regulated for transportation	Non rechargeable Metallic lithium is explosive when exposed to water	Incompatible with 3Rs Immature recycling/ reclamation technology Alternatives: Few
Mercuric Oxide	Implanted medical devices, special environment instrument applications (explosive environments, mines)	Highly reliable Long service life No outgassing	Contains heavy metal Heavily regulated worldwide Non-rechargeable	Mercury is toxic Costly recycling/reclamation Alternative: Zn-Air or $LiMnO_2$
Silver Oxide	Calculators, Hearing aids	Higher voltage than Zinc-Air	More expensive than Zn-Air	Alternatives: Zn-Air or $LiMnO_2$
Zinc Air	Hearing Aids, Electric vehicles	Coin Cells are direct replacement for mercuric oxide nontoxic electrodes and electrolyte		Recycling technology under development Alternatives: Coin: $LiMnO_2$ Elect Veh: LiION, NiMH
Zinc Carbon	Consumer and Commercial products requiring low cost, reliable power	Lowest cost	Relatively quick discharge Comparatively short life Heavy metal content regulated worldwide	Incompatible with Reuse (non-rechargeable) Alternative: Rechargeable Alkaline

continuous review and are revised often, it's beyond the scope of this brief chapter to cover these things. With the information obtained here, however, product designers will be much better equipped when they seek legal or staff support to understand the most current legal requirements affecting batteries.

Ease of Removal Considerations

Consistent with good environmental design principles, batteries must be easy to remove from the host product. Conventional interpretation of *ease of removal* is that the batteries can be removed using no more than common hand tools: screw-driver, pliers, and the like. On the other side of the spectrum, batteries attached to circuit boards by solder or sealed into an assembly typically are considered *not* easy to remove. This principle also addresses the need to make it easy to put batteries into their own recycling streams at the end of product life, different stream from plastics, metals, or other materials.

Marking Considerations

Applying the environmental design principles to batteries necessarily includes the need to identify battery cells and battery packs so that they can be properly managed at the end of the product's life. For the end user of a product containing batteries or for a disposal contractor to properly route spent batteries, they clearly have to know what they are handling. It is a practical requirement that each battery cell or battery pack be legibly and correctly marked to identify its fundamental chemistry to facilitate environmentally correct, inexpensive processing.

Legally mandated marking applies to all batteries and battery packs included in products or sold as spare replacement batteries in the Netherlands. The Dutch battery law distinguishes between "directive batteries" and "nondirective batteries," a reference to European Union directives 91-157 and 93-86, which govern heavy metal content and marking respectively. U.S. law also specifies unique marking for batteries containing mercury, cadmium, or lead in excess of the previously specified limits.

Recycling Considerations

Good environmental design practice takes into account the third R, recycling, whether the product is reusable or not. Ultimately, most products reach a point in their life cycle when the user wishes to dispose of the product. Selection of batteries based on available recycling technology and collection infrastructure is another factor in the overall design equation. Selecting a battery that cannot be economically recycled generally is undesirable because it irretrievably removes the battery material from the reclamation and recycling streams at the end of the product's life.

Generally, collection programs exist for all battery types in Europe. All industrialized countries have developed collection and recycling streams for batteries containing toxic heavy metals, such as lead-acid, nickel-cadmium, and mercuric oxide. Recyclability by battery type is covered in depth by Yender (1998).

Energy Efficiency

Efficient use of energy is covered by the *reduce* design principle. High energy-density batteries are a first choice but may be inappropriate for inexpensive host products. Selecting rechargeable batteries instead of primary batteries always should be a consideration. Battery properties such as self-discharge rate, number of recharge cycles, and power requirements for recharging should be part of the decision. The battery application engineer representing the cell or pack manufacturer usually is the best resource to assist with selecting the most energy-efficient option.

"Smart Battery" Technology

An important way to reduce the resources consumed by batteries is to extend their service life. Making a rechargeable battery able to sustain twice as many charge cycles cuts the replacement rate in half—and consequently halves the waste stream. With some battery chemistries, their life can be significantly extended with careful attention to monitoring and controlling the discharge rate, temperature, voltage, and recharge rates. With some of the newer, more exotic battery chemistries, this is a necessity, and improper management of these parameters can result in serious loss of capacity and reduced life cycle. To meet these challenges, designers are increasingly turning to "smart batteries," which include sensing and switching circuitry as part of the battery pack. Recharge rate and power level in particular must be monitored and managed to prevent too rapid a recharge or overvoltage recharges. With some battery types, temperature is tracked as an indirect measure of recharge state.

The advent of sub-$1 microcontrollers and low-cost sensors is rapidly moving this technology toward being affordable and practical for many consumer items, such as camcorder and portable computer batteries. Several companies offer custom designs, including engineering software to assist with the design of "smart" circuitry, either integrated in the battery pack or remotely mounted in the host product circuitry.

Future Outlook

Demand for portable power is expected to continue in a steady, single-digit growth rate through the year 2000. As more of the world can afford electronic products, battery volume will increase. Likewise, conventional appliances will continue to be replaced by cordless versions relying on battery packs for power. All these factors point to an increased environmental burden, consuming more of the earth's raw materials and potentially adding to the end-of-life waste stream. However, with intelligent application of environmental design principles, the burden can be managed. In particular, development of new battery technologies will increase power density. Lithium and nickel hydrogen technologies appear to be the most promising. The parallel development of recycling technology will reclaim a higher percentage of battery materials for reuse, slowing the depletion of the earth's raw materials. Finding alternatives to toxic materials could reduce the cost of controls during raw material processing and end-of-life reclamation.

References

"Exide and the Environment." Available at www.exideworld.com/environ.htm, 1998.

Fishbein, Bette. "Industry Program to Collect Nickel-Cadmium (Ni-Cd) Batteries." A case study for INFORM, Inc., 120 Wall St. New York, NY 10005-4001, 1997.

Vincent, Colin. "Recent Developments in Battery Technology." *Chemistry and Industry* (September 16, 1996).

Yender, George. "Battery Recycling Technology and Collection Processes." IEEE International Symposium on Electronics and the Environment, Chicago, IL, 1998.

Part V

Electronic Manufacturing Processes and the Environment

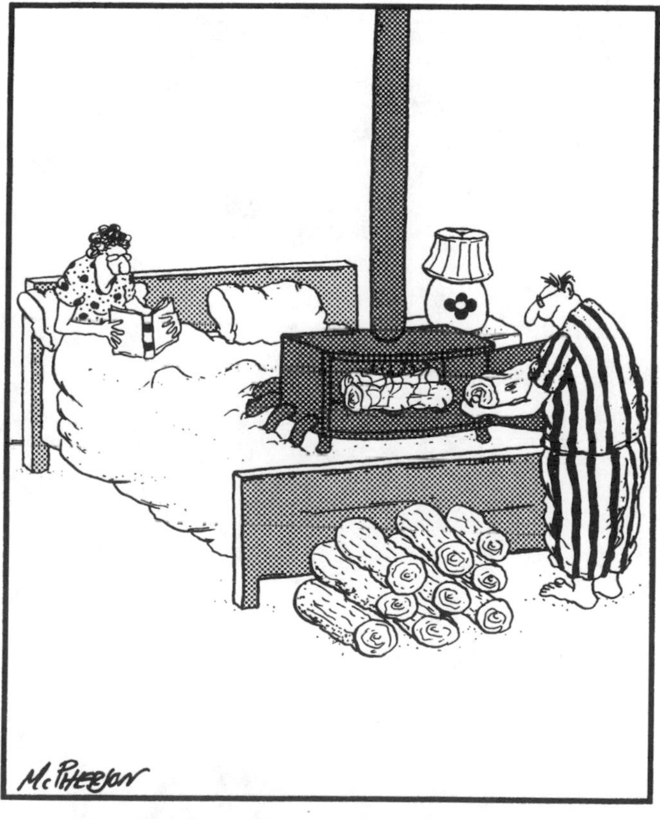

After hearing that electric blankets emit harmful electromagnetic waves, Norm and Sheila switched to a wood-fired blanket.

CHAPTER **13**

Implementing Green Printed Wiring Board Manufacturing

HOLLY EVANS

Director of Environmental and Safety Programs, Institute for Interconnecting and Packaging Electronic Circuits

JOHN W. LOTT

Senior Technical Consultant—Environmental, DuPont Photopolymer and Electronic Materials

The U.S. printed wiring board (PWB) industry has significantly improved its environmental performance over the past 20 years. The industry, with the potential to be a major polluting industry, has consciously altered its processes and practices to minimize its toxic output. While PWB manufacturers once viewed the effects of environmental regulations as a threat to their long-term growth, they reversed this effect. One of the best examples of this remarkable turnaround is how they actively became partners with regulatory agency programs such as the U.S. Environmental Protection Agency (EPA) Design for the Environment program. The industry continues to work with these agencies to assess the performance, cost, and environmental impact of alternatives to traditional PWB manufacturing methods.[1] Despite the great advances within the PWB industry, environmentally conscious designers can further reduce the impact of the products they design by being aware of the consequences of design on processes and material.

The concept of connecting design decisions to environmental consequences further down the supply chain is referred to as *design for the environment* (DfE). It means, for example, that requiring a solder surface on finished printed wiring boards (PWBs) to be shipped to an assembler has more environmental consequences than allowing the PWB manufacturer to use an alternative finish such as tin. To more clearly appreciate this concept let's review the process of making a circuit board.

Process

There are several types of PWBs or circuit boards, depending on the use, operational environment, and cost constraints.

The simplest type of board is single sided, with no holes for connections to other layers; these typically are made out of inexpensive laminate material and used for consumer products where there is little electronic sophistication and cost is the driver. A copper-clad dielectric is coated with a resist material, which is patterned to protect the areas where circuitry will be formed and the remaining copper etched away. This is referred to as the *print and etch* process. The chief waste products are etchant, consumed resist, and scrap or excess board material. The dielectric material can be either a rigid plastic (typically paper phenolic or glass, epoxy) or flexible plastic (for example, certain nylons or polyesters).

The second type of board is double sided, with plated through holes. This board also is in common use. Because of the need to plate the dielectric on the walls of the holes connecting both sides, either electroless copper or more recently direct plating chemistries are used to make the surface conductive. Once the surface is conductive, the walls typically are plated using standard electroplating copper baths. This means that the surface of the board also is plated either as a sheet of copper (panel plating) or as resist-defined circuit areas (pattern plating). In either case, the copper between circuit lines must be removed by etching. In pattern plating, of course, the background copper is much thinner than the circuit lines. The dielectric again can be rigid or flexible.

Most sophisticated boards, requiring complicated circuit routing to accommodate interconnecting integrated circuit chips, usually are multilayer boards. These boards traditionally have been manufactured by building "inner layers" using the print and etch process. These inner layers then are stacked in register and laminated together with partially polymerized dielectric between the layers along with outer layers of plain copper sheet. The outer layer then typically has been drilled with through holes to connect the various layers. The outer layers are either panel or pattern plated after coating the hole walls using electroless or direct metallization. Again the dielectric can be rigid, flexible, or a combination of the two.

The various processes used to make these types of boards have undergone changes during the past few years, and the most significant are listed in the next section. All these changes have had a significant effect on reducing the environmental impact of this industry.

Process Changes

The Switch from Chromic-Based Etchants

Beginning in the late 1970s and continuing through the early 1990s, alternatives were being developed to replace chromic-based etchants. This happened because chromic-based etchants were not easy to regenerate, etched at a slow rate, and had a low limit of dissolved copper.[2] They also were being regulated by environmental and health and safety agencies due to the hexavalent species, which was considered carcinogenic. The copper chloride and ammoniacal etchants, which have now replaced chromic etchants in the PWB industry, overcame all these disadvantages and were cheaper. The changes also significantly reduced the volume of etchant used by the industry and, therefore, its generation of spent etchant. Unlike chromic-based etchants, spent ammoniacal and cupric chloride etchants can be regenerated, reclaimed, or reused in other manufacturing operations.[3]

Elimination of Chlorinated Solvents

With the invention of solvent-developable dry film photoresists in the late 1960s, the PWB industry used significant amounts of 1,1,1, Trichloroethane (TCA) and methylene chloride to develop and strip them. In the late 1970s and early 1980s, aqueous and semiaqueous processable resists were developed, using either bicarbonate/hydroxide or butyl carbitol/cellosolve as developers or strippers.

TCA continued to be used as a cleaning solvent until 1990, when it was found to contribute to stratospheric ozone depletion. During the ensuing decade, it was virtually eliminated from use when the EPA adopted a phase-out program for all ozone-depleting substances (ODS) in Title VI of the Clean Air Act amendments.[4] Other cleaning solvents categorized as ODSs, for example, HCFC-141(b), also were eliminated when the industry switched to alternatives, such as citrus-based terpenes and aqueous-based cleaners.

Improved Process Control

Some of the industry's most successful environmental improvements include the widespread adoption of simple "housekeeping" measures that minimize waste generation and improve process control. Examples of such improvements include taking steps to reduce chemical loss, increase process bath life, and recover materials that otherwise would be disposed.[5]

These steps often included better bath control through improved use of sensors and control equipment. In addition, total quality management (TQM) systems can produce improved environmental as well as economic results. Adoption of a TQM program can reduce facility scrap rates and result in process changes that reduce chemical losses or conserve process baths.

Reduced Use of Tin-Lead as Etch Resist

For many years, electroplated tin-lead was the most common PWB metal etch resist used in pattern plating. Its widespread use also is due to the requirement of many upstream customers to be able to use reflowed tin or lead as the PWB surface finish of choice. The industry began to switch to lead-free etch metal resists due to technical constraints associated with tin-lead etch resists.[6] In addition, the industry saw widespread use of hot-air solder leveling (HASL) as the predominant PWB surface finish prior to adding components. Typically, any tin-lead *plating* had to be stripped off prior to the HASL process, thereby generating a lead-containing hazardous waste. Facilities that switched to HASL began to look for an etch resist that, when stripped, would not be an environmental hazard. Tin was the most logical alternative. As an etch resist, tin performs just as well as tin-lead; however, tin is not considered a hazardous waste and does not represent the worker safety issues associated with lead.[7]

Increased Use of an Alternative Metal-Bonding Surface Finish

To be effective, a PWB surface finish must prevent copper oxidization, facilitate solderability, and prevent defects during assembly. For many years, the reflowed tin-lead surface finish, which applies tin-lead solder to all exposed PWB traces, was the predominant PWB surface finish. Currently, HASL, which applies tin-lead solder only to PWB through holes and pads, has significantly reduced the industry's use of lead.

Despite its advantages, HASL still poses several drawbacks; for example, unless its waste solder dross is recycled, it must be managed as a hazardous waste. HASL also results in domed solder surfaces, whereas new and more complex packaging designs require flat surfaces.[8]

Among its other problems, HASL does not effectively cover the electroless nickel immersion gold process, which has grown in use due to the ease of bonding wire semiconductors to it. Also it has difficulty in adapting to the increased miniaturization of component attachment points.

The IPC currently is assessing lead-free alternatives to HASL through the EPA DfE PWB Project. The project will assess the economic, environmental, and performance characteristics of the following HASL alternatives: organic solder protectorates, immersion tin and silver, electroless nickel/immersion gold, immersion palladium, and electroless nickel/immersion palladium.

Improved End-of-Pipe Pollution Control Practices

In the 1970s, conventional metal precipitation systems were the most common type of wastewater treatment utilized by the industry. Although precipitation remains very common, some facilities are supplementing or replacing such systems with ion exchange and electrowinnowing technologies. For most facilities, copper, lead, and nickel are the only metal ions present in significant concentrations, all of which are amenable to ion exchange and electrowinnowing. Furthermore, these techniques result in salable forms of metals, which can produce economic revenue for the company as well as a "cleaner" waste-treatment sludge that may not be subject to RCRA hazardous waste regulations.

The use of nonchelated process chemistries also has reduced the generation of wastewater treatment sludge. Reduced sludge generation means cost savings, since the avoided cost of managing this sludge, which EPA considers a listed hazardous waste (e.g., F006) in most cases, can be significant.

Increased Reuse and Recycling of Manufacturing By-Products

The circuit formation processes noted already are subtractive and, in many cases, the most reliable and cost-effective ways to manufacture PWBs. The subtractive method generates large amounts of copper-bearing waste streams. Approximately 60% of the copper is removed in the typical etching process, resulting in a significant amount of copper leaving the facility as waste.

Fortunately, the industry recycles a majority of its manufacturing by-products (e.g., wastewater treatment sludge, etchant, off-specification boards, frames, and solder dross). Recycling extracts copper for reuse, reducing the need for virgin copper ore to be mined and reducing potential groundwater contamination (which could occur if copper-containing waste or incinerator ash is left in a landfill). PWB manufacturers can use on-site recycling methods, such as electrowinnowing, to remove metallic ions from spent process solutions, ion exchange regenerant, and concentrated rinse waters; or they can send their manufacturing by-products off site to facilities where the valuable constituents are reused or reclaimed.

Currently, the following materials are not subject to the RCRA hazardous waste restrictions and rules when they are reclaimed: scrap boards, scrap trim, router dust, solder baths and dumps, and solder dross. In addition, some states have ruled that spent etchant, when shipped to specific facilities that use the etchant as a direct feed stock in manufacturing operations, is not subject to RCRA.

Increased Use of Direct Metallization

As noted, the electroless copper process has been used to make drilled through holes conductive. Electroless copper uses large quantities of water, formaldehyde, and chelators, such as ethylene diaminetetraacetic acid (EDTA). These chelators also chelate metal waste streams, complicating their treatment.

The EPA and the IPC, under a DfE project, assessed a number of direct metallization alternatives—carbon, graphite, palladium, and conductive polymers—and found that all of them cost less, perform as well, and have less environmental impact (no formaldehyde or EDTA and less water use) than electroless copper.[9] In addition, facilities that switched to alternatives have found that these alternatives often are less hazardous to use, increase production flow, decrease maintenance requirements, and reduce cycle time, operating costs, and water usage, increasing the facilities' bottom lines.[10]

Increased Water Reuse and Recycling

The PWB industry is dependent on the use of large quantities of high-quality water, which is used primarily to rinse circuit boards between process steps. PWB facilities now increasingly use water reuse and recycling technologies to extend process bath life and decrease their reliance on municipal water, which may be costly and, in some cases, of poor quality. Facilities located in areas where water supplies are scarce may face flow restrictions from municipal water authorities.

The installation of on-site water recycling systems and the use of simple water use reduction methods (e.g., flow restrictors, conductivity controls, flow meters, counterflow rinse tanks, and spray rinse systems) have resulted in large water-use reductions for a number of PWB facilities. Fortunately, the adoption of water conservation practices often results in economic gain.

Future Opportunities for Pollution Prevention

There are additional opportunities for improved environmental impact. These might include

- 100% beneficial reuse and recycling of *all* hazardous by-products.
- Use of raw materials from sustainable sources (e.g., copper foil from recycled copper, laminate from biobased or recycled plastic sources).
- Zero water discharge manufacturing processes.
- Systematic management of EHS compliance and performance (ISO 14001 and EMAS).[11]
- Development of technically acceptable lead-free solder.
- Standardization and implementation of design for reuse and disassembly practices.
- Development and implementation of energy efficient manufacturing operations.
- Integration of environmental cost and activity-based cost accounting tools into traditional accounting methods.

Current Technology Trends Can Improve Environmental Impact

Since the industry is being driven to produce lighter, denser, cheaper circuits, designers must take advantage of these technologies. Many of the newer processes utilize less material, produce less waste, and are more energy efficient. For example, the two major approaches to microvias (vias on the order of 1–3 mils) utilize either lasers to make vias without drilling or photodielectric materials. While both these approaches can produce vias that connect only layer to layer where physically needed, this immediately increases the circuit density and reduces material usage. Photodielectrics, on the other hand, also can produce circuit "channels" as well as vias, which in combination with additive metallization would further significantly reduce waste.

In addition to being used to make vias, lasers also are being utilized more seriously to actually pattern resists used in making the circuit traces. Laser direct imaging allows the circuit design to go directly from the digital output of the design to the board itself without utilizing a phototool. This eliminates the phototool and its waste streams. In the case of a photodielectric, it may even be possible to image the vias and "channels" directly into the dielectric.

Electrical Design Effects on Environmental Impact

As can be seen from the improvements both at the chemical usage and the technology levels, it is possible to utilize materials and processes to significantly reduce the environmental impact of a circuit board. However, this can happen only if the PWB manufacturer is allowed to pick the best process and materials and not be hampered by outmoded specifications that might call for some specific chemical usage. For example, if electroless copper in the vias or holes is specified, then the manufacturer cannot utilize direct metallization processes to do the same process. Thinner copper and utilization of polymer thick-film (PTF) conductors for via metallization, shielding, and even conductor metallization can save much waste, since either less copper is used or, in the case of PTFs, the process is strictly additive.

In addition, newer technology should be implemented where possible. For example, microvia technologies can be used to significantly reduce layer count or board size. This freedom to trade off layer count for board size can be significant, especially if the original board dimensions do not fit well into the standard panel sizes used in the industry. Unused panel areas that end up as edge trim scrap typically must go through all the process steps as the final board. This means that all that processing and material is wasted and accounts for a significant portion of the scrap. Using mixed flex-rigid boards, thinner flexible materials can be used in place of rigid materials to not only carry circuitry but also function as an interboard connector.

The key to utilizing the right materials and processes is to work with and consult closely your PWB manufacturers. Decisions can be arrived at that both meet technical specifications and have the least environmental impact. Many people currently are working on methods to incorporate design for the environment in design algorithms, but direct discussions with your suppliers often will serve the same function. Many PWB fabricators also now have in-house design capabilities and can suggest alternatives to a given design.

Summary

The PWB has made great strides in reducing its environmental impact by stepping up its pollution-prevention efforts. Additional improvements have been made by improving the processes and materials utilized. Still other ongoing efforts may reduce the environmental burden even further. While the manufacturers themselves can implement much of this, cooperation along the electronic supply chain is critical. Those asking for specific materials and design considerations must be aware of the consequences of those design decisions. Despite the number of efforts to implement DfE mechanisms to make this process easier, it is just as important to work directly with suppliers to understand the constraints that design decisions impose and the opportunities for improvement should other choices be made.

Notes

1. The industry has been a lead partner in EPA's Design for the Environment Printed Wiring Board (DfE PWB) Project since 1994. This project identifies, evaluates, and disseminates information on viable pollution-prevention opportunities for the PWB industry. The project's work product, which includes eight case studies and four technical documents, can be found on the Internet at http://www.epa.gov/opptintr/dfe/pwb/pwb.html.
2. See Clyde F. Coombs, Jr., *Printed Circuit Handbook*, 3rd ed. (New York: McGraw-Hill, 1988).
3. PWB Project Case Study 2, On-Site Etchant Regeneration, EPA744-F-95-005, July 1995.
4. FR 42 USC Section 7671(c).
5. PWB Project Case Study 1, Pollution Prevention Work Practices, EPA 744-F-95-004.
6. U.S. EPA, "Printed Wiring Board Industry and Use Cluster Profile," EPA 744-R-95-005, (September 1995), pp. 2–38.
7. 29 CFR 1910.1025 requires employers to perform exposure monitoring for employees exposed to lead and to develop plans depending on the level of exposure to safeguard employees.
8. IPC Surface Mount Council White Paper, "PWB Surface Finishes," SMC-WP-005, April 1997.
9. U.S. EPA, "Implementing Cleaner Technologies in the Printed Wiring Board Industry: Making Holes Conductive," EPA 744-R-97-001 (February 1997).
10. Ibid.
11. ISO 14000 is the international standard for environmental management systems. EMAS is a similar standard that was developed in the European community.

CHAPTER **14**

No-Lead Solder Assembly

William Trumble
Retired from Nortel Networks, Nepean, Canada

Lead compounds, such as those formulated in paint, have been proven to have toxic effects when ingested or inhaled. How this toxicity was extended to lead metals or lead alloys involves a science that often is questioned. Be that as it may, public and regulatory pressure against the use of lead in any form in products is increasing, especially in Europe. Much of the regulatory pressure is focused on solder and the solder in electronic products, probably due to its high commercial profile. This situation has led to a search for alternatives in the electronics industry.

There are replacements for tin lead solder and for some applications a drop-in replacement, but for the electronics industry, there is no easy drop-in replacement, mainly because the structure of the electronic printed circuit board (PCB) is built around the duet of copper and tin lead solder. Other issues that constrain an electronics designer in the search for a new solder are

- Higher signal speeds usually mean lower signal voltages, which place stronger requirements on a solder's conductivity characteristics.
- Smaller solder pads are needed on PCBs.
- Boards and systems are operating at higher temperatures, which can stress solders.
- Lead solder sites are becoming narrower and closer together.
- More electronics are operating in an unprotected environment.
- New lead finishes such as palladium nickel are appearing.
- Alloy 42 (nickel-iron) alloy lead solders are being used.
- The industry demands faster board assembly time.
- Component lead configuration (e.g., BGA) is becoming more complex.

Experimental projects have demonstrated that a search for a *universal* drop-in replacement for tin lead solder is a long and often frustrating process. To take the first step, it is better to start with a relatively simple printed circuit assembly (PCA) and then characterize the solder joint.

A solder joint has three components: the solder pad, the solder and the component finish. The nonjoint players are the solder profile, solder the atmosphere, flux and cleaning.

Solder Pad Characteristics

The solder pad on a printed circuit board usually is composed of pure copper metal. There can be other pad materials but copper metal is the most common. To keep the pads so that solder would wet and adhere to them, a finish is applied to the pads and all exposed copper on the board. One finish on copper pads is tin lead (hot-air solder leveling, or HASL). This finish must be replaced for a no-lead solder joint. Several metal replacements for HASL are being tested or used presently. Among these are tin immersion and gold over nickel, but other metal finishes also are supplied by the solder manufacturers.

Another finish for the bond pad is called *organic solder protect* (OSP), composed of a polymeric copper antioxidant that is designed to leave the bond pad as the solder comes in contact with it. There are reports that the OSP is only good for one or two passes in a reflow oven, but experiments demonstrate that this fate is conditioned by the solder atmosphere.

Solder

The selection of the solder is critical to the quality of the solder joint. The present design of the solder joint, the pad size, lead configuration, and geometric relation of the lead to the pad are designed to maximize the performance of tin lead solder. To select a nonlead solder as a replacement, the following guidelines must be observed.

- The temperature of the solder at soldering temperatures must not exceed the recommended maximum stability temperature of any of the components.
- The cost of the solder must be within a measurable margin of the present cost.
- The solder must be applicable in three modes of application: reflow (surface mount technology, or SMT), wave solder (plated through hole, or PTI), and hand solder (repair).
- Solder must have a narrow plastic range, preferably a eutectic melt.
- Solder must have adequate wetting properties for all surface finishes on the components (no lead) and on the PCB using all three modes of application.
- Solder must have applicable physical properties equal to or better than tin lead solder.

- The application of the solder must not involve the capital expense of new or developmental solder process machines. The thermal profile of the solder should be in the operating range of the present tin lead equipment.
- Assembly with the new solder must be accomplished using the present workforce with a minimum of training.
- To minimize metallurgy complications in operation, the solder should be a binary alloy.
- The solder should have an adequate shelf life under reasonable or instructed storage conditions.
- The solder paste, when applied to the board, must have a reasonable time of stability to factory conditions before thermal processing.
- The solder joints from all three applications should have a thermal fatigue resistance appropriate to the design intent of the product.
- When fused, the solder must have a thermal and electrical conductivity equal to tin lead solder.
- The solder should be flexible with the present-day flux technology.
- The solder or solder paste should be composed so that it presents no toxic threat to workers.
- The solder must not constitute an environmental hazard when disposed of alone or on products into the public domain.
- The solder must not be made of metals that involve an environmental hazard when extracted or processed; that is, to get bismuth, lead has to be mined.
- The solder should form very little dross when used in wave solder assembly.

In spite of the restrictions in these guidelines, a number of alloys have been tested and are determined to be adequate replacements for tin lead.

Solders on Appropriate Applications

The International Tin Research Institute in consort with Multicore Cor, GEC, Nortel, and others evaluated a series of solder alloys using the preceding guidelines. Their research demonstrated that two alloys, 96.5% tin, 3.5% silver and 99.3% tin, 0.7% copper most nearly fit the criteria. Alpha Metals performed similar research and concluded the two solder alloys, tin-silver and tin-copper, fit best the design and environmental criteria for a direct replacement for 63% tin, 37% lead solder.

Both the tin-silver and the tin-copper solder alloys have a melting point above tin-lead (63%/3.7%) solder (222° and 227°C, respectively, versus 183°C). This results in the usual soldering temperature for the tin-lead solder being 220°C versus about 245° and 255°C for the no-lead alloys. Manufacturing process test runs indicate that none of the components on the tested PCB that were normally surface mounted or wave soldered were adversely affected by the soldering temperature. However, the solder selected must fit the robustness requirements of the board and components.

Component Lead Finishes

The types of component lead solders are expanding. Among others are leadless solder, the various configurations of leaded solder (e.g., gull wing, J-lead), and the flip chip and BGHA lead solders. For the sake of simplicity and to better explain the metallurgical relationship between solder and the component lead finish, we confine our attention to the classical leads and leadless components. Some of the finishes and component leads commonly used in addition to tin-lead are tin, tin-copper, tin-silver, silver-palladium, gold on nickel, copper, nickel, palladium, and nickel. The art and science enters in matching the solder to the finish to minimize damage to intermetallic voids and cracking during installed operation.

Whatever the lead finish, the composition of the finish and the underlying metal must be identified. A lead finish often is diffused into the solder and some combination of the finish and solder comes in contact with, wets, and adheres to the underlying metal surface. Contaminants can affect the efficiency and integrity of any of these actions. Iron in a nickel finish, for example, can cause a very harmful intermetallic formation at the interface. Metal contamination in the solder joint is a major cause of solder joint failure. There are caveats to the use of several component finishes, which are described next.

Nickel

Nickel can be used as a component finish but it must be used very soon after the component is manufactured. Unless environmentally packaged, the nickel forms an oxide very quickly that cannot be removed with flux or any other oxide removal process. Nickel-finished components must be used within a month of production.

Tin

The use of tin has been avoided because of its reputed tendency to grow tin whiskers. All the experimental literature describes whiskering as associated with electroplated tin, especially that with organic leveling agents. The whiskering is attendant to the compressive forces from electroplating and the loss of the organic leveling agent. This barrier to the use of tin can be overcome by

- Eliminating the use of organic leveling agents.
- Annealing the electroplated tin-finished components to relieve stress.
- Installing tin-finish components where the system operating temperature never gets near or exceeds 50°C.
- Using a high melt solder such as tin-silver or tin-copper where the soldering temperature (245° to 255°C) exceeds the tin melting temperature (231°C).
- Installing the tin in systems whose operating temperature always exceeds 150°C.

Gold

Gold finishes exceeding 50 microinches can cause delamination at the solder lead finish interface.

Other Considerations for No-Lead Solder Assembly

Fluxes

The suppliers of solders have fluxes appropriate for each solder for every solder format: no clean, low Volatile Organic Compounds (VOC), no VOC, and the like. The supplier of each solder will be of great assistance in matching flux with solder for a specific application.

Inert Gas Atmosphere Solder Operations

Much debate has concerned the value versus the cost of the use of nitrogen-shielded solder reflow ovens and wave solder machines. Solders having a soldering temperature below that of tin lead solder (such as the bismuth alloys) *may* be activated effectively and efficiently with no inert atmosphere depending on their drossing tendencies. But, for solders that have a soldering temperature above that of tin-lead, such as the 99.7/3 in. copper or the 96.5/3.5 tin-silver alloys, an inert gas atmosphere is a must. The advantages of the inert gas atmosphere include less tin drossing, less thermal stress on flux, and less thermal oxidative stress on the component finishes, plastic housings of the components, and the organic solder protection. Reduced stress on the solder protection makes it practical for more than one or two solder passes. For these reasons, the inert gas atmosphere must be evaluated as part of the process on any no-lead solder assembly program.

Conductive Adhesive Printed Circuit Assembly

An alternative method to production of printed circuit assemblies is to use conductive adhesives such as silver-filled epoxies to join the components to the substrate. These adhesives have progressed rapidly in terms of cost/joint, processing time, and component "green" and cured adhesion to the substrate. They enjoy several advantages over solders:

- The adhesive is activated between 125° and 150°C, which puts less thermal stress on the components.
- The adhesive is thermosetting; there is plastic movement before 300°C if at all.
- Some conductive adhesives can be activated by exposure to UV light, so less energy.

- Very little interaction takes place with component lead or substrate finishes except those of tin-lead.
- They are the best joining material for flexible circuits.
- The recommended maximum long-term stability temperature is 300°C (epoxies).

Adhesive solders also have disadvantages:

- The coefficient of thermal expansion triples a thermal point called the *glass transition temperature*.
- The glass transition temperature can vary from 25° to 125°C, depending on processing conditions.
- It takes 24 hours for the adhesive to achieve its full mechanical properties.
- The conductive material is silver or silver-plated carbon; there may be some electromagnetic issues in humid environments.
- The coefficient of thermal expansion of the most common epoxy conductive adhesive is twice that of copper.

Whether a no-lead solder or a conductive adhesive is used, a successful result can be achieved if the project is planned carefully. Among those operations that will fulfill the desired result are

- Carefully writing out the system requirements for the solder.
- Selecting the component lead finishes that work with the solder.
- Designing a test program to measure the solder performance with the system requirements.
- With the supplier, selecting solder and flux and configuring a solder profile.
- Applying the solder to the product substrate as recommended.
- Testing and evaluating various solder joints.

Summary of Solder Testing

Both the eutectic tin-lead solder and eutectic tin-copper solder exhibited excellent wetting to a variety of surface finishes on surface mount components when a nitrogen-inerted environment was used for reflow. A maximum reflow temperature as low as 250°C appears adequate to achieve acceptable reflow conditions with the tin-copper solder alloy. The resulting tin-copper solder joints are rougher in texture than the corresponding tin-lead solder joints but still relatively shiny in luster.

The printed circuit board materials and most surface mount and through-hole components could withstand the higher process temperatures associated with the tin-copper alloy. However, certain component types—namely, electrolytic capacitors, brittle through-hole components, and components constructed of lower-melting-temperature materials—should be avoided when using the lead-free solder alloy.

The microstructure of the eutectic tin-copper solder alloy consists of a matrix of tin grains with dispersed Cu6Sn5 intermetallic particles located at the tin-tin grain boundaries. As a result of thermal cycling, both the tin grain size and the intermetallic grain size increase significantly, although the overall grain size is slightly less than observed for eutectic tin-lead.

During soldering, the eutectic tin-copper solder reacts with the substrate or the plating materials to form the same intermetallic species observed for tin-lead solder. However, the intermetallics that form with the tin-copper solder typically are larger, due to the higher process temperatures and the abundance of tin. The larger size of the intermetallics appears to have no negative impact on the overall integrity of the solder joints.

The internal void content in the tin-copper surface mount solder joints was significantly higher than observed in the corresponding tin-lead solder joints. These voids frequently were sites of crack initiation and growth during thermal cycling.

Cracking was observed in the surface mount and the through-hole tin-copper solder joints after 2,000 thermal cycles from 0° to 100°C (see Figure 14–1). These cracks continued to grow in length and severity with further cycling up to 6,000 thermal cycles. The number of cracks per solder joint, the severity of the cracks, and the length of the cracks all were lower for the tin-copper surface-mount solder joints than tin-lead joints after 2,000 thermal cycles. After 4,000 thermal cycles, the relative performance of the two alloys reversed, with the tin-lead solder outperforming the tin-copper solder up to 6,000 thermal cycles.

Virtually all the cracking in the eutectic tin-copper solder joints was intergranular in nature. The cracks propagated along the tin-tin grain boundaries regardless of the components' lead style, the solderable finish, or the overall stress state.

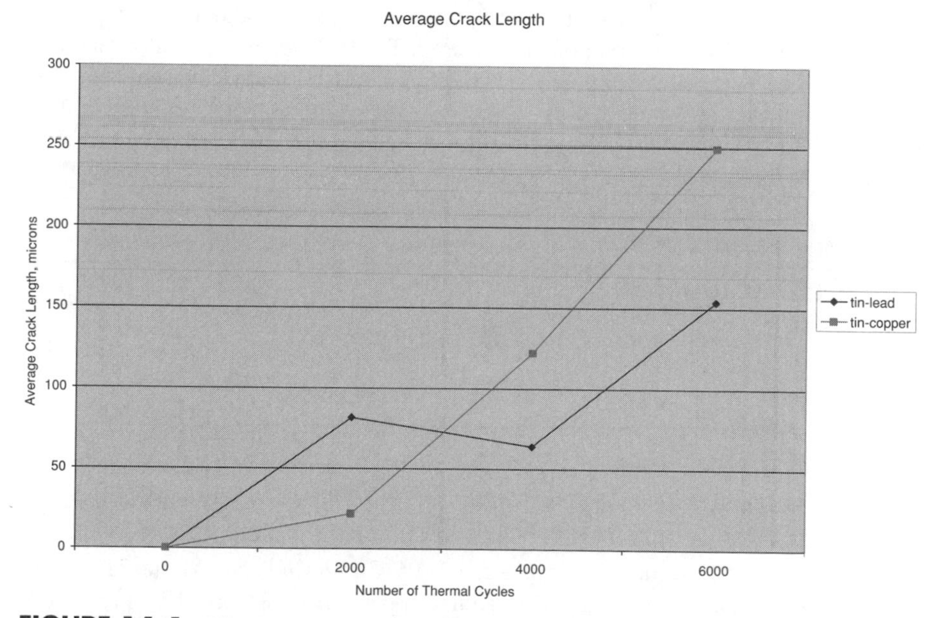

FIGURE 14–1 Crack length in solder joints is directly related to their exposure in thermal cycling.

The mechanical properties of the eutectic tin-copper solder joints appear to be similar to eutectic tin-lead solder joints. Microhardness tests indicate that the tin-copper alloy might be slightly stronger than the tin-lead alloy. Shear strength tests on 1206 chip capacitors indicate that the solder joint strengths are almost the same for both solder alloys up to 4,000 thermal cycles. At 6,000 cycles, the tin-copper solder joints exhibit a lower strength than the tin-lead solder joints.

Conclusions

The eutectic tin-copper alloy is a viable alternative to eutectic tin-lead solder for some applications.

There are limitations to the types of components that can be used, due to the higher melting temperature of the tin-copper alloy, but it appears that standard SMT assembly equipment can be used to process the lead-free alloy. The only unique requirement is a nitrogen-inerted atmosphere for soldering.

Component lead finishes that are very thick and react with tin to form intermetallics should be avoided for use with the eutectic tin-copper solder alloy. The recommended finishes for use with this alloy are tin or tin-copper.

The thermal fatigue performance of the tin-copper alloy is actually superior to tin-lead up to 2,000 thermal cycles from 0° to 100°C. Beyond 4,000 thermal cycles, however, the inherent brittleness of the tin-tin grain boundaries in the tin-copper solder limits its ability to resist crack growth.

Based on the results of this analysis, the tin-copper solder alloy can be used successfully on assemblies that are required to withstand up to 2,000 thermal cycles as long as no incompatible components are used. The tin-copper solder also might be used in applications that are required to withstand 4,000 thermal cycles, but extensive product testing is recommended to ensure reliability. The eutectic tin-copper alloy probably is not appropriate for applications that require the solder joints to withstand 6,000 thermal cycles.

Acknowledgment

This work was performed under IEC sales order 70855.

References

ASTM Metals. *Metallography, Structures and Phase Diagrams*, vol. 8, eighth ed. ASTM Metals, Philadelphia, PA, 1973.

Bader, W. "Dissolution of Au, Ag, Pd, Pt, Cu and Ni in a Molten Tin-Lead Solder." *Welding Journal* (Research Supplement) 48, no. 12 (1969), pp. 551s–557s.

Fretterolf, T. "99C Wavesoldering Evaluation with No Clean on Copper/Entek." Multicore Laboratory Report 609012, 1996.

Nortel Networks. "Acceptability of Electronic Assemblies," IPC-A-610B, Kanata, Canada, 1994.

Nortel Networks. "Lead-Free 8009 Manufacturing Assembly Trials." EC30, Kanata, Canada, 1996.

Nortel Networks. "Workmanship PCBA Surface Mount." Nortel workmanship standard 150.09, Kanata, Canada, 1996.

Porter, D., and K. Easterling. *Phase Transformation in Metals and Alloys*. New York: Van Nostrand Reinhold, 1981.

Pratt, R. "Fracture and Deformation Behavior of Eutectic Pb-Sn Solder Joints." MS thesis, University of Rochester, 1991.

Pratt, R. "The Effect of Noble Metal Contamination on the Mechanical Properties of Eutectic Tin-Lead Solder Joints." Ph.D. thesis, University of Rochester, 1994.

Pratt, R. "Bell Northern Research A0649450 lead-Free Assembly Process Details." IEC Technical Report RP-25-96, Bell Northern Research, Ottawa, Canada, August 1996.

Pratt, R. "Mircrostructural Analysis of Eutectic Sn-Cu Alloy Solder Joints." IEC Technical Report RP-26-97, Bell Northern Research, Ottawa, Canada, August 1997.

Pratt, R. "Microstructural Analysis of Eutectic Sn-Cu Alloy Solder Joints after 2000 Thermal Cycles, 0°C–100°C." IEC Technical Report RP-28-97, Bell Northern Research, Ottawa, Canada, September 1997.

Pratt, R. "Microstructural Analysis of Eutectic Sn-Cu Alloy Solder Joints after 4000 Thermal Cycles, 0°C–100°C." IEC Technical Report RP-01-98, Bell Northern Research, Ottawa, Canada, January 1998.

Pratt, R., E. Stromswold, and D. Quesnel. "Effect of Solid-State Intermetallic Growth on the Fracture Thoughness of Cu/63Sn-37Pb Solder Joints." *IEEE Transactions on Components, Hybrids, and Manufacturing Technology*, vol. CHMT-19 (1996), pp, 134–141.

Romig, A., P.D. Bristow, and David E. Fowler. "Physical Metallurgy of Solder-Substrate Reactions." In *Solder Mechanics: A State of the Art Assessment*. NewYork: TMS Publications, 1991.

Smith, W. *Principles of Materials Science and Engineering*. New York: McGraw-Hill, 1989.

Stromswold, E., R. Pratt, and D. Quesnel. "The Mechanical Properties of Cu/96.5Sn-3.5Ag Solder Joints with Comparisons to Cu/63Sn-37Pb Solder Joints." SAND93-7102, Sandia Laboratories, White Sands, NM, 1993.

Trumble, B., and J. Brydges. "World's First Lead Free Circuit Telephone." IPCWorks 1997, Washington, DC, October 5–9, 1997.

Warwick M., and S. Muckett. "Observations on the Growth and Impact of Intermetallic Compounds on Tin-Coated Substrates." *Circuit World* 9, no. 4 (1983).

CHAPTER **15**

Chemical Conversion Coatings on Electronic Equipment

WILLIAM TRUMBLE

Retired from Nortel Networks, Nepean, Canada

Chemical conversion coatings are used throughout the electronics industry to protect the base metal (zinc-plated steel, magnesium, aluminum, iron, etc.) of enclosures, housings, and other assemblies from the oxidative effects of the environment. One of the most historically popular conversion coatings has used chromate-based compounds, thanks to their ease of application and relatively low cost. Over the past several years, increasing environmental awareness throughout the electronic industry has identified chromate conversion coating as a process that creates excessive toxic wastes in all phases of the product cycle and causes problems with the recycling of metal parts at the end of their life.

In Europe, the political pressure derived from these environmental concerns extends to the point that returned equipment treated with chromate is not allowed to be disposed in landfill, but must be stored in a dangerous goods storage site. The European council is initiating action to force vendors to take back electronic equipment at the end of its useful life and incur the expense of disposal by the year 2002.

Fortunately, alternatives are now available that have much less environmental impact and electrical properties better suited to the demands of high-speed digital equipment. Since you, the reader, are most likely an electrical engineer or technical manager who may not be familiar with this aspect of electronics manufacturing, we take a quick look at the topic of conversion coatings in general before looking into chromate coatings and their alternatives.

Conversion Coatings 101

Fundamentally, the mechanism that conversion coatings employ is to potentially oxidize the base metal in a controlled manner to form a coating that helps it resist corrosive forces. Some of the more commonly used conversion coating methods include anodizing, phosphating, chromating, and controlled oxidizing. The protection provided by these conversion coatings is not permanent, since environmental forces such as heat, light, air, moisture, and temperature change work alone and together to gradually deteriorate the conversion coating. The protection provided by the conversion coating usually is extended by an overlay of paint.

Other ways to protect the base metal against the effects of the environment are metal plating (such as nickel plating) and substituting a corrosion-resistant metal for the base metal. These responses may not be very rewarding because each plating method has some environmental flaw. Both alternatives are expensive, and despite alloys, some metals cannot be sufficiently corrosion resistant to assure their integrity for the full service life of the product. This makes conversion coatings very attractive, since they are much less expensive and often easier to apply. They are effective when used within their design parameters, and their functional life can be extended by an appropriate protective overlay (e.g., paint). Fundamentally, the proper conversion coating or other environmental protection can be selected by answering three questions:

1. What do you want the product to do?
2. How long do you want it to function?
3. Under what conditions will the product be operating?

Much of the metal used in the electronics industry ends up in enclosures for electronic equipment. These enclosures usually are made of zinc-plated steel or aluminum and used to array the electronics, dissipate some of the heat given off by the circuitry, and protect the electronic equipment from mechanical damage. Additionally, a metal case can serve to protect the electronic equipment from electromagnetic interference (EMI) and confine the EMI generated by the protected circuitry. The EMI protection that is integral to the electronic enclosure imposes another requirement on the conversion coating: electrical conductivity. Electrical conductivity includes surface conductivity (as measured by surface resistance) and contact conductivity (as measured by four-wire contact resistance). This requirement for electrical conductivity eliminates many potentially useful conversion coatings as candidates for electronics equipment.

Breaking the Chromate Tradition

The hexavalent chromate conversion coating has been in use for at least 50 years. It has a good track record for corrosion protection of the base metal even in tropical zones. Telephone equipment manufacturers adopted it for switching and other call-handling equipment for the following reasons:

- Chromate's electrical conductivity was adequate to give the appropriate EMI protection at the time.
- Electromechanical switching did not use much EMI protection, if any.

- Chromating the zinc-plated steel substrates was spontaneous and required no electricity. The operator merely had to immerse the part in the chromate solution for a time appropriate for the desired corrosion protection.
- Chromate provided an economic useful life without painting in the protected central office environment.
- The chromate solution was reasonably robust to small amounts of metal contaminants.
- The capital outlay for equipment to apply chromate to zinc-plated steel was minimal: a chromate tank and a rinse tank.
- The chromated surfaces could be painted after a certain cure time with simple paint technology.
- Chromating was fast, typically 5–45 seconds.
- The process control to attain a suitable coating was simple: temperature and pH acidity.

Chromate conversion coating was used on the telephone equipment and other equipment with no real reflection until the 1990s. Two forces caused an examination of the use of chromate conversion coating: the demands of high-speed digital electronic switching or computing equipment and rising concern over the environment.

Chromate conversion coating no longer was acceptable because

- Chromates were a health hazard both in processing and products.
- The chromate process and the end-of-life products were environmentally damaging.
- The contact resistance and surface resistivity of chromate on the zinc-plated steel was too high for the needed EMI protection.
- The contact resistance and surface resistivity could not be held steady within a plated batch of substrates and sometimes not within a given part.
- Because of the innate resistivity of the chromate, tin-lead-plated beryllium-copper gaskets were needed to attain acceptable EMI protection. Both lead and beryllium are environmentally questionable.
- The chromate conversion coating has a thermal stability threshold of 66°C. This limitation prevented using the powder coating, electrostatic spray-baking method. While the solvent-free powder-coat process is environmentally preferable to traditional solvent-based paints, the high-temperature bake required to set the powder exceeds the chromate coating's stability threshold.
- If low-solvent paints are used, a 72-hour cure time is required for the chromate before the coating can be applied. This increases the work-in-progress cost.
- The coating was applied in a solution that had a pH of 2 (very acid), requiring considerable expense to neutralize to a pH of 5.6 for disposal.
- Chromate concentrates are considered dangerous. They must be disposed of in a hazardous waste site at considerable expense.

Alternative Conversion Coatings

Anodizing

Anodizing is a method to impart corrosion of a base metal by converting the base metal to its oxide in a controlled manner. The anodization, especially in the case of aluminum, is very stable to the environmental forces that cause corrosion. These metal oxides are not very conductive electrically. The oxide coating is powder and so porous. Sealer is applied to the anodize coat to prevent moisture intrusion through the protection. This makes the coating even less electrically conductive. Anodizing is great for architectural metals but not for electronic enclosures.

Phosphatizing

Phosphatizing is a method to impart corrosion resistance by converting the base metal to one of its phosphates. The metal phosphates are much more conductive than the oxides but not very weatherproof, because some of the phosphates of the metal are soluble in water and the process of application does not produce all the insolubles in soluble phosphates if the metal has any at all. The phosphates make an excellent base for applying paint, so most metal phosphates are painted.

Group IV Metal Oxides

Group IV metals are high-valence metals like manganese, molybdenum, vanadium, and tungsten. Like chromium, they have oxides that are very strong oxidation agents and react with active metals such as zinc, aluminum, and magnesium to form an environmentally stable coating. Some of the metals are more dangerous than chromate; others are considerably more expensive. Three of the oxides—zirconium oxide, manganese oxide, and molybdenum oxide—in the highest oxidation state are being investigated as a replacement for chromium oxide. They are not really on the market for some reason.

Molybdenum and Other Acid Phosphates

A more recent entry into the conversion coating field is molybdenum phosphate, specifically an oxide salt (e.g., molybdenum oxide) mixed with a phosphoric acid system. The acid system contains phosphoric acid among other ingredients to control the coating reaction. The cleaned, descaled metal (e.g., zinc) is immersed in the molybdate phosphoric acid solution for a controlled time. When completed, the surface is a matrix of molybdenum and zinc phosphate. In this case, the molybdenum, which is a metal more passive to oxidation than zinc, retards the oxidative reaction of the environment. Theoretically, this action can be accomplished with other high-valence (which implies rich in oxygen) metals such as vanadium, chromium, and tungsten, but molybdenum is the most environmentally friendly of these metals. A case study of this conversion coating is at the end of this chapter.

Environment

Some adverse comments have been made about the environmental impact of applying any kind of conversion coating to a metal. But, if the application of the coating extends the product's useful life from three years to ten years, delaying refabrication of the product 22-fold, the attendant environmental impact of recycling the old and remaking the new will be saved.

Section III
Management Issues

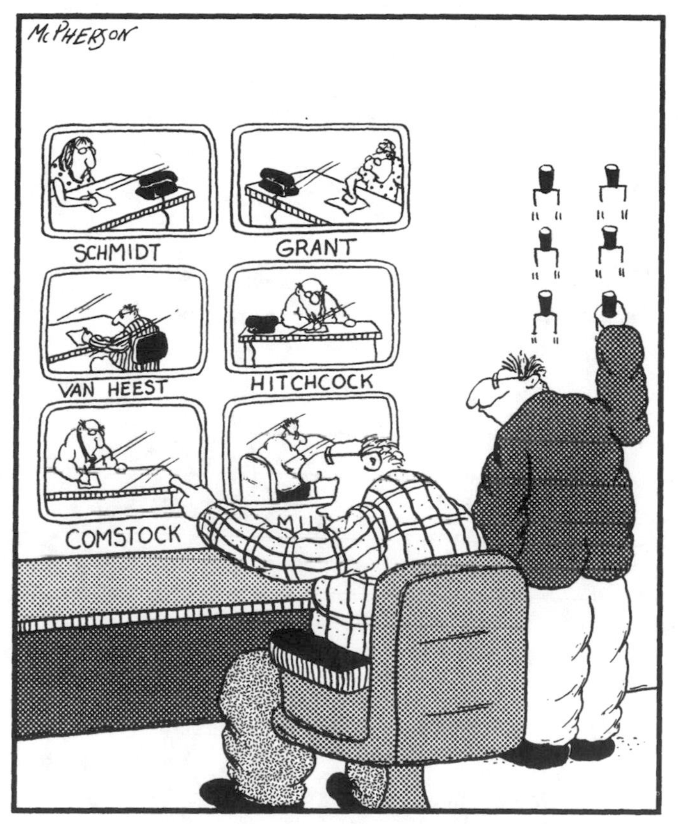

"Comstock's moving a little slow on that Megatron Industries proposal. Give him seventy-five volts for five seconds. What the heck, make that ten seconds."

Introduction: Musings Before a New Dawn

TED D. POLAKOWSKI
Environment, Health and Safety Officer, Microelectronics Group, Lucent Semiconductor, Murry Hill, New Jersey

The clock by the bed reads 4:07 AM. It's dark in this hotel room as I huddle in the pale glow of my laptop's screen. Despite my body's urgings to the contrary, I have given in to my brain's repeated demands to get up, turn on the computer, and start this introduction. For some unknown reason, I awoke little more than an hour ago with thoughts running through my head as to the perfect way to structure it. For a while, I debated about whether I had to get out of bed to formally write down this stuff or, in the worst case, turn on the computer to officially start writing. I thought wistfully about using the ever-present note pad and pen to jot down some pertinent outline topics. In a last-ditch effort to salve my conscience and sink back to unconsciousness, I tried to assure myself that I would remember everything that I have been thinking about for the past hour when I awoke later this morning. Even I didn't believe that last argument; so here I am, waiting for my computer to boot up, promising myself I will just spend a few minutes entering the pertinent items and get back to bed.

I hate when this happens to me. Anyone who's ever traveled for business knows that empty, "Huh? Where-am-I, and why-am-I-here?" feeling you get when you semi-awaken in an unfamiliar place. That's how I started this adventure, in a completely darkened room with only an eerie red glow several inches from my face reading 3:04 AM. It took a little while to remember that I was in Orlando, Florida, for my business group's Environmental Action Team's second annual strategic planning meeting. This get-together is one of the activities prescribed in our ISO 14001-based environmental management system, EMS.

Yes, as strange as it may sound, in several hours I will preside over a meeting that brings together people who normally don't interact to take a long look into the future and think about what our business will be like then. We will have product marketers, process developers, academia, applied R&D folks, and people representing the role of the environmental regulatory community together with my business group's facility-based environmental managers and engineers. The intent of this meeting is to review and discuss potential product demands and the process requirements needed to satisfy those demands over a horizon of three to five years. The regulators are here to tell us how they think legislative action will proceed in the United States and Europe over this planning horizon.

The expected outcome of this strategic planning meeting is twofold. First, we hope to gain a better understanding of where the business will be going in the future. Then, we plan to debate where we, as the company's environmental specialists, will need to work with these business and regulatory folks to help make these expectations successful from both the business and environmental performance perspectives. Through these proactive preparatory exercises, we learn that the concepts of business success and superior environmental performance most often are not mutually exclusive. In fact, by being proactive, we find that we can help add to the company's profitability and productivity. This contrasts sharply with the traditional stereotype of environmental management as a cost adder and a hindrance to almost any phase of a project.

Maybe some kind of weird mind meld also is going on within me as I sit in front of this computer keying thoughts onto the screen. Perhaps it's just disorientation from the late hour, but I seem to feel an uncanny synergy between my thoughts on today's meeting with its portent of initial EMS success and this writing exercise. About a year ago, when Lee Goldberg and I started discussing the rationale for getting involved with environmental management systems, we found we both were after the same outcome but were coming at it from different directions.

If I might take a stab at paraphrasing our conversation, it went something like this. Lee explained how he thought an EMS would be a good tool for technologists. He felt it would be a method of delivering a discipline for engineers to use and, by doing so, guide their actions in a way that would positively affect the environmental performance of a company. An engineer at heart, Lee saw this sort of bottoms-up approach for this book.

I told him I agreed that his approach was useful and necessary but that it would not go far enough. To be truly effective, the corporate culture itself must change to embrace environmental principles as fundamental elements of its mission and to begin to practice industrial ecology. To better define this concept I believe that business must strive to practice industrial ecology with an ultimate goal of sustainable development. I told Lee that I thought the bottoms-up approach was self-limiting. A revolution in the lab does not necessarily grant access to the core cabal of business decision makers, who are defining the principles and operational culture that the company will practice in the future. Bottoms-up might be sufficient to positively effect that which is happening now, within the existing corporate framework, but it does not drive the changing and recalibration of the institutional memory at the very core of a company's business approach.

I explained that, to get accepted into this seemingly mystical core decision-making process, an EMS must seek to gain recognition from the key reason for corporate existence, the customer. I also tried to show Lee that, to receive and maintain customer interest, an EMS would need to have credibility and acceptance outside the organization. For this reason, I insisted, an EMS program must be certified by an accredited third party registrar. Finally, I told him that, to be effective and credible, a EMS must follow the teachings of an internationally accepted EMS scheme, such as ISO 14001 or EMAS, to be truly accepted.

One of the most important changes in our environmental management philosophy requires that the EMS be focused on product as much as the traditional fixation on manufacturing process. All the preceding thrusts mean that, to practice what we preach, we must become part of the product realization process—and the earlier in the process the better. If a company constructs its EMS around the concepts just outlined, I think it will be well on the way toward reinventing itself to meet the economic and environmental challenges of tomorrow. It then has a chance to prove that integrating environmental thought into product deliberations is a sound, vital business strategy. Therefore, I believe my arguments for this holistic approach are the reason Lee chose to include Section III of this book.

The beauty of the ISO 14001 EMS standard is that it allows a company to set its environmental policy and future vision statement and, therefore its EMS, in a way that will allow for this new paradigm in approach. What follows in this section are some examples of how individual organizations are making the move from reactive to proactive management techniques. They are learning how to reinvent themselves and integrate their jobs to meet the demands of the future. A primary force accelerating these advances is the advent of the internationally accepted EMS standards based on continual improvement.

Huh? What's that? Oh, it's just the alarm clock. I guess I'll "get up" and go to my strategic planning meeting. I hope you enjoy this section of the book and take away from reading it a passion to change.

Part VI
DfE for Engineering Managers

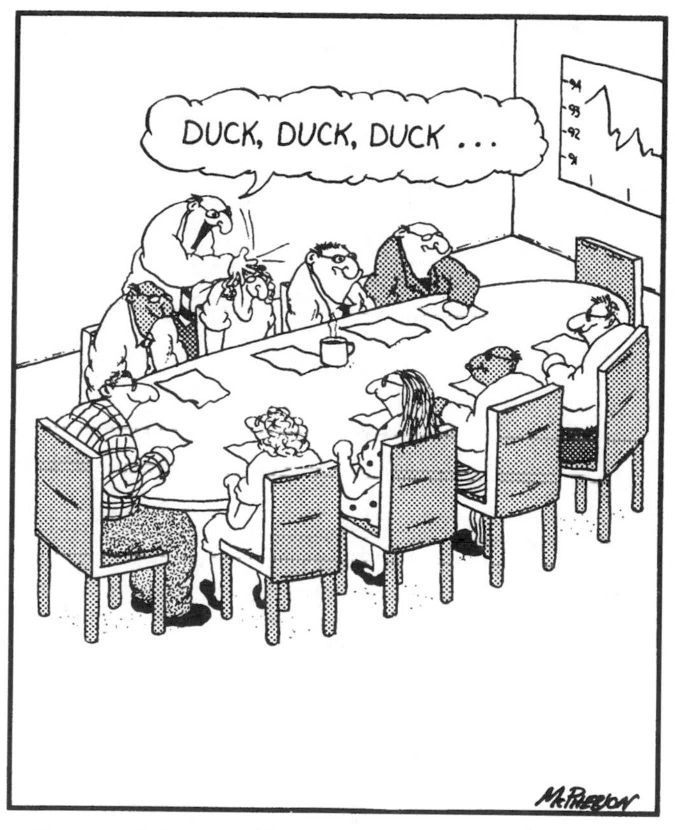

Successful executives know the importance of unwinding after a high-pressure meeting.

CHAPTER 16

DfE for Engineering Managers: Making It Count—DfE and the Bottom Line

JILL MATZKE

Apple Computer, Cupertino, CA

Introduction

It is easy to assume that designing products to be friendlier to the environment is a good thing. In a business, the question becomes much more complicated. Two primary reasons for this are that it often is not obvious which choices in product design are true environmental improvements, and if there is a greener choice to pursue, it often is unclear whether the choice offers any advantage to the firm seeking to adopt it.

From a pure business perspective, it is possible to ignore the true environmental value, at least in the short run. After all, if the green alternative offers business advantages, then it is worth doing in its own right. This sometimes happens with trendy or well-marketed "green" stunts. But, in the long run, any environmentally preferable product design must be a credible one, and so companies adopting DfE also must take care to be sure that they are making a positive difference.

These issues make the job of the engineering manager seeking to "green" a product quite difficult. And this complexity must be managed while assuring that product performance, time to market, and price are not compromised. Although this holds considerable challenge, some ways to approach these problems can maximize the potential gain in both environmental performance and the corporate bottom line.

How Green Is My Product, Really?

As we find in everyday life when asked "Paper or plastic?" environmental preferences in a product often are difficult to assess. The difficulty comes in large part from the variety of ways that a product can affect the environment. This is accompanied by the need to consider all aspects of a product and the material used to make it, going back in the supply chain and forward through the complete life cycle of the product.

Generally, environmental impact is broken down into three types:

- *Use of limited or nonrenewable resources.* The very existence of a product implies that resources are used to make it. This means that some transformation of material has been made that may result in the material becoming unavailable for future generations. The best-known example of this is fossil fuel, which is associated with virtually every product on the basis of transportation alone.
- *Toxicity.* Transformation of material into new forms may either create substances that cause harm, as in the case of certain organic materials, or move toxic substances to places where they can do harm, as in the case of heavy metals.
- *Destruction of ecosystems.* The classic issue here is destruction of natural environments such as rain forests. It is important to remember here that the facilities used to manufacture a product involve this impact and, in fact, can represent one of the more serious aspects of environmental impact by a product.

Beyond these different types of impact is the problem of looking at the entire life cycle of a product. To do this accurately means going back all to way to the original mining operations that produced the raw metals, oil, and any ceramics or glass used to make product components. Similarly, the life cycle of the product moving from design and manufacturing into use and ultimate disposal also must be assessed.

Other parts of this book go into great detail on the means for evaluating these types of environmental impact. From such tools as life-cycle analysis or similar methods, it is possible to come up with some sense of what is environmentally better. However, looking at these models, two things are clear. First, they entail value judgments. For example, a liquid crystal display (LCD) offers greater energy efficiency than a cathode ray tube (CRT) device. However, this benefit may be offset by the toxicity of the mercury and other chemicals that make up the LCD device (of course, the CRT also has lead in its glass screen). The trade-off pits the environmental impact attributed to a watt of energy against that associated with a microgram of mercury. That is, the value of the resources used and harm done to create that watt of energy are being weighed against the harmful toxic effects from mercury. There is no explicit way to normalize these very different types of impact, so in taking on an assessment of alternatives, it is important to look at the judgments involved.

Perhaps the more obvious problem with such assessments is that they are expensive to perform on a product as complicated as most electronic products. Imagine all of the components of LCDs and CRTs, and all of the types of impact from resource use, toxicity, and ecosystem for these components. The expense of such analyses is apparent.

These problems have led many electronics firms to avoid such analyses altogether and instead rely on standards developed by third parties. Historically, the complexity of making environmental trade-offs has led such standards to take the form of government regulation. In fact, the management of the environment by government is moving swiftly into the territory of product design, through such actions as material bans (e.g., ozone depleting chemicals such as CFCs) and material handling requirements (e.g., hazardous material disposal or product take-back laws). However voluntary standards also are growing in popularity, as a tool of government as well as a tool for industry and other environmentally motivated groups. A brief discussion of these follows.

Legally Mandated DfE

While DfE often is seen as a largely voluntary activity, no engineering manager today can ignore the fact that legal requirements are creeping into the product design process. Governments throughout the world have recognized that the most effective means for improving the environment is to move away from regulating smokestacks and work upstream to change the way products are designed and manufactured. Some examples of where regulatory developments are likely to affect product design now and into the early 21st century include the following.

- Material bans and restrictions:
  Bans on lead, mercury, and other toxic metals.
  Bans on ozone depleting substances.
  Efforts to ban halogen-containing substances.
  Use of recyclable materials for containers and packaging.
  Restrictions on endocrine-disrupting substances.
- Product handling regulations:
  Manufacturer take-back laws for packaging, batteries, and products.
  Restrictions on movement of waste for recycling or disposal.
  Disposal bans, such as the banning of CRT disposal in landfills.
- Others:
  Product labeling requirements such as disposal warnings.
  Designation of numerous substances as toxic.
  Public disclosure requirements for wastes and toxic substances used.
  Carbon taxes associated with efforts to reduce global warming.

It is beyond the scope of this chapter to elaborate on all aspects of the emerging regulatory picture, but it is critical for all companies to keep a close watch on such developments to avoid missing a critical item that could force changes in a product at a point where it is expensive to do so or, worse, cause a company to be subject to legal action and negative public image as a result of simply not being aware of a requirement.

Ecolabels

Voluntary Standards for Design

The idea that product design is the origin of many types of environmental impact has led governments and others to develop a set of environmental design standards that, taken together, constitute what are called *ecolabels*. Generally, these are voluntary standards applied to a product and a label the firm may associate with the product for marketing purposes after verification of conformance to the standard either by the company itself or a third party.

The last ten years has seen a proliferation of ecolabeling programs throughout the United States, Europe, and more recently, Asia. Increasingly, these programs have targeted electronic products as a reaction to the growing importance of these products in our daily lives. Some of the more prominent programs are listed in Table 16–1. While these programs do not target every electronic product, their guidelines generally are transferable from one product to another, given the similarity in basic components that all electronic products share.

Industry Driven Standards

While ecolabel programs offer a convenient means to approach design for environment, disagreement has centered on the validity of some of these standards

TABLE 16–1 Examples of Ecolabel Programs with Standards for Electronic Products

PROGRAM	SPONSOR/APPLICABILITY	COMMENTS
Energy Star	U.S. government, also adopted by Japan and other countries and used as basis for other energy standards	Deals only with energy efficiency; one of the most widely recognized labels
Blue Angel	German government	Widely recognized in Europe and beyond; focus is on design for recyclability
Nordic Swan	Norwegian government	Recognized in Nordic countries; one of the most stringent standards
EU Ecolabel	European Union	Newer program intended to replace member state programs; so far it has not affected German, Nordic, Swiss, and other European programs
Green Seal	U.S. nongovernment organization	Few participants
TCO 92, 95, 99	Swedish labor organization	Office products only; widely adopted for video display terminals and similar devices; strong focus on worker safety features plus environmental attributes

as well as how they are applied. In some cases, the requirement for lengthy third-party verification has been a deterrent to companies in terms of time to market. And often the organization responsible for developing the standard lacks the technical knowledge to fully judge the feasibility of the standard. As a result, there are a few movements to develop industry-sponsored standards.

One example is the European Computer Manufacturer's Association (1997), which is developing a declaration standard for computers and other electronic products. Also, the International Standards Organization (ISO) is working on a standard for ecolabeling programs in an attempt to assure fair, valid standards.

Corporate Standards and Specific Problem-Solving Efforts

In adopting standards, companies are accepting both the scientific evaluation and the judgment of the standards organization, even though they may not fully agree with them. Some firms have taken the approach of developing their own standard as part of a corporate commitment to the environment.

In addition, many have focused on making design changes in specific areas where a known environmental problem exists. Such efforts often are associated with some of the more innovative aspects of DfE. Examples include design of product enclosures for recycling, replacements for lead use in PWB solder, replacements for mercury-containing backlights in LCDs, and less toxic batteries.

Whether following a standard or innovating on its own, the assumption being made by companies here is that design for environment is better, or at least will be perceived as better and thus offer some benefit to the firm adopting it. More often than not, this benefit is not so obvious.

What Green Alternatives Are Worth the Investment?

Firms seeking to invest in environmental improvements in their products also must ensure that these investments will meet the needs of corporate shareholders in some way. If there is no connection between a green design and the bottom line, such design efforts will fail in the long run. Thinking about the ways that product features are linked to the bottom line means that an environmentally preferable design must either decrease the cost or risk to the firm in producing the product or increase the value of the product in the eyes of the customer. There are several ways in which DfE meets these objectives, although some are far less certain than others.

Decreased Costs and Risks

While the potential for a green design to result in increased product sales or profit margins may be tenuous, the benefit of lower cost is easy to see. Admittedly, applying DfE principles could result in higher, not lower, product cost, as more expensive materials or more features (e.g., energy-saving modes) are added. Still, some designs offer savings, not only in product cost-of-goods, but in the total life-cycle cost of the product as well.

Some examples of where a product can be made more cheaply by DfE are

- *Design for recycling and design for manufacturing are compatible.* Products designed to be recycled often are easier to make and service, in addition to being more cost effective to handle at end of life. For example, recycle-friendly snap-fit parts require fewer fasteners and are quicker to assemble, reducing manufacturing costs.
- *Dematerialization saves in two ways.* Using less material means less material paid for to make a product. If the mass or volume reductions are substantial, significant savings may emerge in transportation and handling costs as well.
- *Design for recyclability leads to fewer types of materials and common parts.* The discounts from increased purchase lot size can yield significant cost advantages in some cases.
- *Reduction of toxic components is cost effective.* Reduction of toxic components means that, when the product is disposed of at the end of its service life, the user may not be subject to the increased costs associated with hazardous waste handling.
- *Manufacturing efficiency can be gained by careful choice of specification tolerances.* These practices can assure that scrap is minimized without compromising quality.
- *Improved energy efficiency results not only in energy cost savings but also in lower heat production.* This can reduce the need for expensive cooling fans in the product and lower cooling costs for the user.

Note that some of cost savings here are not attributable to the manufacturer but to the service provider or customer. While this sort of savings is valid in terms of lower cost of ownership, it may be more difficult to attach a corporate benefit to the product design. However, as governments and customers demand that producers take responsibility for products throughout their useful life, more of these savings will come back directly to the bottom line. Those companies with the forethought to design with this in mind may reap the benefits later on.

Some DfE endeavors are founded on the prediction that future costs or risk of regulatory impact may affect a company's future performance. For example, some countries are seeking to ban lead in products and so a firm with access to lead-free manufacturing technology will be at an advantage if such laws come into wide adoption. Similarly, future liability owing to product safety or waste disposal may be mitigated if design alternatives take this into account. Because environmental issues are complex and require that the needs of many parties be considered, environmental performance increasingly will be the target of regulatory authorities throughout the world, as well as that of insurance and financial institutions who have a stake in a company's future performance.

Cost savings and risk reduction always are desirable, but these factors alone are not enough to drive the level of environmental improvement being pursued today by electronics firms. More critical is the ability of a green product to enhance revenues and profit margins through increased customer value.

Increased Customer Value

Increased customer value means that either the customer will pay a premium for the green product or will give preference to that product, other things being equal. Market research in this area suggests that some customers say they are willing to pay extra for green products, but most often, they are willing to give preference among equivalent products (Environmental Research Associates, 1998). This, of course, assumes that the greenness of the product is apparent to the buyer—something that requires both a clear environmental message and appropriate exploitation of that message through marketing.

Earlier, the adoption of standards or ecolabels was described as a common approach to managing green design. In addition to simplifying the process of identifying and validating green alternatives, these standards offer the credibility of third-party endorsement and are more easily recognized by customers. In some cases, consumers give these standards preference and thus firms who adopt them have the edge when purchasing decisions are made. For example, the U.S. federal government is mandated to purchase Energy-Star-compliant office equipment and some parts of the German government prefer Blue-Angel-labeled equipment.

Still the very nature of standards is that they can be adopted by many firms, and this limits the potential competitive advantage. It follows that nearly all major computer manufacturers offer Energy-Star- and Blue-Angel-labeled products.

Adding to the demand for ecolabels are specific customer demands for such attributes as energy efficiency or recyclability, which have relatively obvious user benefits. Governments throughout the world, large institutions, and private corporations are among the customers who most often include specific environmental requirements in their purchase criteria, and the firms that understand these needs and are prepared to address them can be at significant advantage.

Finally, many investments in green design are made with the hope that enhanced brand image will result. This type of investment has been more common in such industries as energy, petrochemicals, and automobiles but is also the reason "of last resort" when investment in doing good simply feels like the right thing to do. While this benefit may be the least quantifiable, it is surprising how many corporate environmental efforts, including design for environment, are founded primarily on this basis.

Beyond Making a "Better Box"— Using DfE to Rethink Entire Products and Services

While redesigning products is the major focus of this book, it is worth mentioning that redesign of business processes is an important strategy being explored by electronics firms. For example, some companies have invested in development of take-back infrastructures, betting on the trend toward producer responsibility and that having such infrastructure will provide competitive advantages. There also are other forms of what is termed *reverse logistics*, where companies seek to find customers for materials that they produce as a by-product of their operations. One example is the recycling of plastic case materials for automobile parts.

The assumptions made so far in this discussion are that we are taking a given product and either redesigning or substituting parts of it to reduce its environmental impact or offering services to handle the wastes produced during the life of the product. A much more fundamental approach is to go back to the core features and benefits that a product is meant to provide and totally rethink how those benefits might be delivered in a far more environmentally conscious way. This perhaps is the most risky yet most potentially profitable approach to design for environment, and few firms have ventured into this arena. One very modest example of this is leasing versus purchase as a business model. Firms that lease products rather than sell them are motivated to maximize the service provided at minimum product cost. They also are motivated to reduce end-of-life costs through better up-front design, since they will endure all life cycle costs for the product.

Finally, there is the environmental impact of a product as it performs its functions in the larger scheme of society as a whole. Electronic products, perhaps more than any other class of products in the late 20th century, have altered the lives of everyone from office workers in North America to cell-phone users in remote locales in developing nations. In the process of changing our lives, electronic products produce ancillary types of environmental impact that can be either positive or negative. For example, computers held the promise of the "paperless office" and yet they've contributed more to the increased use of paper than its elimination so far. The recent trend toward electronic telecommunication holds the promise of reducing transportation as people have less need to travel to the office or to faraway destinations to perform the functions of daily life.

All these aspects of electronic products hold vast opportunities in designing a better future (Day, 1998). While few if any electronics companies have taken DfE to the point of redefining their business on the basis of environmental performance, such efforts may offer the most dramatic returns in the future and undoubtedly are being explored by progressive firms concerned about their long-term success.

References

Day, Robert M. (World Resources Institute). "Beyond Eco-Efficiency: Sustainability as a Driver for Innovation." At http://www.wri.org/wri/meb/sei/beyond.html, March 1998.

Environmental Research Associates, Inc. *The Environmental Report* 15 (1998).

European Computer Manufacturer's Association. "Declaration of the Environmental Aspects of Computer Products." Technical report 70, 1997.

CHAPTER 17

Making It Happen—DfE Implementation

JILL MATZKE

Apple Computer, Cupertino, CA

While much of this book deals with strategic and technological choices in the pursuit of design for environment, the management of DfE within the complex organizations of most companies offers its own challenges. For DfE to be successful, it must be accomplished without compromising core business imperatives that characterize the electronics industry: performance, time to market, and cost. Combine this with the extensive reach of DfE into nearly every facet of the organization, and the management complexity is apparent.

Organizing Around DfE

Most firms do not have the luxury of forming an "environmental business unit," and it's probably a good thing they don't. For DfE to be effectively practiced, it should be integrated into existing business processes and, ideally, adopted by everyone in his or her daily work. Still, specialized knowledge must be acquired and used for this new discipline and so, in practice, DfE often is the domain of a few professionals who seek to affect the design process as effectively as they can.

While a growing number of firms are employing DfE specialists, most still rely on more traditional environmental specialists or engineers who take on this additional role. Frequently, the Environmental Health and Safety (EH&S) function, which historically handled such tasks as hazardous waste management and worker safety, is seen as the best source of specialized information on environmental regulations, industry standards, and voluntary labeling programs affecting product design. However, these folks generally are not accustomed to working within the R&D process and so are in no position to accomplish DfE as effectively as they could.

Further, successful DfE also must involve corporate sales and marketing, both in the process of evaluating the business value in pursuing green alternatives and in promoting such features once they are achieved.

Integrating DfE into the Product Development Process

In developing new products, most companies use some variation on a typical product design process (Figure 17–1), where product features are defined, the design work occurs, and the product is tested against these features then goes into production.

Theoretically, DfE goals can be achieved simply by communicating the environmental performance needed during the conceptual phases of the project and checking along the way until the product is introduced to the marketplace. In practice, however, this is not nearly enough. First, the organizational structure of many electronics manufacturers is fast changing and quite informal. Second, the long list of environmental criteria for any given product may be too extensive to be evaluated by everyone affected. Equally important is that many product attributes are determined outside the core R&D process for a given product. For example,

- Long-term supplier contracts dictate materials choices throughout product lines.
- Common part policies for cost reduction determine many components.
- Design leverage means most products are evolutionary, based on previous designs.
- Core technology, product architecture, and industrial design decisions often precede product concepts.

Failure to address the issues that operate outside the core design and development process increases the cost and decreases the chances for success in achieving environmental product goals.

Figure 17–2 illustrates a more complete scenario of the practical considerations in implementing DfE. Note that the players include everyone in departments from sales and marketing to procurement and manufacturing and that the environmental specialist or designated expert takes action every step along the way.

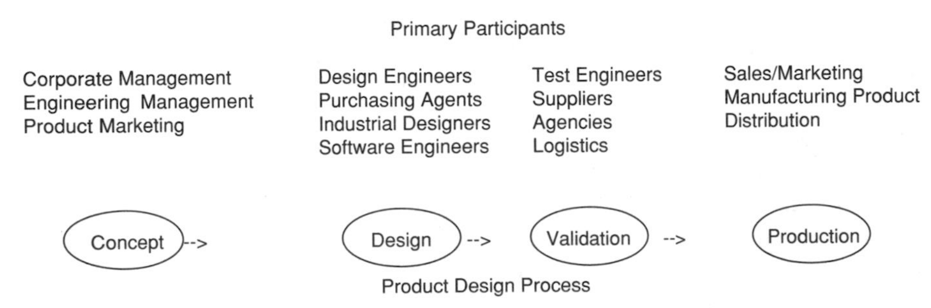

FIGURE 17–1 Basic product development process typical of an electronics firm.

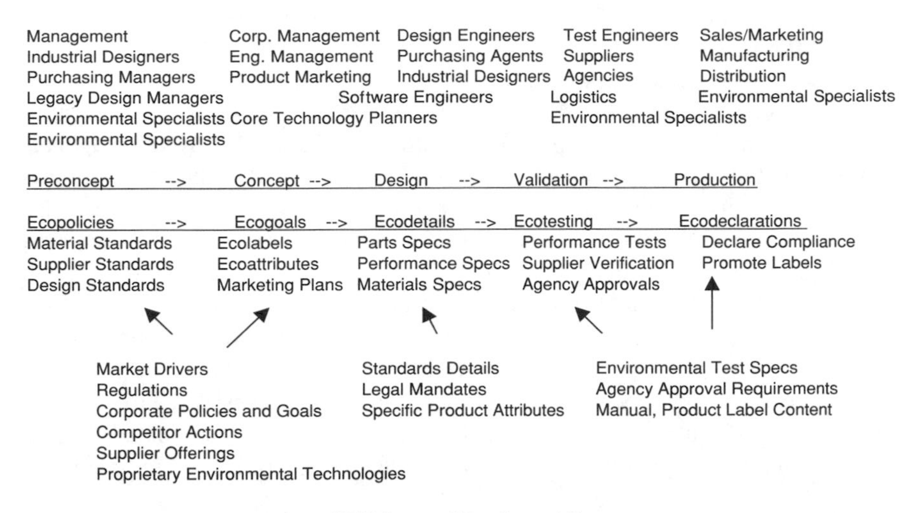

FIGURE 17–2 Practical view of the product development process and its participants, showing the ties to DfE drivers and processes (Source: Adapted from Matzke, Chew, and Wu, 1998).

The complexity of this picture illustrates both the management challenges in executing on DfE and the many activities that must be integrated into the design process. The decisions of all the various participants must be aligned to further the product environmental goals. That said, it also should be acknowledged that in this complexity is some strength, as some players may be in a unique position to contribute to DfE where the specialists cannot. For instance, a marketing manager may be aware of an environmental product feature being adopted by a competitor. Or a purchasing manager may become aware of a new, greener material or know when green alternatives move from the theoretical to the practical in terms of the supply chain. And software engineers may be involved in efforts to develop power management systems that can be leveraged for greater energy efficiency.

Additional resources for the DfE effort lie beyond the strict organizational lines of the electronics firm. Such partners as suppliers, product recyclers, and customers offer unique information on new developments, legal or sales requirements, and even competitor's offerings.

Practical Information Management for DfE

Looking at the large number of players and business processes that must be accommodated in DfE, the management challenge is obvious. And, because DfE information comes from many sources, it is impractical to expect all players to sort through the volumes of regulations, standards, and design alternatives in support of the DfE effort. These factors place a premium on information management as a tool in developing an effective DfE system. Information must be managed in a way that is compatible with the needs of all decision makers, expressed in actionable terms that can be applied directly in their work.

At Apple Computer (Matzke et al., 1998), a database tool was developed to manage this complexity. Using this tool, customized input can be given to suppliers, procurement managers, engineers, marketing managers, and technical specialists. And, to support potential innovation on the part of any player, the system also has a direct tie between technical specifications and the environmental goals they support. But perhaps the most useful aspect of the system is that it sorts through overlapping regulations and standards to give clear direction on product attributes (Figure 17–3). For example, at least four energy efficiency standards can apply to a computer, each of which has unique aspects. A decision (shown as a corporate goal) must be made as to which standards will be supported, and this decision must be translated into an actionable product specification. At Apple, over 100 such specifications are included in this system to cover all of the products and attributes that are part of its DfE program.

Other Management System Changes to Drive Environmental Improvement

Beyond the adaptation of DfE activities to fit the idiosyncrasies of an organization, it is possible to improve the outcome of DfE through organizational efforts that can bring more effective decision making and execution.

Making DfE Specialists Core Members of the Development Team

In many electronics firms, the folks in the organization that may be in the best position to track the sorts of standards, regulations, and evaluation techniques for DfE are located well outside the engineering groups. For example, a common struc-

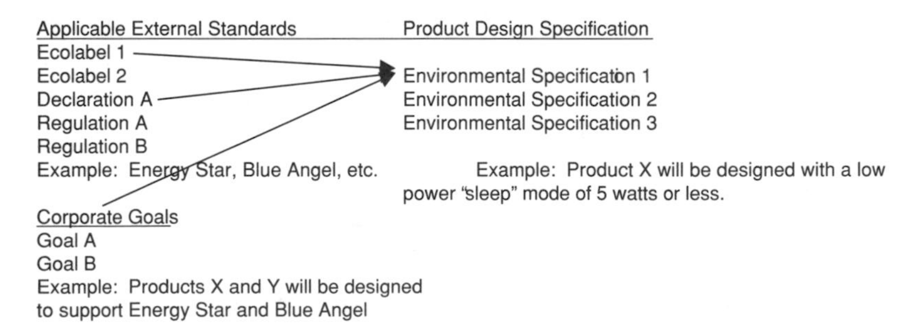

FIGURE 17–3 Use of a database tool to support DfE efforts as applied to theoretical product X at Apple Computer (Source: Matzke et al., 1998).

ture puts environmental health and safety professionals in the facilities organization, in keeping with their traditional role in managing facility-generated wastes and worker safety issues. More recently, the trend has been to either relocate certain EH&S specialists into the R&D world in some way or to hire environmental professionals specifically for DfE within the engineering department.

Whichever alternative is chosen, the individual charged with assuring that DfE goals are developed and achieved must be tightly integrated into the development process to assure that all aspects of product decision making are made with DfE at the table.

Make the Business Case

Often, green design efforts are viewed as a nonessential luxury, something nice to do if the resources can be spared. No corporate function will succeed for long on this basis, especially in the increasingly competitive electronics industry. As described elsewhere in this book, the business case for DfE can be every bit as compelling as other product features and must be treated in the same manner, using market research, cost-benefit analysis, and traditional financial decision-making tools such as internal rates of return or return on investment. Given that many design decisions in electronics firms are made with little or no business analysis, the DfE practitioner who comes to the table armed with a solid business case will build credibility and support for both current and future efforts.

Leveraging the Other DfXs

Individuals working to green the product development process often may find their needs superseded by other considerations, especially as cost and time-to-market pressures grow. For example, if there is a choice between investing engineering resources in a green alternative (say, energy efficiency) and adding an additional product feature, the new feature often wins. But DfE is one of many DfXs, where downstream issues are addressed as early as possible through concurrent engineering processes. So, while the case for DfE alone may not be enough to sway the organization into adopting an environmentally desirable change, often others would benefit as well. Designs that support recyclability and product longevity through upgrade also are easier to build and service, for example. The DfE practitioner who recognizes and exploits these synergies will have greater success in seeing green designs adopted.

Internal Evangelism

In line with the need to understand environmental impact is the need to communicate such information internally. Most folks want to feel that they are doing what they can to help the environment. For example, engineers who hear how many barrels of oil went into the production, distribution, and use of their product may be more inclined to support initiatives aimed at reducing product energy consumption.

By ensuring that everyone in the organization understands the environmental impact of the firm and what is being done or could be done to minimize this impact, the circle of support for DfE activities will grow and innovative ideas may come forward from unexpected places.

Generating a Green Corporate Culture

Few firms today have made a wholesale commitment to the environment as a core value. This is understandable, given that society as a whole has not yet gotten to the point where environmental considerations are integrated into many decisions. However, with increasing focus on global environmental issues and increasing concern on the part of consumers, this is likely to change in the future (Hawken, 1993). As a result, corporations that lag behind society in greening their culture will suffer increasingly negative consequences. Steps can be taken to start the process of change in preparation for this future possibility.

Adapt Cost Accounting Systems to Facilitate DfE Decisions

As described in more detail elsewhere in this book, accounting systems in companies rarely take into account the full fiscal impact of many corporate decisions. For the environment, design decisions may lead to unnecessary waste or avoidable costs as the product cycle moves into production and distribution to the customer. For example, a design specification may lead to increased scrap as parts that fail to meet the spec are discarded. While such specifications often are crucial to maintaining the quality of the product, they may be set without consideration of the waste costs they produce.

In addition to the internalized costs associated with the environmental impact of a product are the external costs borne by the sales and distribution channel and customers through the life cycle of the product. Such costs are not as easily integrated into corporate decision making, but the need for this will increase as producer responsibility (product take-back) laws grow in number.

Walk the Talk— Understand the Ecoimpact of Your Own Operations

While DfE can be a critical driver for environmental improvements in a firm, it commonly is practiced in isolation from other environmental issues associated with a company's products and operations. If efforts are made to green products while ignoring obvious corporate environmental impact (even that as simple as leaving on lights and computer screens continuously), a mixed message is sent. Next, the sense of corporate commitment fades, taking with it the inspiration for employees to support DfE through adherence to principles and standards as well as innovation.

Measure and Publicly Communicate Environmental Progress

Internal communication and evangelism efforts for DfE will hold the most promise if they are backed up by both qualitative facts and quantitative measures that describe a firm's environmental progress. Everyone loves data, but qualitative (or semi-quantitative) facts should not be ignored, because often the cost of obtaining data on environmental impact is prohibitive and sometimes a good story does the best communications job.

There is nothing like public disclosure to focus the discipline of the firm on an issue like the environment. Conversely, little benefit is accrued to a firm in making environmental improvements unless these are communicated to corporate stakeholders. Companies increasingly are participating in public communication of environmental performance through such activities as publishing annual environmental reports, maintaining public environmental Web sites, responding to surveys, and participating in partnerships with environmentally oriented groups (Krut, 1997). These efforts so far have dealt almost exclusively with the traditional end-of-pipe environmental impact. As DfE takes its place at the forefront of environmental management, such efforts also must be prominently communicated.

Design for environment appears to be a business process that is here to stay in the electronics industry. While most firms have made a commitment to some form of design for the environment, only those firms that build the capability to execute on DfE will be able to capitalize on its benefits.

References

Hawken, Paul. *The Ecology of Commerce: A Declaration of Sustainability.* New York: HarperCollins Publishers, 1993.

Krut, Riva. "Sustainable Industrial Development: A Benchmark Evaluation of Public Environmental Policies and Reporting in the Electronics Industry." Washington, DC: EPA Office of Policy Planning and Evaluation, Industry Strategies Division, November 1997.

Matkze, Judy, Corky Chew, and Tse-Sung Wu. "A Simple Tool to Facilitate Design for the Environment at Apple Computer." Proceedings of the IEEE Conference on Electronics and the Environment, Chicago, May 1998.

CHAPTER **18**

Getting the Math Right: Accurate Costing Through Product Life Cycles

KELLY WEINSCHENK
Corbet Consulting

The world we have created today as a result of our thinking thus far has problems which cannot be solved by thinking the way we did when we created them.

—*Albert Einstein*

Introduction

Design has more influence on total cost than any other aspect of product creation. Companies now are realizing that "green" features should be incorporated during design stages for maximum cost effectiveness. However, these added eco-characteristics often are perceived as too expensive. This is largely a misperception, generated because few firms properly account for the long-term costs and benefits of their products.

As a result, environmental progress is being suboptimized by imperfect quantitative analysis, leading to unclaimed opportunities for enhanced profitability.

Of course, companies believe they are tracing the costs correctly; but the changing nature of inputs to production—as well as changing regulatory parameters—have drained the old system of its ability to "get the math right." If companies were better at tracking costs, they probably would design for the longer run and find it more profitable, too. As the saying goes, "What gets measured gets managed."

This is particularly true for electronics firms, where quarterly results might reflect an entire product generation. Such three-month thrusts leave little time or inclination for exploring various cost-capturing tools like life-cycle- and activity-based costing. It is a prime example of "the urgent versus the important." Sadly, the urgent usually wins.

The emergence of electronic waste take-back regulation in Europe and Asia, and now even in the United States, is forcing firms to take a longer-term perspective in costing strategies. Rather than disappearing from the balance sheets at the point of sale, many products will now be returned to the OEM after the consumer is finished with them.

Current accounting and financial models disregard the serious cost ramifications of these policy and preference shifts. They will demand a broader and more inclusive costing analysis than was required in pre-take-back days. This chapter can help prepare you for that eventuality.

Background

The term *design for environment* (DfE), though not distinctly defined, is an important step in controlling environmental impact. On its own, however, DfE fails to incorporate common business considerations, a blind spot that limits its potential acceptance and power within companies. To sell a concept internally, it is best to use terms and ideas that managers already understand. While mainstream corporate decision makers often do not relate well to environmental issues overall or the more ephemeral ideas behind DfE, they do understand accounting and cost reduction. To get their attention, state the benefits of green design in terms of money; cash flow, bottom line. Those concepts "hit 'em where they live, " giving you an opportunity to uncover hidden costs—including environmental costs—by applying broadly accepted business tools, using money as the primary unit of measure.

To be really successful, environmentally dedicated concepts need to be integrated with other business concepts, which make them valuable to business managers. By looking at environmental activities from a business perspective, environmental professionals can move from compliance to strategic thinking; taking their department from cost to a center to a value-added performer within the company.

Basically, cost should become a proxy for environmental performance. The more you are spending on things like hazardous disposal, training, and personal protective equipment, for example, the more you probably are polluting.

Life-cycle costing and activity-based thinking, as introduced here, provide designers tools and information they've never had before. Together, they offer environmental managers greater insight to business concepts and provide business managers greater understanding of real environmental—and other—costs. Ultimately, getting the math right offers companies options for greatly improved decision making at each stage of product existence, not just the end of the line.

Three basic cost confinement ideas are explored here: life-cycle costing, product-function expandability, and activity-based thinking.[1] Each should be considered as early as the product design stage. Each concept is important in understanding and maximizing product value, not just through one product "incarnation" but through many. Using these tools, designers should be able to more clearly assess the financial benefits of their environmental enhancements. This will make "selling" the ideas within the company far more palatable and understandable.

Life-cycle costing incorporates the costs and benefits of retrieving and perhaps recycling a product. In the life-cycle perspective, costs do not "begin" at the point of raw materials purchase nor do they "end" when the product is shipped off the premises. It is based, as the name implies, on a cycle. Therefore, by starting the process at a particular point—R & D, for example—decision makers ultimately are led back to that starting point with a greater knowledge of design needs and the like, based on having assessed a continuum that now includes reuse, recycling, or waste.

Product expandability, the partner concept to life-cycle costing, can demonstrate the potential profits from expanding the model beyond a product's typical useful lifespan and application. Xerox has successfully developed this way of thinking and created "blended unit manufacturing costs" that reflect the true costs to the firm of a product or part throughout its many manifestations.

Activity-based thinking carries the broad-based concepts of the life cycle and takes them deeper. This means applying the costs of manufacturing, distributing, and such activities directly to the products produced. It sounds reasonable, but it is not what usually happens in modern accounting.

Current accounting practices apply the standard measuring inputs of labor, raw materials, and "overhead." But cost parameters have changed substantially since this type of accounting was developed. That's why numbers are misleading, particularly when it comes to "environmental" costs. Often charges for hazardous waste disposal and other miscellaneous environmental costs are relegated to—and lost in—"overhead." Thus hidden, they remain unmanaged. Activity-based thinking brings those costs to light.

For example, assume a firm produces 1,000 widgets annually—500 blue widgets and 500 gold widgets. In this case, it might automatically divide overhead in a 50/50 ratio. If, however, the gold widgets require much more energy to produce, create more toxic waste, and impose a need for greater regulatory governance, it is not likely that their true share of overhead is just 50%. In fact, it is quite likely that the blue widgets are inadvertently subsidizing the gold widgets. This is why it is so important that costs be applied to the products according to the activities each generates.

Life-Cycle Costing

Life-cycle costing is the practice of establishing costs of a product over its entire existence. Given new regulatory requirements for electronic waste take-back, costs may now extend to include old product retrieval and, perhaps, to disposal, recycling, or reuse. Now that items are beginning to come back to the maker, either by law or customer preference, a new dimension is added to the balance sheet.

This new environment requires that a more comprehensive inventory of costs should be incorporated into the decision-making process. In addition to research and development, things like product design, storage, inspection and maintenance, administrative and program management, disposal, insurance, potential clean-up, and potential liability costs related to environmental impact should be included in a project's total cost assessment

Life-cycle costing requires an expanded model of product materialization capabilities, as well. As an example, Figure 18–1 shows how an electronic good is

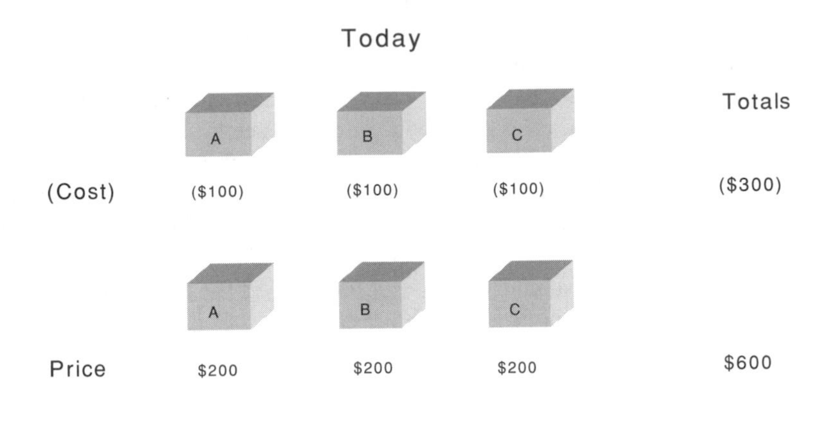

FIGURE 18–1 Scenario A: Doing business using traditional accounting practices.

produced at a cost of $100, and sold for $200, the present value of the profits is $100. Most managers would be relatively pleased with those margins. Before electronic waste take-back laws, the product life cycle went like this: make, sell, then never have to see the product again. The firm will realize the financial benefits of its product once and only once. Since the product is not designed to "come back," no accounting or logistics systems deal with the product even if it is returned.

As regulations or consumer preferences start to require product take-back, the entire profitability equation changes. Depending on financial preparatory work, it could change for the worse or the better.

To understand this changing environment, let's contrast the following scenarios: Scenario A, selling a product without designed-in longevity, and Scenario B, selling a product with the idea that it will come back one day.

With a traditional accounting structure (Scenario A), a product makes a single pass from the manufacturer to the consumer, to the landfill. Here, the prospect of taking back products appears to be a liability rather than an asset.

Scenario B illustrates the advent of two important life-cycle considerations: designed-in longevity and tracking the costs over more than a single materialization. In this case, the product has been planned with the intent to reuse it.[2] For the sake of illustration and argument, the new manufacturing cost has been increased by 10% over the original cost. This could be due to better materials or design improvements that provide the product with worth to the manufacturer on its return. After take-back and reconditioning, it will have a second (or third) revenue potential when it is resold or leased.

As illustrated in Figure 18–2, the first incarnation sales show a slightly decreased profit, from $100 per unit to $90 per unit. It will not necessarily be the case that environmental upgrades or life-cycle considerations will yield a higher-priced product. Although it is often just the opposite case, it is good to envision a

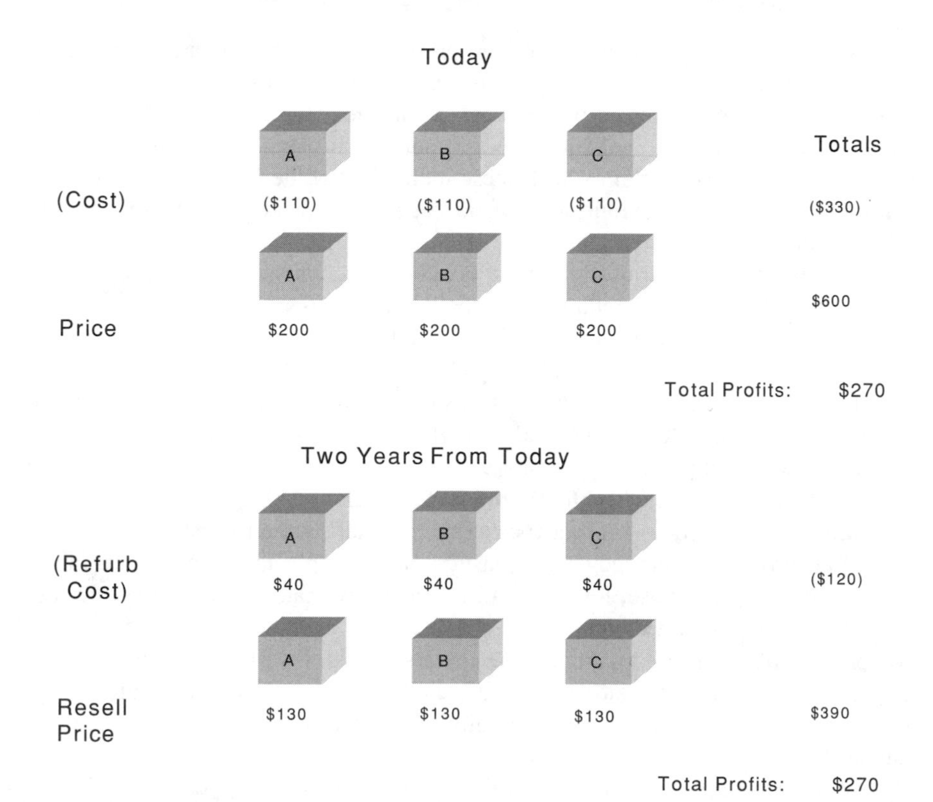

FIGURE 18–2 Scenario B: Doing business using life-cycle accounting and extended product life design practices.

conservative scenario by assuming some additional cost to lengthen the scope of the design:

Profits from a single-use life cycle:	$300
Combined first and second sales profits:	$540

When the customer is finished with the product and it is time for the company to retake it, it is assumed that the refurbishing costs, including storage and retrieval, will be $40. Of course, the original sales price and the price of the used good are determined by the marketplace, with the resell price assumed to be less than the new product. We can estimate a reasonable price for a reconditioned product at 65% of the original cost, $130.

Basically, by selling the same or a similar product twice,[3] the profits grow by $240, from $300 to $540. In a more detailed analysis, we would certainly incorporate a discount rate, say 10% to account for the time value of money during the two years prior to refurbishing and reselling the products.[4] A net present value (NPV) for the second scenario shows that profits in today's dollars would still be $488.70, or 62.9% greater than in a predesign, pre-take-back scenario.

When undertaking analyses like these, it is important to look at the range possibilities: conduct sensitivity analyses. In the case here, even if the refurbishing costs were increased and the resale prices were diminished, the net present value still would be positive in most realistic cases. Although you won't be able to predict all future costs with exact certainty with these methods, you definitely will be able to gain more insight and proximity than if no costs were tracked throughout the life cycle of a given product.

The extended scenario offers more qualitative benefits. Although they do not add up quite so neatly as dollars, they should not be disregarded. For example, intrinsic recyclability may be a prerequisite to selling a product in certain countries. Thus, by designing in broader terms, entry to potentially restricted markets might be gained. Perhaps using a certain type of easily recyclable plastic,[5] although more expensive than others to purchase, also might enable sales in certain geographic regions that were not previously possible.

Another less tangible benefit of product life-cycle thinking is the possibility of using the first generation of a product as a raw material source for the second generation of the product. Using recyclable plastic as an example again, the effects might include reduced energy use, less demand for new raw material, and therefore less pollution. This could be valuable in cost terms, as well as providing a more positive, environmentally proactive image to stakeholders watching corporate environmental performance. Although a positive image is a challenging variable to measure, a negative image can be—and has been—readily measured in terms of stock price, for instance.[6]

Myriad examples of unexpected life-cycle benefits can appear as well. One such benefit occurred in a camera company. Responding to European legislation on packaging reduction, the firm fortified the actual camera. This was done to accommodate a less protective package, but the results went beyond packaging. Because the camera body was strengthened, it was brought in less frequently for warranty repairs. So, by looking at the entire life of the product (rather than treating packaging as one completely separate aspect and product design as another), the manufacturer was able to achieve several benefits: (1) maintaining the possibility of selling into the European market, (2) reducing packaging costs, and (3) limiting warranty repair costs. Had the firm not kept close watch over its life-cycle costs, it would not have recognized this and perhaps erroneously believed that the extra material required for the improved camera design was not worth the cost.

In general, by thinking in a life-cycle framework, managers can benefit by gaining information to help produce the following:

- Tools for improved environmental design choices.
- Identification of cross-media shifts (such as solid waste incineration costs).
- Screens for new product and process development.
- Fact-based assessments of investment options and trade-offs.
- Improved understanding of competitive assets and liabilities.

Product Expandability

There is a companion benefit to implementing life-cycle tracking: One name for it is *product expandability.* When companies start paying attention to their product life cycles, they actually can create value in the end-of-life (EOL) pieces. In one case, managers of an equipment manufacturer had been frustrated by the lost revenue and quality control issues that arose because their products were being refurbished and serviced by unauthorized third parties. Spurred by European environmental regulations and a few demanding U.S. customers, the company initiated a take-back program. Having reclaimed its EOL products, it suddenly had the "ingredients" to sell used products to a different realm of customer, thus expanding its market.

Much to its surprise, the firm found the margins on the used products were much higher than for new products; and the third parties did not—as it had feared—cannibalize its new goods market. With a larger inventory of parts, it also found it was better able to service its contract maintenance customers. Both benefits were unexpected side effects of their electronic waste take-back policy. The company's previous accounting practices had led it to believe this practice would not be profitable.

Extending the life—or lives—of a product, therefore, requires much bigger thinking than in earlier days. The previous Xerox example of "blended unit manufacturing costs" illustrates that Xerox had the opportunity to use parts creatively: as service parts, as raw materials for new products, and so forth.

Another very well-known electronics company, in fact, has done this in Europe. It recycled keyboards by using old units as the polymer source for new ones, with no decrease in quality, just a decrease in cost. Before it could use recycled plastic, however, it had to overcome prejudices of recycled quality.[7] It also had to think of product possibilities in ways it never had before.

Opportunities for product expandability are numerous, almost unlimited. For instance, who is to say that a panel of one product could not be designed to be completely compatible with another, non-functionally related product? If established during the design stages, it is not inconceivable that a recycling scenario like the following could happen.

Activity-Based Thinking

In addition to tracking life-cycle costs, expenses should be applied internally to the manufacturing process (in other words, go wide and deep). Many firms have undertaken the detail-intensive process called *activity-based costing* (ABC) to highlight and decouple overhead costs.

ABC can be a valuable process, but its thorough application can also be time consuming and burdensome. For this reason, it is often better to apply costs in a more general, less detailed manner. We refer to this modified version as *activity-based thinking*. (At this point it is healthy to invoke the ABC adage, "Closeness is better than precision.")

In its most simple terms, activity-based thinking applies production costs to the activities that go into making a product. The activities create the costs. After establishing this connection, activities are aligned to their output. The ultimate cost of each activity then can be designated through the output figures. The two main tenets behind activity-based costing or thinking can be broadly described as (1) identifying activities and their relative costs and (2) assessing those activities through cost drivers.[8]

Activity-based thinking is an excellent step toward accounting for true production costs. Like traditional accounting, it is truncated in terms of time and location and does not incorporate adequate cross-functionality. For example, when the price of a product is determined, the price makers seldom reach back into R&D costs or forward into environmental liabilities or disposal costs. To truly understand costs, managers need to adopt a fuller costing perspective, both in time and location.

This is a very different concept from conventional accounting, which evenly divides overhead costs among all products, regardless of their demand on a company's resources. This was relatively accurate when the majority of overhead costs actually were labor and raw materials. Modern manufacturing practices have changed costs such that labor often is a much smaller fraction, leaving factors such as design, marketing, and waste disposal to consume a greater proportion. These variations in resource consumption go largely unnoticed in traditional accounting.

Not only does traditional accounting incorrectly assign costs to products, it also captures primarily historical rather than current inventory information. This often is not the most important information to have while planning strategically for international competition.

Activity-based thinking specifies product activities in ways that can help managers understand not only which activities place the highest demands on corporate resources but also why the resources are used. It further helps identify value-added versus non-value-added activities to better eliminate waste. Initially, ABC was not intended to uncover environmental costs, but by bringing to light the individual cost contributors, it becomes obvious that many "environmental" costs have gone unaccounted for.

Some benefits of activity-based thinking are shown in the following example. A manufacturer, Seemore Company, produces one product (magnifying glasses) in two finishes (gilded and natural). Seemore makes 10,000 units of each magnifying glass per run. Because they are created in equal volumes, overhead costs are distributed evenly.

As you can see in Tables 18–1 and 18–2, for the golden magnifying glass, the per-piece profit is $3.77, according to traditional accounting methodology. The natural finished glasses seem to offer profits of only $0.73, so the management had been considering ceasing production.

Employing activity-based costing, however, it was able to reveal the hidden costs obscured in traditional overhead expenses. The finish on the gold magnifying glasses requires special plating, and because it can not be soldered together (due to

TABLE 18–1 Gilded Magnifying Glass: Traditional Costing versus Activity-Based Costing

	Traditional Costing	ABC
Raw materials	$15.00	$15.00
Direct labor	$10.50	$10.50
General overhead	$25.20	$25.20
Environmental overhead	$5.53	$10.74
Cost	$56.23	$61.44
Price	$60.00	$60.00
Profit/loss [price – cost]	$ 3.77	($1.44)

the finish), it requires specialty adhesives. Therefore, the gold magnifying glasses require the following extra costs:

- Hazardous waste disposal: solvents and toxic adhesives.
- Storage permits for hazardous substances.
- Storage space for hazardous substances.
- Environmental site audits.
- Special ventilation systems.

In the tables, notice the differences between what the executives at Seemore Co. thought was profitable, and what they thought was not profitable. The environmental costs such as plating chemicals and solvents, personal protective equipment, and solid waste disposal are much greater for the gold magnifying glasses than the regular ones. Had they ceased production of the natural finish line, they would have been producing one money-losing magnifying glass. Because they had been dividing undetailed overhead costs by mere production numbers, the profit-intending managers at Seemore inadvertently had been subsidizing the gold line through the natural finished magnifying glasses.

On the other hand, by carefully applying costs to all the activities required to manufacture the natural finish magnifying glass, they were able to uncover a greater

TABLE 18–2 Natural Finish Magnifying Glass: Traditional Costing versus Activity-Based Costing

	Traditional Costing	ABC
Raw materials	$10.00	$10.00
Direct labor	$10.00	$10.00
General overhead	$24.00	$24.00
Environmental overhead	$5.27	$0.06
Cost	$49.27	$44.06
Price	$50.00	$50.00
Profit/loss [price – cost]	$ 0.73	$ 5.94

profit margin than they had assumed in the traditional costing model. In this case, the profits emerged as $5.94, rather than $0.73, a significant difference. Without accounting for these environmental costs in an activity-based way, the firm would never have been able to determine the true costs of each type of magnifying glass.

As stated, activity-based thinking helps identify the activities associated with the production of a good and assign costs to those activities. One of the best ways to do this is by applying costs to an actual process flow diagram. Almost every engineer feels comfortable with the familiarity of a process map. The difference in adding activity-based thinking to the map is that more information will be added around the perimeters. A process map, a subsection of which is shown in Figure 18–3, is the first step.

Through such a process map, you can begin to identify activities and outcomes not generally enumerated such as "nonsellable" inputs and outputs. Experienced process mappers expect to discover areas of duplication and non-value-added steps. They also might expect these insights to help lead them to the root causes of certain problems. What they are not accustomed to, however, is the inclusion of "nonsellable input" and "nonsellable output." "Nonsellable" or "nonproduct" input is something within the process that does not end up as part of the product. Chemicals used to degrease metal parts, contaminated rinse water, and heat used for drying are examples of nonproduct input and output. Traditionally, these have not been considered part of the manufacturing process, even though they are integral and certainly add costs.

The next step is to apply costs to the activities (remember not to let perfect ruin good; you will probably never have exact figures). Note the cost drivers in Figure 18–4 (again, a subsection).

It is important to identify nonproduct costs, because many products demand a high degree of environmental time (e.g., personnel to obtain permitting) and unrecognized costs (e.g., the high cost of disposing of certain chemicals). So, when drawing the process map, every loss potential, including air, water, solid wastes, leaks and spills, accidents, mistakes, scrap, yield, and energy should be included.

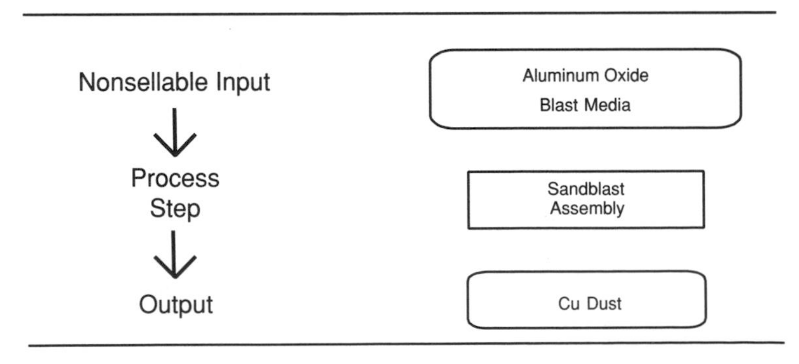

FIGURE 18–3 Process map subsection.

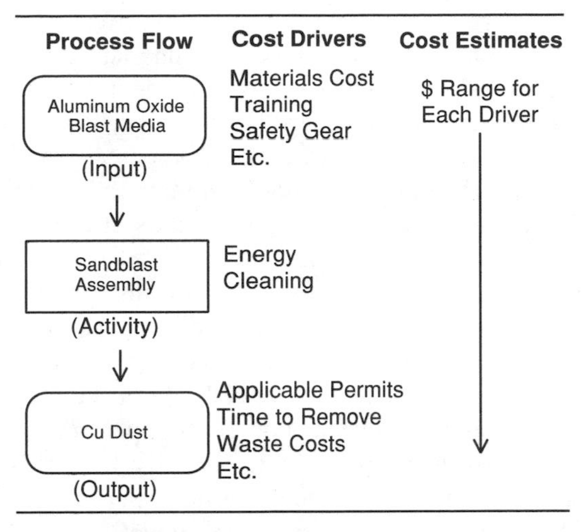

FIGURE 18–4 Applying costs to the process map.

When the process map is complete, you can begin to apply approximate costs to each activity in the map. This is referred to as *activity-based life-cycle costing* because it is a way to begin to see costs as they apply to each cost-driving activity in the process, through the entire life of the product. The individual most knowledgeable about the distinct costs should provide a range of costs for that activity. In this stage, it is valuable for costs that are not known precisely to be given in ranges.[9] These ranges provide a beginning point for information and keep team members from debating exact numbers.

This process is not "rocket science." It is, however, relatively new, so that you probably will be able to find a lot of previously obscured costs the first few times you undertake this entire exercise in your company. So far, I have never worked with a company that has not been able to find significant opportunities for cost and liability improvements. That is a good-news, bad-news situation: On the one hand, it means that you can affect significant change. On the other hand, it means the amount of waste and pollution going unchecked is larger than anyone probably suspects.

Probably the most challenging part of the entire process is getting people to change. Processes remain intact because "we've always done it that way," and there is a certain comfort level in that. Inspiring change will require patience and well-documented reasons for changing.

Teamwork

It is not possible to implement life-cycle costing and activity-based thinking through environmental personnel alone: Concepts must be channeled through multidepartmental efforts. This can be extremely effective because it draws together the expertise of procurement and production managers, accountants, asset management personnel, design engineers, environmental professionals, and the like to yield cost-minimizing solutions.

The cross-functional team creates an environmental "knowledge web" that ensures important comprehensive pieces don't slip through the cracks. Because the experts in each area are active in explaining their parts of the puzzle, they bring to light previously confusing or unnoticed issues.

In addition, they also become an integral part of improving the environmental process over the long run: They "buy in" and develop a level of ownership. All parties gain a new understanding of what is really needed, what is feasible, and so on. This can be an eye-opening, financially beneficial experience.

It is important to point out that support from upper management is a critical element in successful cost-tracking implementation. While such concepts can be pushed through from the middle ranks, they are far easier to implement with blessings from above. Driving new ideas up an organizational chart is difficult for a mid-level manager, no matter how valuable the idea. There are many stories about the manager who tried to decrease defects or improve production through implementing what we now call TQM (total quality management). Often he or she was laughed out of meetings or ignored. However, (almost) nobody laughs when a CEO or vice president initiates or supports innovative programs.

Some Final Points

Once the priority goals have been set, and before embarking on improvement, it is important to measure and document the current costs. This may sound insultingly intuitive, but based on the number of times it has been forgotten, repeating its importance might prove valuable. Baselines are essential for measuring progress, obviously, but they also are important in "proving" the value of environmental considerations in common business decisions.

Because these costing systems newly integrate business concepts into the Environment, Health, and Safety (EH&S) realm, some environmental managers have been reticent to undertake this path. The ideas make sense, but the world of EH&S compliance never had to think so proactively and rarely did it have to consider the business implications of compliance. This new strategic arena can be intimidating for many EH&S professionals. Yet pursuing it, armed with knowledge, can provide invaluable input for corporate planning and international competitiveness.

Understanding and minimizing environmental impact and costs also is becoming a matter of stakeholder demands. Companies now are reporting increased customer inquiries regarding environmental performance. This could become a competitive issue, as a deciding factor for consumers might be the firm's environmental image. Knowing the "real" numbers will be important in this new reporting phase.

In devising costing models and possibilities, it is important to keep an open mind. As Shunryu Suzuki said, "In the beginner's mind there are many possibilities, but in the expert's mind there are few." Consider a broad range of possibilities. Even if they seem ridiculous.

Conclusion

Firms with a tighter grasp on their costing are better able to make intelligent and strategic choices. Most environmental costs within firms remain unknown or ignored. By employing life-cycle and activity-based tools to unveil, and subsequently manage, environmental costs, firms can not only improve designs for their processes and products but their bottom lines as well.

Myriad examples demonstrate the vast opportunities for improvement being missed. Pollution of any sort is just another term for inefficiency. Inefficiency demonstrates suboptimization of a product or process. By strategically implementing proper costing models, companies will receive benefits for many years to come. In addition, environmental professionals will move from the perception of compliance and Band-Aids to being seen as a value-added center for the company.

Common benefits from having costed out the product correctly can include the following:

- Improved quality.
- Faster time to market.
- Improved processes.
- Reduced health and safety risks.
- Reduced environmental costs.
- Improved access to markets.
- Reduced capital expenditures.
- Reduced liabilities.
- Improved product pricing.
- Better competitive advantage.

Products—and their concomitant processes—seldom are devised in a manner that extracts and sustains maximum value for the manufacturer or the consumer. What we need now, instead of planned obsolescence, is planned longevity.

Notes

1. Most sources refer to the system of activity-based costing (ABC) but it is important to grasp and apply the general concepts before diving into a detailed ABC system. Hence, activity-based thinking.
2. Note that reuse can manifest in many ways. If the product were sold to a consumer initially, on its return, it could be refurbished, used in the field, become service parts for leased goods, and so forth. In this example, the second generation of product always must be identified as used on subsequent lease or sale.

3. When selling a used product—or a product that contains used parts—it is absolutely vital to identify that status. One electronics company failed to do so early on and has since received bad publicity and fines.
4. Discounting shows the value of tomorrow's dollars in today's currency. Think of it as interest in reverse. In these situations, using the net present value provides "apples to apples" numbers. It is worthwhile to discount in a life-cycle cost/benefit analysis, to bring all the financial conclusions into current dollar figures.
5. Certain plastics with fire resistant qualities have become quite controversial in parts of Europe, for example.
6. For instance, firms like Nike have suffered greatly for their poor environmental and "socially unresponsive" records.
7. In many cases, the quality of recycled products actually is higher than their original manifestation. This phenomenon might be attributed to any number of different factors; for example, perhaps eliminating the issue of infant mortality rates in electronic parts or the chemical bonding of a recycled polymer becoming stronger the second time around.
8. A cost driver could be the number of times an activity is required. For example, number of times an object must be dipped in cleaning solution.
9. For some stages, activities and their costs will need to be subgrouped, as not all costs and activities can be expressed on every process map. Subgrouping will depend on the process being analyzed, its complexity, and its goals.

CHAPTER 19

Design for Environment—A European Logistics Perspective

CARSTEN NAGEL
Fraunhofer Institute for Material Flows and Logistics IML, Dortmund, Germany

Producer Responsibility Legislation in Europe

A Short History

Waste from electrical and electronic equipment (WEEE) was part of the European Union's (EU) high-priority program in the early 1990s, designed to find out general ways to set up regulations for waste streams. Waste was included in this program due to its large volume (e.g., waste from packaging materials or demolition waste) and its hazardous potential. The total output of WEEE has been estimated to be "only" 6.5 to 7.5 million tons per year, which is less than 1% of the EU's solid waste and about 4% of the municipal solid waste (AEA, 1997). More recent calculations of the European Commission's Directorate General (DG XI) found the latter actually to be 5% (IPTS, 1998).

Parallel to these activities, authorities of several EU member-states started working on national legislation. In Germany, for example, the first draft of an "Electronic-Scrap Ordinance" was published in July 1991, covering the whole range of WEEE. Since then, there have been years of heavy discussion among all the stakeholders involved. This lead to changing approaches and different positions almost every year and, until now, no final solution, a situation sure to satisfy nobody.

Status Quo

While the first member states already have issued producer responsibility legislation, others have not yet done so. They seem to maintain a "wait and see" attitude, while they attempt to ascertain what's going on in their neighborhoods. It may well be that they are waiting for general guidelines to be issued by the EU. Table 19–1 shows the current status of the EU member states' legislation on take-back of WEEE.

TABLE 19–1 Status of European Take-Back Legislation, An Overview

Countries with (draft) legislation already produced or adopted:
Austria, Denmark, Germany, The Netherlands, Sweden, Switzerland
Countries with legislation yet to be produced:
Belgium, Finland, France, Italy , Norway, United Kingdom
Countries having taken no significant official steps:
Greece, Ireland, Portugal, Spain

Whereas some (draft) legislation covers the whole range of WEEE, other legislation focuses on certain product categories. In Germany, for example, an ordinance restricted only to IT appliances currently is under discussion.

A Look Into The Future

Harmony of legislation within the EU is very likely for the next millenium, as it is already standard in other sectors of waste management legislation. For example, all member states were "forced" to adopt the EU's waste definition, which led to several significant changes in waste legislation at the national level.

As a first approach in this field, in October 1997, the European Commission's Directorate General XI (Environment, Nuclear Safety, and Civil Protection) came up with a "Working Paper on the Management of Waste from Electrical and Electronic Equipment" (EC DG XI, 1997). On April 21, 1998, DG XI released the first version and, on July 7, 1998, the second draft of a new EU directive on waste from electrical and electronic equipment (EC DG XI, 1998a and 1998b). This directive is not expected to be published earlier than the year 2000 or to be effective earlier than 2002 or 2003, due to discussions and transformation at the national level.

The directive follows the three guiding principles of the initiative on end of life (EOL) of the electrical and electronic equipment:

1. Reduce the volume of waste through prevention and reuse, recycling, or recovery.
2. Reduce the hazard posed by waste by decreasing the use of hazardous substances and components.
3. Treat the waste in an environmentally sound manner, in particular hazardous parts and components.

These environmental aims should be reached by several distinct regulations, such as

1. A ban on the heavy metals lead, mercury, cadmium and hexavalent chromium.
2. A take-back obligation, free of charge to the final user, financed by an upfront fee added to the new product's price, preferably on the basis of a shared-responsibility approach.
3. Specific collection, reuse, and recycling targets[1] and the use of a minimum of 5% of recycled plastics inside the EEE.

Learning from practice

Take-Back Pilot Projects, an Overview

In the last couple of years a significant number of individual collection trials[2] have been conducted—and more are still being carried out—most of them by community or regional authorities with more or less private companies involved, especially recyclers. Some of these studies have been scientifically supported by research institutes, universities, or private consulting firms. The trials' exact objectives varied, among others, between

- Having a decision basis with regard to national WEEE legislation.
- Analysis of economical viability.
- Learning to understand the final user's behavior.
- Comparing the effectiveness of different logistic strategies.
- Having an idea of the amounts of WEEE to be collected in practice.
- Looking at the WEEEs "quality," their "real" recycling or reuse potential.

The resulting inhomogenity led to different points of interest and, therefore, different data have been collected and examined. For example, product categories have not been the same, either because of the lack of accepted (and therefore varying) definitions of WEEE or because of definitely different types of WEEE collected in each trial. Even more, overall parameters, like size of collection area, number of inhabitants, duration, and collected amount of goods, varied within wide ranges (see Figure 19–1).

Therefore, key numbers cannot be compared with each other. For example, it is difficult to estimate "the quantity of WEEE collected per inhabitant, per year," as it is typical behavior for many people to dispose of all their accumulated WEEE as soon as the collection starts. Of course, this leads to significantly higher average return numbers at the beginning (skewing the overall figures for short-time trials).

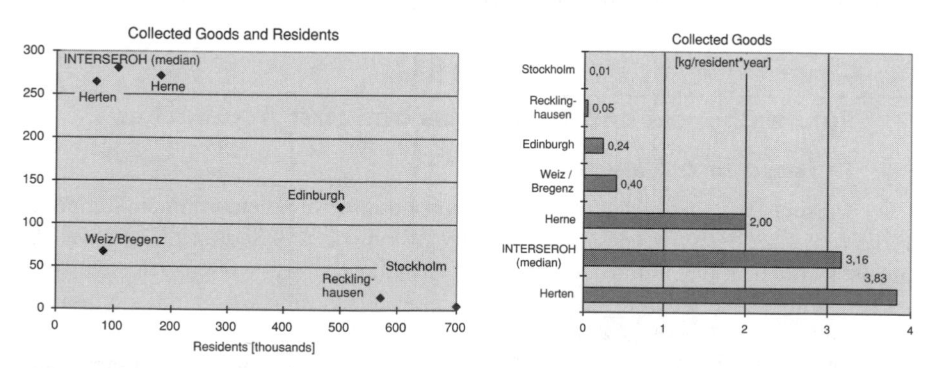

FIGURE 19–1 Varying parameters of collection trials.

Although a study that profoundly compares the results of all (or at least most) of these trials has yet to be produced,[3] the findings tend to be reach some remarkably similar conclusions:

- Collection of items at a municipal collection point or by retailers (when a new item is purchased) is the most favorable and the least expensive.
- The cost of recovery is very high at the moment; even for community based schemes these are 450-850 ECU/ton.
- 30–50% of all costs are caused by collection and disassembly or dismantling.

Consequences

Take-back schemes will be compulsory in the (very) near future, at least for Europe. We also can expect corresponding legislative actions in Japan and Taiwan and some parts of the Asian market. Perhaps there will be room for voluntary take-back activities organized by industry, but as far as the technical challenges of developing effective take-back strategies are concerned, that makes little difference—there definitely is no way out.

When designing take-back schemes, great attention must to be paid to precisely defining their objectives. This is because there are big differences between establishing and operating a countrywide take-back program (for all sorts of WEEE) and setting up a take-back program along product or brand (e.g., photocopiers from Xerox) lines. As of today, the economies of scale still are low and so the costs are high, especially for reprocessing.

As soon as buying a green product (including free take-back) means a real additional value for most consumers, the economics and logistics situation should improve markedly. Once this happens, companies really will start thinking about how to efficiently close a product's life cycle. This, in turn, will resolve the economy of scale problem, as more and more consumers will buy these products. Although much of the success of such a scenario depends on developing easily recyclable products, it also depends on developing cost-efficient solutions for take-back. To assure the greatest chance for success, both tasks must be performed with a deep look into the experiences gathered so far.

Future Chances and Challenges and First Approaches

In Need of a New Approach

Current DfE approaches focus primarily on integrating environmental metrics in the *technical* design process, the majority of which are based on LCA concepts, and lack direct applicability to real-world situations. Only a few try to take into account things like existing links between DfE and design for manufacturability, assembly, reliability, and the like.[4]

Obviously, this is not enough. To be successful, a new, *holistic* DfE approach seems to be necessary. To achieve this, we have to recognize "E" as an integral part of the whole product *management* process. This must include the product definition (i.e., consumer needs[5]), the technical design process, the supply chain, production, distribution, and last but not least, everything that addresses after-sales activities. In this aftersale arena, the "right" EOL strategy[6] plays an important role.

Reverse logistics play an important role within EOL strategies. Several studies clearly have shown that it is much more difficult to design an economically viable EOL solution than simply to be ecologically viable. One significant barrier to cost-effective take-back systems is the high percentage of the budget that must be dedicated to logistic costs, up to 50%. This is five to ten times higher than on the supply chain and can be a deciding factor in the success or failure of a reprocessing operation. This and other factors clearly underline the importance of strategies for logistically optimizing EOL. Paying attention to real-world logistic issues becomes even more critical if we are thinking about linking EOL to the supply chain, which really would be closing life cycles (see, e.g., Jünemann et al., 1996; Nagel, 1997)

With a look at experiences gathered in this field, we have to state that existing take-back activities lack systematic analysis[7] and planning, efficient supportive tools, and intelligent and suitable logistic components.

The next two sections discuss some recent approaches that have been developed within Fraunhofer IMLs applied research activities.

Cost-Optimized Take-Back and Recovery Systems

Talking about the cost effectiveness of schemes for take-back and product recovery is difficult and useless to do without looking at the whole process chain. This involves combining the logistics aspects of transport and collection with those associated with recovery. Furthermore, it is not possible to make a sound decision without a close look at critical factors such as

- Collection area, population density, and household equipment ratio.[8]
- The spectrum of products being recovered (white goods, brown goods, without CRT, IT appliances, etc.).
- Product life-cycle times.[9]
- Product characteristics and recycling potential.
- The existing recycling infrastructure, especially existing processing[10] facilities.
- Costs.

To support the planning of integrated, cost-optimized take-back and recovery systems, Fraunhofer IML developed a methodology and a corresponding software tool, EDS-RLog. The main objective is to develop tailored take-back systems, whether for manufacturers, retailers, logistic service providers, or waste management companies (private or municipal) with respect to the whole process chain of EOL management. EDS-RLog aids in a stepwise planning and evaluation of different system scenarios with variable degrees of detail for a variety of typical logistics problems.

A project starts with an in-depth analysis of the criteria just mentioned. Analysis is made on the basis of the "geographical" data (→ A), the "chosen" product (→ B, C), and correction factors based on empirical data and long-term experience. When these factors are combined with data on the amount of products to be collected within a specific period of time at a specific location,[11] the total activity within the entire collection area can be predicted.

Depending on the optimization task (whether planning a totally new operation or optimizing the existing infrastructure) the facility-location problem or the allocation-problem can be solved, too. The decision is based on costs for all relevant processes—collection, transport, handling, storing, sorting, disassembling—as well as revenues expected from the specific recycling processes taken into account (→ D, E, F).[12]

This analysis technique also makes it is possible to develop optimized vehicle routing and scheduling for the collection and transport of reclaimed WEEE. Various planning and installation projects already have revealed the great extent of exploitable optimizing potentials.

New Logistic Components: The Lobster Project

However, the focus should be not only on strategies for reverse logistics, as already addressed in the chapter. A very important aspect and major impediment today is the lack of suitable equipment for operating efficient collection and recycling systems. Looking at current solutions, it is clear that the whole process chain is far from optimal. The containers used for collection of WEEE seem to be especially Stone Age. This is true for big 40 m^3 containers, preferably used in recycling yards as well as for collecting WEEE on a van's loading platform or at retail outlets. In both cases, all equipment has to be handled again and again as it is readied for disassembly. Furthermore, many old-fashioned containers provide no protection against mechanical impact, so that used but still functional components tend to break during collection and transportation.

Within the Lobster Project (Logistik bei Sammlung und Transport für das Elektronik-Recycling; logistics for collection and transport for the recycling of electrical and electronic equipment), the Fraunhofer IML researchers developed a totally new hardware concept for the collection of WEEE. This project was a joint venture carried out in close cooperation with a large waste management company (AGR Abfallentsorgungsgesellschaft Ruhrgebiet mbH, Essen), vehicle construction and machine factories (Girke Fahrzeug- und Stahlbau GmbH, Bochum; Maschinenfabrik Ernst Hese GmbH, Gelsenkirchen), and the Anwenderzentrum Herne GmbH. The new Lobster collection vehicle (see Figure 19–2) enables the simultaneous but separate collection of up to nine different fractions on one tour. This is accomplished with the help of a revolutionary container system and a horizontal-paternoster like storage mechanism that employs nine containers on a circular conveyor belt, which easily can be mechanically loaded and unloaded from the vehicle. In this way, the operator can load and unload containers or sort incoming waste into different categories with a minimum of time and effort.

The new containers have been designed so they can be dropped off at retail outlets to serve as collection bins as well as for collection "on tour" and storing the

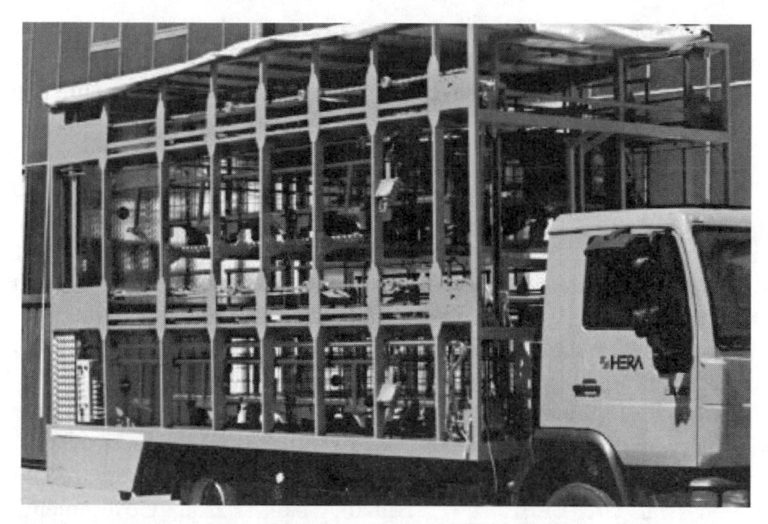

FIGURE 19–2 The Lobster collection vehicle (Hauser, 1998).

used equipment on the transport. Once offloaded at the disassembly facility, the same containers are used to transport materials inside the plant.

As a result of this new technology, handling times along the whole process chain of collection and transportation could be reduced by more than 20% and the vehicle can be operated by one person (compared to two people for the classic system). This system is successfully being operated in the city of Herne, Germany.

Conclusions

Tools and methodologies for analyzing, describing and optimizing EOL systems are still far from satisfactory. Despite decades of research and almost innumerable practical experiences in the field of supply chain management, the situation is totally different for resource recovery. Nobody can really disagree with the fact that we are almost at the beginning of a very long and hard road toward sustainability. To make this goal viable within a capitalist economic framework, we must develop systems capable of generating profit at a product's rear end. Toward this end, we must develop the same standards the same performance and professionalism as in the classical areas. Without them, the task of achieving an economically viable closed-loop resource cycle becomes significantly more difficult or even impossible.

Despite the accomplishments described here and others, we probably have to employ a double-edged compromise strategy for at least the next decade. This will involve taking back and recycling non-DfE products while designing, taking back, and recycling DfE products at the same time. With a look at average life cycles compared to the automotive industry, the electronics industry has a much better position, especially in the rapidly developing IT sector.

In conclusion, a lot of work has been done so far by a lot of companies, but we cannot be satisfied with the state of the art. There is still a lot to do, and in order to succeed, we should heed the advice of a famous athletic supply company… Just do it!

Notes

1. Whereas the working paper and first draft contained detailed collection and recycling quotas for each type of WEEE, the second draft demands a yearly *collection* total of 4 kg of WEEE per capita from private households and, on this basis, a *recycling* quota in the range 70–90% until January 1, 2004.
2. For example, Eindhoven, the Netherlands (Ploos van Amstel et al., 1997); Bregenz, Austria (Salhofer and Gabriel, 1996) and Weiz, Austria (Nelles et al., 1996); the ICER Collection Trial, UK (ICER, 1996); the LEEP Collection Trial, UK (LEEP, 1997); Bilbao, Spain (Basque Government, 1996); Rhône-Alpes, France (FIEE, 1997); INTERSEROH, Germany (Gallenkemper et al., 1997).
3. The best studies available so far have been elaborated for the European Commission (AEA, 1997; Ökopol, 1998) and try to summarize the experiences gathered in the major collection trials as well as examine the feasibility of establishing collection targets. I am involved in more detailed activities going beyond those investigations (Nagel, 1998; Nagel, Nilsson, and Boks, 1999).
4. An excellent example here is the methodology and the corresponding tool developed recently by MCC (e.g., Murphy et al. 1998).
5. Why not sell the benefit instead of the product? Of course, to a certain extent this means changing consumer behavior, but companies like Xerox clearly show that there is a growing market segment here.
6. Whatever this will be. This could address approaches like design for non-disassembly, design for upgrading, and (much) more.
7. There is an intense need for a systems analysis approach toward EOL processing. The basic thoughts and the general approach can be found in Nagel and Meyer (1999) and shall not be discussed in this paper.
8. The penetration ratio describes the average percentage of households being equipped with a special type of electrical or electronic equipment, such as the number of personal computers per household or per capita.
9. How long is a special type of equipment used before being discarded?
10. Processing shall include all EOL processes like disassembly, shreddering, and smelting.
11. The location usually is described by using ZIP code areas. Depending on the accuracy needed three-digit to five-digit ZIP codes are taken as a basis.
12. A database providing these costs and revenues is part of the software tools and permanately being updated.

References

AEA. (1997). "Recovery of WEE: Economic & Environmental Impacts Final Report." A report produced for European Commission DG XI by AEA Technology National Environmental Technology Center. Brussels: European Commission DG XI, 1997.

Basque Government. (1996). *Collection and Treatment of End-of-life Electrical and Electronic Equipment: Domestic flow, Enterprise flow A Mixed Experience*. Bilbao: Basque Government, Ministry of Territory, Housing & Environment, December 1996.

EC DG XI. (1997). "Working Paper on the Management of Waste from Electrical and Electronical Equipment." Brussels, 9 October 1997.

EC DG XI. (1998a). First Draft: Proposal for a Directive on Waste from Electrical and Electronical Equipment. Brussels, 21 April 1998.

EC DG XI. (1998b). Second Draft: Proposal for a Directive on Waste from Electrical and Electronical Equipment. Brussels, 07 July 1998.

FEEI. (1996). *Systemvergleich für Elektro- und Elektronikaltgerte (EAG) Sammlung/ Verwertung/Entsorgung, volkswirtschaftliche Auswirkungen.* Wien: Fachverband der Elektro- und Elektronikindustrie, July 1996.

FIEE. (1997). *Produits Electriques et Electroniques non Portables en fin de vie en Region Rhone-Alpes*. FIEE; January 1997.

Gallenkemper, et al. (1997). *Wissenschaftliche Begleitung des Pilotprojektes der Interseroh AG zur Erfassung von Elektroaltgerten.* Cologne, Interseroh, April 1997.

Hauser, H. and A. Krawczik. (1998). "A New System for Collection and Transportation of Waste Electrical and Electronic Equipment". *CARE Innovation 98-Eco-Efficient Concepts for the Electronics Industry Towards Sustainability.* 2nd International Symposium. Vienna, November 16–19, 1998, Proceedings. Vienna: International CARE "Vision 2000" Office, 1998, pp. 283–289.

ICER. (1996). *Producer Responsibility for EEE: Facing the Challenge, Tapping the Potential*. London: ICER, November 1996.

IPTS. (1998). "Towards a European solution for the management of waste from electrical and electronical equipment." First Draft. A report prepared by the IPTS for the Comittee on environment, Public Health and Consumer Protection of the European Parliament. Seville: Institute for Prospective Technological Studies IPTS, September 1998.

Jünemann, R., U. Hansen, and C. Nagel. (1996). "Innovatives Stoffstrommanagement." *Fraunhofer-Institut für Chemische Technologie ICT (Hrsg.): Neue Technologien für die Kreislaufwirtschaf.* Symposium Strategien für die Produktion im 21. Jahrhundert, Karlsruhe, May 21–22, 1996. Proceedings. Karlsruhe: DWS Werbeagentur und Verlag, 1996, S. 8.18.26.

LEEP. (1997). *Unplugging Electrical & Electronic Waste: The Findings of the LEEP Collection Trial*. LEEP/EMERG, February 1997.

Murphy, C.F., C. Mizuki, and P.A. Sandborn. (1998). "Implementation of DFE in the Electronics Industry Using Simple Metrics for Cost, Quality, and Environmental Merit." *Institute of Electrical and Electronics Engineers IEEE (Hrsg.): IEEE International Symposium on Electronics and the Environment 1998, Proceedings*. Oak Brook, Ill., May 4–6, 1998. Piscataway, NJ: IEEE Service Center, 1998, pp. 25-29.

Nagel, C. (1997). "Reverse Logistics Basic Step towards (Eco-)efficient Recycling." *Eco-Efficient Concepts for the Electronics Industry Towards Sustainability. CARE Innovation 96 Proceedings of the International Congress*. Frankfurt, 18–20 November 1996, Hotel Intercontinental. Technology Publishing Ltd., London, 1997, pp. 247–249.

Nagel, C., J. Nilsson, and C. Boks. (1999). "European End-of-Life Systems for Electrical and Electronic Equipment." Yoshikawa, H., R. Yamamoto, F. Kimura, T. Suga, Y. Umeda. (Eds.) *EcoDesign '99 1st International Symposium on Environmentally Conscious Design and Inverse Manufacturing, Proceedings*. Tokyo, February 13, 1999. IEEE Computer Society: Los Alamitos, CA, 1999, pp. 197–203.

Nagel, C. and P. Meyer. (1999). "Caught between Ecology and Economy End-of-Life Aspects of Environmentally Conscious Manufacturing." *Computers & Industrial Engineering. Special issue on 'Operational Issues in Environmentally Conscious Manufacturing'" (in preparation)*.

Nelles, M., M. Harant, J. Hochhuber, and K. Lorber. (1996). *Modellversuch zur Sammlung, Demontage und Verwertung von Elektro- und Elektronikalgerten (EAG) im Bezirk Weiz*. Leoben: Montanuniversitt Leoben, April 1996.

Ökopol. (1998). "Collection Targets for Waste from Electrical and Electronic Equipment (WEEE)." Final Report compiled for the Directorate General (DG XI) of the Commission of the European Communities. Hamburg: kopol Institut für kologie und Politik GmbH, May 1998.

Ploos van Amstel, J.J.A., et al. (1997). *Back to the beginning: National pilot project, for collecting, recycling and repairing electrical and electronic equipment in the district of Eindhoven Apparetour*. Eindhoven: Ploos van Amstel Milieu Consulting B.V., September 1997.

Salhofer, S. and R. Gabriel. (1996). *Bregenz Pilot Project: Waste from Electrical & Electronic Equipment*. Wien: Universitt für Bodenkultur, April 1996.

Part VII

ISO 14001—The Environment Standard for Industry

REMEMBER, THE STAPLER SHOULD ALWAYS BE PARALLEL TO THE LEFT EDGE OF THE DESK AND THE POST-IT NOTES GO ON THE RIGHT EDGE.
WHEN YOU'RE MAKING YOUR Q's, FIRST MAKE A NICE BIG O AND THEN ADD THE LITTLE TAIL. SEE?
McPHEESON

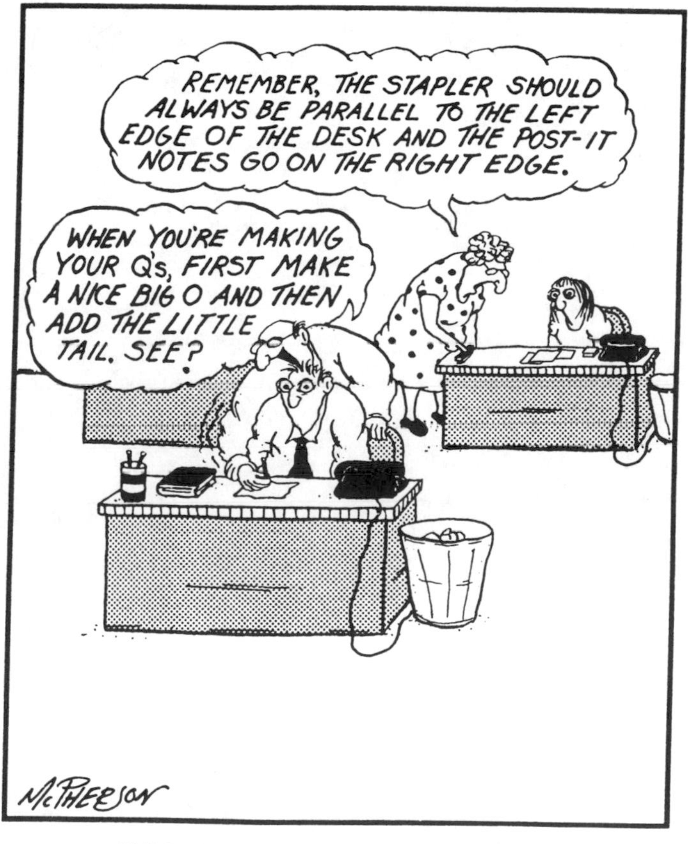

TLS Industries had a tendency to overmanage its employees.

CHAPTER 20

Meeting the Letter and Spirit of Environmental Management Using the ISO 14001 Standard

JAMES LAMPRECHT

What Is Environmental Management?

Over the years, countless definitions of *environmental management* and *environmental management system* have been proposed. Comparing these definitions, one notices some similarities and, yet, significant differences in tone or emphasis. For example, the international standard on environmental management, ISO 14001, offers the following definition:

> Environmental management system: That part of the overall management system which includes organizational structure, planning activities, responsibilities, practices, procedures, processes and resources for developing, implementing, achieving, reviewing and maintaining the environmental policy.

Although adequate, the definition is incomplete. Indeed, one must go back to the early 1980s, in an age when few dared challenge the rationality of regulatory enforcement, to find perhaps one of the most complete definitions of an environmental management system:

> An environmental management system is the framework for or method of guiding an organization to achieve and sustain performance in accordance with established goals and in response to constantly changing regulations, social, financial, economic, and competitive pressures, and environmental risks. When operating effectively, a corporate environmental management system provides management and the board of directors with the knowledge that;
>
> The corporation is in compliance with federal, state, and local environmental laws and regulations.

Policies and procedures are clearly defined and promulgated throughout the organization.
Corporate risks resulting from environmental risks are being acknowledged and brought under control.
The company has the right resources and staff for environmental work, is applying those resources and is in control of its future. (Greeno et al., 1985, p. 6)

The definition concludes by stating that the environmental management system provides a basis for guiding, measuring, and evaluating performance to ensure that "a company's operations are carried out in a manner consistent with a support of applicable regulations and corporate policy." Although it is true that the preceding definition is longer than those offered by ISO 14001 or the French standard (NF X 30-200), it nevertheless encompasses all the key elements of an environmental management system. With this in mind, we examine the ISO 14001 standard to see how it can be used as a tool to meet the spirit of this larger definition.

The ISO 14001 Standard

Most individuals familiar with the ISO 9000 series of standards will recognize that, although not perfect, the ISO 14001 standard and its associated appendix is less ambiguous and more concise than the ISO 9001 standard. Certainly, improvements will be made over the next few years.

Of the 20 or so documents that eventually will constitute the ISO 14000 series over the next two to three years (see Table 20–1), the ISO 14001 standard, Environmental Management Systems—Specification with Guidance for Use, is the most important. This is because it is the reference standard to be used by organizations that wish to have their environmental management system officially certified or registered by a third-party registration body. Issued in 1996 and derived from the British Standard Institution's 7750 document, Environmental Management System (1992), the ISO 14001 Standard, Environmental Management Systems—Specification with Guidance for Use, traces its heritage to earlier environmental management systems developed in the United States during the late 1970s and early 1980s.[1]

The standard is based on the fundamental concepts of quality assurance and total quality management (TQM) developed over the past several decades. It is summarized in the successful ISO series of quality assurance and management standards known as the ISO 9000 series (issued in 1987, revised in 1994, and due for its next revision in late 2000).[2]

To better understand the fundamental premise of the ISO 14001 standard, one should read the standard from the perspective of total quality environmental management (TQEM). In the world of TQEM, one does not take the acronym CEO as the usual, but limited meaning of chief executive officer but, rather, the broader context of chief environmental officer. Viewed from a TQEM perspective, environmental management takes on a different meaning. As Joel Makower so aptly observes,

TABLE 20–1 The ISO 14000 Series

ISO 14001: Environmental Management Systems—Specification with Guidance for Use
ISO 14004: Environmental management systems—General Guidelines on Principles, and Supporting Techniques
ISO 14010: Guidelines for Environmental Auditing—General Principles of Environmental Auditing
ISO 14011/1: Guidelines for Environmental Auditing—Auditing Procedures
ISO 14012: Guidelines for Environmental Auditing—Qualification Criteria for Environmental Auditors
ISO 14013: Management of Environmental Audit Programs
ISO 14014: Initial Reviews
ISO 14015: Environmental Site Assessments
ISO 14020: Environmental Labeling—General Principles
ISO 14021: Terms and Definitions for Self-Declaration Environmental Claims
ISO 14022: Environmental Labeling—Symbols
ISO 14023: Environmental Labeling—Testing and Verification Methodologies
ISO 14024: Environmental labeling—Guiding principles, practices and criteria for multiple criteria based practitioner programs—Guide for certification procedures
ISO 14031: Evaluation of the environmental performance
ISO 14040: Environmental Management—Life-Cycle Assessment—Principles and Guidelines
ISO 14041: Environmental Management—Life-Cycle Assessment—Goal and Definitions/ Scope and Inventory Analysis
ISO 14042: Environmental Management—Life-Cycle Assessment—Life-Cycle Impact Assessment
ISO 14043: Environmental Management—Life-Cycle Assessment—Interpretation
ISO 14050: Terms and Definitions—Guide on the Principles for ISO/TC207/SC6 Terminology Work
ISO 14060: Guide for the Inclusion of Environmental Aspects in Product Standard

"Considering that waste and pollution are defects (in that they result from inefficiencies in the system), it follows that an ultimate goal of environmental quality is to achieve zero waste and pollution" (1994, pp. 6–7). These objectives certainly are in line with the fundamental premise of the ISO 14001 standard.

Finally, one must note that ISO 14001 applies to all companies, large and small, and its geographical scope, in the case of multinationals (or so-called transnational corporations), could extend to several regions.

ISO 14001: What It Is and Is Not

A valuable feature of the ISO 14001 standard is that it includes a good informative annex, which acts as a supporting document to clarify the standard. In an attempt to perhaps avoid earlier misinterpretations regarding the purpose of guidelines (so prevalent with the ISO 9000 series), the opening paragraph of the annex (Annex A: Guidance on the Use of the Specification) is careful to point out that the annex "does not add to or subtract from the content of" the standard.

As for the purpose and scope of the ISO 14001 standard, it is stated within the first two opening sections: Introduction and Scope. Not surprisingly, the scope of 14001 is very broad and is intended for "all types and sizes of organizations." In the event that the reader may have missed the point, the following sentence is repeated:

> The standard is applicable to any organization that wishes to:
>
> implement, maintain and improve an environmental management system; and/or
> assure itself of its conformance with its stated environmental policy; and/or
> demonstrate such conformance to others; and/or
> seek certification/registration to its environmental management system by an external organization; and/or
> make a self determination and declaration of conformance with the standard.

Having defined its all-encompassing scope, the standard's opening paragraphs emphasize the following general objectives:

- The overall aim of the standard is to support environmental protection in balance with socioeconomic needs.
- The environmental management system can be integrated with other management requirements as found in the ISO 9000 series, for example.
- The standard contains only those system elements that may be objectively audited for certification or registration purposes or self-declaration purposes.[3]
- The standard requires an organization to formulate an environmental policy and set objectives, taking into account legislative requirements and information about any significant environmental impact. In addition to complying with applicable legislation and regulations, the organization must demonstrate its commitment to continuous improvement (as it relates to environmental issues and policies).
- To achieve environmental objectives, the environmental management system should encourage organizations to consider implementation of best available technology where appropriate and economically viable. The cost effectiveness of such technology should be taken into account fully.

What the standard is *not*:

- The standard is not intended to address and does not include requirements for aspects of occupational health and safety management; however, it does not seek to discourage an organization from developing integration of such management system elements.
- The standard does not state specific environmental performance criteria.

Also note that a vague reference to sustainable development (which is not defined) is made in the first paragraph of the standard.[4]

A Quick Look at the Standard Through Some Key Sentences

The most frequently used verbs found throughout the standard are *establish* and *maintain*. These verbs are invariably associated with the word *procedure* as in "establish and maintain procedure." However, the ISO 14001 standard is significantly different from the ISO 9001, ISO 9002, or ISO 9003 standards in that the term *documented procedure* is excluded from most paragraphs. Although one could argue that it would be difficult to establish and maintain procedures without documenting them (thus relying on verbal means of communication favored by most small- to medium-size organizations), the obsession with the need to document everything, typical of the ISO 9000 series, so far, nonetheless is tactfully and intelligently by-passed in ISO 14001.

Exceptions to the preceding rule include the following:

- "The organization shall establish and maintain documented environmental objectives and targets, at each relevant function and level within the organization" (4.2.3 Objectives and Targets).
- "Roles, responsibility and authorities shall be defined, documented, and communicated in order to facilitate effective environmental management" (4.3.1 Structure and Responsibility).
- "The organization shall establish and maintain documented procedures to monitor and measure on a regular basis the key characteristics of its operations and activities that can have a significant impact on the environment" (4.4.1 Monitoring and Measurement).[5]

In addition to these requirements, the following "shall sentences" define the overall purpose of the standard. In the majority of cases, all shall sentences must be addressed, unless of course particular conditions make it either irrelevant or not applicable to a company. However, even in such cases, it is recommended that the company briefly explain why the sentence(s) or clause(s) is not applicable. Before describing the requirements of each clause, let us look at what any organization shall have to do if it wants to implement an environmental system that will comply to the ISO 14001 standard.

An organization:

Shall define its environmental policy.

Shall establish and maintain procedure(s) to identify potential for accidents and emergency situations, and how the organization shall respond to these situations.

Shall determine [those activities] which can have significant impact on the environment. . . whether or not the environmental system conforms to planned arrangements.

Shall ensure that these impacts are considered in setting the organization's objectives.

Shall keep information up-to-date.
Shall consider legal and other requirements when reviewing objectives.
Shall provide resources essential to the implementation and control of the environmental management system.
Shall appoint management representatives who shall have the authority to ensure that the environmental management system is established, implemented and maintained and who shall report on the performance of said system.
Shall require that all personnel [who have an impact on the environment] shall be competent on the basis of education, appropriate training and/or experience and have received appropriate training (as required).
Shall consider processes for external communication on its significant environmental aspects and record its decision.
Shall review and revise emergency preparedness and response procedures.
Shall monitor and measure the key characteristics of its operations and activities that can have a significant impact on the environment.
Shall calibrate and maintain monitoring equipment [and maintain records].
Shall evaluate compliance with relevant environmental legislation and regulations.
Shall take action to mitigate any [environmental] impacts caused by nonconformances.
Shall implement and record changes in procedures.
Shall store and disposition records to demonstrate conformance to the requirements of this standard.
[Management] shall review the environmental system to ensure that it is effective and address possible need for changes to policy, objectives or other elements.

ISO 14001: Environmental Management System

This surprisingly short standard consists of only five major paragraphs, generally broken down into several subparagraphs. A description of each of the paragraphs follows. The association with the ISO 9001 standard is demonstrated by referring (in parenthesis) to the closest ISO 9001 paragraph.

Environmental Policy (ISO 9001 §4.1)

This paragraph requires the organization to define its environmental policy. To prevent organizations from either copying someone else's environmental policy or write flowery policies with little substance, the standard also requires that the organization ensure that its environmental policy satisfies several important conditions:

> The policy must be appropriate to the nature, scale and environmental impacts of its activities, products or services. In other words, the environmental policy of a chemical plant which may produce several tons a day of a variety of potentially hazardous chemicals should be different in scope from the policy of a small manufacturing assembly plant which may use 50–100 lbs of chemicals a day.
>
> In addition, a commitment must be stated with regard to: continuous improvement, pollution prevention, compliance to relevant environmental legislation and regulations or other requirements to which the organization subscribes. These requirements are rather clear:
>
> Any organization who wishes to be compliant with the ISO 14001 standard must ensure that it not only satisfies all local (national) laws and regulations, it must also apply fundamental principals of total quality management to demonstrate its commitment and/or intent to continuously improve the quality of the environment by preventing pollution. It is important to understand that an ISO 14001 audit will not be a compliance audit whose purpose will be to ensure that all relevant laws are complied with. Rather, the primary task of ISO 14001 auditors will be to verify that the organization has an effective management system that conforms to ISO 14001 and is designed to ensure that all relevant local and/or national laws are adequately addressed.

The commitments specified previously must be set within well-defined objectives and targets. This requirement is important for it prevents organizations from making vague statements such as "we will improve our waste management program by focusing on waste reduction." The standard wants to know what are the company's objectives and how it will quantify (set targets) these objectives to measure its effectiveness in achieving your goals stated in the policy (see other paragraphs later).

Finally, the organization's environmental policy must be documented, implemented, maintained, and communicated to all employees and available to the public.

Planning

Environmental Aspects (Nearly Equivalent to ISO 9001 §4.2.3)

The choice of the word *aspects* is most unfortunate for it conveys no clear meaning. In this instance, by merely repeating the word *aspects*, the usually informative appendix offers little assistance. The ISO 14001 standard defines *environmental aspects* as the "Element of an organization's activities—products or services which can interact with the environment." The problem is that such a broad definition may not be very helpful. Indeed, if an organization is to operate within a well-defined geographical boundary known as *the environment*, by the very nature of its existence, it must interact with that environment (air, soil, water). In turn, such (organization-environmental) interactions are likely to lead to some form of impact on the environment.

Nevertheless, one can deduce the probable intended meaning. The organization must establish, document, and keep up-to-date a procedure that will identify its activities, products, or services that can have significant impact on the environment (e.g., air, soil, and water pollution or even noise pollution, which generally is covered by urban zoning regulations). For countries that have environmental laws, most of these activities, products, and services already have been defined and continue to be reviewed and updated in a multitude of national or provincial laws, congressional acts, city or county ordinances, and a myriad of regulations (e.g., health and safety regulations, transportation regulations for hazardous chemicals, hazardous waste disposal and storage).

The standard contains, in my opinion, an unfortunate, convoluted sentence that is likely to lead to some confusion and abuse (the appendix tries to clarify the meaning): "The organization shall establish and maintain the environmental aspects of its activities, products or service that it can control and over which it can be expected to have an influence, . . ." Who shall determine whether the organization adequately controls activities over which it is "expected to have influence" remains to be seen.

Legal and Other Requirements (No ISO 9001 Equivalent)

This paragraph requires the organization to have a procedure that will identify or otherwise have access to legal and other requirements applicable to the environmental aspects of its activities, products, or services. This requirement simply states that it is the responsibility of an organization to ensure that it is informed as to all legal and other requirements such as regulatory guidelines.

Objectives and Targets (No ISO 9001 Equivalent Yet)

This is one of the very few places where the word *documented* is used. The organization is required to establish and maintain documented environmental objectives and targets that shall be consistent with the environmental policy and the commitment to pollution prevention. Obviously, one effective way to satisfy this clause is to set quantifiable objectives that will be monitored and, hence, measured periodically. In this regard, the standard seems oddly timid in its approach, for it requires only that the organization consider legal requirements; technological options as well as financial, operational, and business requirements; "and the views of interested parties." In fact, the explanatory notes associated with this paragraph (found in the appendix) emphasize, oddly enough, that organizations are not obliged to use environmental cost accounting methodologies; the very tool that can be most helpful in cases of financial cost assessment.

The use of metrics or indices (also known as *performance goals*), is not new to companies. Some years ago, the Polaroid Corporation developed a toxic use and waste reduction index (TUWR) to measure its "green performance." The TUWR index takes into account not only toxic use and waste reduction but also the consumption of energy and water, pollution from electricity use, as well as lower impact gained from greener product design. Thorn EMI, a music and electronic giant based in London, also establishes green targets and progress toward those targets for each of its business groups. In its 1993 environmental report, "the company promised a 15 percent to 20 percent cutback in energy consumption for its Canadian music unit." The multinational DuPont has set a dozen environmental performance goals to be achieved by certain target dates.[6] The use of so-called green metrics, such as cardboard recycling, food composting, reduced electrical consumption (energy conservation), collecting and monitoring of surface water, to monitor environmental objectives also has been successfully applied by grocery stores such as Larry's Market in Seattle, Washington (Rogers, 1995).

Environmental Management Programs (Similar to ISO 9001 §4.2.3)

Once objectives and targets have been set, a process of implementation must follow. The standard wants to know how the policy and its objectives will be implemented; the time frame involved; what individuals or functions will have the responsibility to manage, review, and plan the whole environmental program from design activities to materials acquisitions, storage and disposal, production, and servicing. This would include new activities such as the construction of a new plant and the eventual decommission of activities.

Implementation and Operation

Structure and Responsibility (ISO 9001 §4.1.2)

This paragraph is very similar to the "resource and management responsibilities" paragraphs found in the ISO 9000 series. The organization must define, document, and communicate to all necessary parties who has the responsibility and authority to implement and control all aspects of the environmental management system. In addition, a manager must be appointed to ensure that the performance of environmental management system, as defined in ISO 14001, is maintained and duly reported to upper management for review.[7]

Training, Awareness and Competence (ISO 9001 §4.18)

All personnel whose work may potentially impact the environment must receive appropriate training to ensure that they are competent. Competency may be determined on the basis of education, appropriate training (in-house or public seminars for example) and/or job experience. The training must be proceduralized to ensure that everyone is made aware of the importance of conforming to the environmental policy and procedures. In addition, all staff concerned with environmental matters must also be made aware of:

- The actual or potential impact of their work activities.
- Their role and responsibility in abiding to procedures defined in the environmental management system including emergency preparedness and response requirements.
- The potential consequences of departure from specified operating procedures.

Records of all training activity will need to be maintained. In the United States, these requirements should be relatively easy to satisfy. OSHA's requirements, specified in 29 CFR 1910.119 (see Table 20.2 for definition of terms), mandate that companies have programs in place to manage process hazards. Over the past two to three years, hundreds of chemical companies have trained thousands of their employees in health and safety, hazardous chemical management, hazard evaluation procedures and operations, and the like.

Communications (No ISO 9001 Equivalent)

With regard to the environmental system and so-called environmental aspects (that is, organizational activities "which can interact with the environment"), a procedure will need to be established to define how the organization communicates information internally among various functions. In addition, the procedure will need to define how the organization receives, documents, and responds to (environmentally) relevant requests from external interested parties such as public authorities or citizens groups. One example of an issue that could be addressed by this paragraph is how the organization communicates with public authorities on matters regarding emergency planning. Records of decisions will have to be kept (perhaps in the form of minutes or formal interdepartmental communication).

An example of external communication from Monsanto follows:

> Monsanto recognized some time ago that the general public is, for the most part, not interested in parts per million of chemicals per cubic centimeters of air but rather, wants to know if and how an emission or discharge to the environment may affect their family. Therefore, in an attempt to effectively communicate with the public at large, the Monsanto company established community advisory councils (CACs) which include as some of their panel members, a cross section of the public (teachers, housewives, businessmen, and local politicians). In addition, Monsanto employees and plant managers receive communication training which allows them to discuss and explain to the community what Monsanto is achieving locally and globally in terms of environmental management. Over the years, Monsanto has learned some valuable lessons on how to interact with community members:

- Don't preach to your audience.
- Be willing to listen to unpleasant accusations and be willing to discuss uncomfortable issues truthfully. Avoid becoming defensive.
- Recruit participants who can be objective. In other words do not only enlist the help of individuals who will be predisposed to a favorable view of the company.
- Encourage all subjects to be discussed.
- Act on legitimate community objections. Do not seek opinions only to ignore them.

Since small- to medium-size companies are not likely to have the same resources as larger corporations, they will need to adjust their efforts accordingly. The periodic publication of brochures, newsletters, or pamphlets may be an effective way to communicate with the public. In some cases, the environmental quality manual, or an abridged version of the manual, also may be used as a means to communicate with the public at large.

Environmental Management Systems Documentation

This paragraph merely states that the environmental management system, which describes how various documents are interrelated, shall be documented either on paper or electronic form.

Document Control (ISO 9001 §4.5)

This paragraph mimics clause 4.5, Document and Data Control, of the ISO 9001 standard (for further clarification, refer to the ISO 9001 standard). Organizations that already have registered to one of the ISO 9000 standards will have no difficulty implementing this clause. A procedure must be established to define how documents relating to the environmental system are controlled. This means that the procedure must ensure that

- Documents are reviewed periodically, revised as necessary, and approved by authorized personnel (the company also needs to identify who has the authority to create and modify documents).
- The allocation of relevant and up-to-date documents is identified.
- Obsolete documents are reviewed for all points of issue.
- Any obsolete documents retained for legal or knowledge preservation purposes are suitably identified.

Operational Control (ISO 9001 §4.9)

The correspondence table found at the end of the 14001 document associates this paragraph with the following ISO 9001 paragraphs: 4.2, Quality System Procedure; 4.3, Contract Review; 4.4, Design Control; 4.6, Purchasing; 4.7, Control of customer supplied product; 4.8, Product identification and traceability; 4.9, Process

Control; 4.15, Handling, Storage, Packaging, Preservation and Delivery; and 4.19, Servicing. Although I have worked with the ISO 9001 standard for over six years, I find it difficult to agree with the correspondence. Paragraph 3.6 is very short paragraph, approximately ten lines. It is difficult to imagine that ten lines could be matched with as many as nine relatively long ISO 9001 paragraphs.

In my opinion, paragraph 3.6 attempts to capture the intent of paragraph 4.9, Process Control, of ISO 9001 without duplicating the text. The result is a somewhat vague and short list of "requirements." Three major objectives must be satisfied:

> Operational procedures must be established to prevent deviations from the environmental policy and its associated objectives and targets. In other words, one cannot have a set of operational procedures that contradicts the essence of the environmental policy and objective.

To satisfy this, it is likely that "operating criteria" will have to be specified for certain procedures. In other words, operating parameters will have to be defined. This already is achieved automatically in most chemical plants, paper mills, steel plants, aluminum plants, and some foundries, for example. These industries often rely on sophisticated and very expensive software to "run" their plants. A different scenario will have to be planned for in other industries, particularly small manufacturers who may not be fully automated.

The standard attempts to include suppliers and contractors in the requirements just stated. The standard appears to be saying that an organization also should ensure that the procedures or products provided by its suppliers and contractors do not violate its environmental policy.

Emergency Preparedness and Response (No ISO 9001 Equivalent)

The title of this paragraph is self-explanatory. The organization shall periodically test, review, and revise, as necessary, its emergency preparedness and response procedures. The purpose of these reviews would be to ensure that all potential emergency situations and preventive responses have been considered.

Checking and Corrective Action

Monitoring and Measurement (ISO 9001 §4.10.5 and §4.11)

To track the performance of objectives and targets set in the environmental policy, the organization must establish and maintain a procedure to monitor, measure, and record, on a regular basis, the key characteristics of its operations and activities that have a significant impact on the environment (as defined in 4.3.6, Operational Control). This requirement is quite logical, how else can a company monitor the effective implementation of continuous environmental improvement measures?

In addition, procedural means to evaluate compliance with relevant environmental legislation and regulations must also be established (see 4.4, Environmental Management System Audit, for suggestions).

Nonconformance and Corrective and Preventive Action (ISO 9001 §4.13 and §4.14)

As with all previous paragraphs, a procedure must be established defining who bears responsibility and authority for investigating environmental nonconformances or, more precisely, nonconformance relating to the environmental management system (which could include for example, accidental spills or releases and unplanned increases in waste production).

> If the corrective and/or preventive action(s) suggest additional (or more specific) training, changes to procedures or processes (and associated training), such changes shall be implemented and recorded. Naturally, appropriate document control will follow as required. For example, obsolete procedures will have to be updated and all old documents will have to be either retrieved from all points of issue or updated.

Records (ISO 9011 §4.16)

Legible records of all activities relating to this international standard (i.e., ISO 14001) must be maintained to demonstrate conformance. A procedure will need to be written stating how records are stored, traced, disposed of, and protected against deterioration or loss. Such a procedure already may exist for companies registered to one of the ISO 9000 standards. The retention time for all records needs to be established. In the United States, the guidelines in Table 20–2 have been suggested.

Environment Management System Audit (ISO 9001 §4.1.3)

The International Chamber of Commerce defines an audit as

> [a] management tool comprising a systematic, documented, periodic and objective evaluation of how well environmental organization, management and equipment are performing with the aim of helping to safeguard the environment by: (i) facilitating management control of environmental practices; (ii) assessing compliance with company policies, which would include meeting regulatory requirements. (1993, p. 60)

The audit procedure shall ensure that the environmental management system is audited periodically.

TABLE 20–2 A Sample of Record Keeping for U.S. Environmental Compliance

Clean Water Act permit records: 3 years from date of sampling, measurement, report, or application (40 CFR 122.41 (j)(2))
Clean Air Act continuous emissions monitoring records: 2 years from the date of reporting for all measurements, source testing, performance evaluations, calibration checks, adjustments, and maintenance (40 CFR 60.7 and 60.13)
Resource Conservation and Recovery Act (RCRA) waste manifest: 3 years from date waste was accepted by the transporter (40 CFR 262.40(a))
Comprehensive Environmental Response, Compensation and Liability Act (CERCLA) emergency notification: Good practice to maintain records indefinitely
Emergency Planning and Community Right-to-Know Act (EPCRA) section 313 Toxic Release Form R reports: 3 years from date the report was due (40 CFR 372.10(a)), which is 4 years from when the releases occurred; good practice to maintain records for additional years to document reductions or defend release increases due to production increases or changes in reporting instructions
Toxic Substances Control Act (TSCA) Comprehensive Assessment Information Rule (CAIR) for importation, manufacture, or process of any of 19 substances: At least 3 years from date report is submitted (40 CFR 704.11)
Occupational Safety and Health Administration (OSHA) 200 recordable occupational injuries and illnesses and 101 supplementary information forms: At least 5 years from the date they cover (29 CFR 1904.5); recommend retention to equal the life of the facility
OSHA employee exposure and medical records: 30 years from date they cover (29 CFR 1919.20(d))

Note: Number in parentheses refers to the U.S. Code of Federal Regulations (CFR): 40 CFR means Title 40 of the Code of Federal Regulations, which is the codification of the general and permanent rules published in the *Federal Register* by the executive departments and agencies of the federal government.

Source: June C. Bolstridge, "Recordkeeping for Environmental Compliance," *Occupational Hazards*, (May 1995), pp. 77–79.

An important difference between the 9000 series and 14001 is that, unlike the 9000 series, 14001 does not require that audits be "carried by personnel independent of those having direct responsibility for the activity being audited." The purpose of environmental audits, which must be documented, is to ensure that the environmental management system addresses the requirements of the ISO 14001 standard and that it is effective. The results of these audits must be reported to management for its review (see 4.5, Management Review).

The concept of internal environmental audits has made many U.S. firms very uneasy. The general feeling is that government agencies such as the EPA will use the results of internal audits to assess additional fines. This is unlikely to happen, however, because under the new audit policy announced by the EPA in 1995, the EPA would offer "reduced penalties and a safe harbor from criminal referrals for companies that voluntarily disclose and fix identified violations found through auditing" ("Audit Privilege Is Incentive," 1995, p. 98).

Management Review

Management Review (ISO 9001 §4.1.3)

This last paragraph is an extension of the previous one in that it requires top management to periodically review the suitability, adequacy, and effectiveness of the environmental management system. The purpose of these management reviews, which must be documented, is to assess whether or not changes need to be made to the policy, objectives, or other elements of the environmental system. The continuous improvement loop is now closed.

As one reviews the five major headings of the ISO 14001 standard, one discovers that the Plan, Do, Check, Action cycle developed by Walter Shewhart during the 1930s (and reintroduced by Dr. Deming during the 1950s) has been adopted by contributors to the ISO 14001 standard. The paragraphs naturally fall into Plan (Planning), Do (Implementation and Operation), Check (Checking and Corrective Action), and Action (Management Review) categories.

The Value of 14001

Except for the real possibility of becoming yet another bureaucracy, I cannot think of any negative aspects associated with ISO 14001 certification. Certainly, some unresolved issues remain, particularly with regard to the question of equivalency. Will an ISO 14001 certificate issued in some developing country be equivalent to a 14001 certificate issued in the Netherlands, Germany, the United Kingdom, or North America? Probably not, unless, of course, the developing country has similar environmental laws and enforcement capabilities as the developing countries. This is unlikely to happen even though, in some developing countries, the ratio of environmental inspectors to industry often is higher than in the United States or European countries.[8]

Still, as with any new process, enough time will need to elapse before any significant and definite conclusions can be reached. There is no doubt that, within the next five years, the ISO 14001 standard will evolve and improve. Differences will be resolved and some of the issues raised in this and other chapters will be either eliminated or, more likely, attenuated. The ISO 14001 standard certainly is an excellent system to bring about global environmental management awareness; it is flexible and easily adaptable to a multitude of situations. Most important, it is not, nor should it be, threatening. The standard will provide a common global reference for environmental management that can be adapted to the respective needs of each country. One of its most important virtues is that ISO 14001 allows each country to adopt the standard according to its current economic needs and limitations. One final appealing feature of 14001 is that, within these national constraints, certification is achievable by all large and small companies.

As Joe Cascio noted:

> ISO 14001 embodies a new approach to environmental protection. In contrast to the prevailing command, control, and punish model, it chal-

lenges each organization to take stock of its environmental aspects, establish its own objectives and targets, commit itself to effective and reliable processes and continual improvement, and brings all employees and managers into a system of shared and enlightened awareness and personal responsibility for the environmental performance of the organization. (1995, p. 24; Cascio chairs the U.S. technical advisory group to ISO TC 207)

Notes

1. In their eagerness to be recognized as environmental leaders, a few companies throughout the world, as early as 1994, already were achieving registration to the near equivalent, but more demanding, British Standard 7750: Environmental Management System (issued by the British Standard Institution in 1992). The rationale for such a strategy was that, when the ISO 14001 standard was published in 1996, these "leaders" rapidly could switch or upgrade (actually downgrade since 7750 is a bit more demanding than 14001) their (BS 7750) certificate to an ISO 14001 certificate.
2. Numerous books have been written about the ISO 9000 series. My own contribution includes the following titles: *ISO 9000: Preparing for Registration* (1992); *Implementing the ISO 9000 Series* (1993), *ISO 9000 and the Service Sector* (1994), and *ISO 9000 for Small Business* (1995).
3. The value of self-declaration is questionable, and it is likely that the market will request third-party certification.
4. The opening paragraph of ISO 14001 reads as follows:

   Organizations of all kinds are increasingly concerned to achieve and demonstrate sound environmental performance by controlling the impact of their activities, product or services on the environment, taking into account their environmental policy and objectives. They do so in the context of increasingly stringent legislation, the development of economic policies and other measures to foster environmental protection, and a general growth of concern from interested parties about environmental matters including *sustainable development*. (Introduction to ISO 14001, ISO/DIS 14001, p. 4, emphasis added)

5. The requirement for documentation was not included in the February version of the draft document, perhaps an oversight.
6. Some examples would include reducing hazardous waste by 35% compared to 1990 levels; reducing toxic air emissions by 60% compared to 1987 levels by 1993; phasing out chlorofluorocarcons (CFCs) by 2000 at the latest, and so forth (see Smart, 1992, p. 189).
7. *Environmental performance* is defined as "Measurable results of the environmental management system, related to an organization's control of its

environmental aspects, based on its environmental policy, objectives and targets" (ISO 14001 definition 3.8).

8. In the state of Sao Paulo, Brazil, officials at the state environmental agency cited as many as 300 inspectors for approximately 40,000 industries, or 3 inspectors per 40 factories—not a bad ratio. I have read of similar ratios for Thailand. Of course, ratios mean nothing if there is no enforcement.

References

"Audit Privilege Is Incentive for Environmental Compliance." *Occupational Hazards* (May 1995), p. 98.

Birchard, Bill. "By the Numbers." *Tomorrow* (1995), pp. 52–53.

Cascio, Joe. "The Carrot Is Sweeter Than the Stick." *International Environmental Systems Update* 2, no. 111 (1995), p. 24.

Greeno, J. Ladd, Gilbert S. Hedstrom, and Maryanne DiBerto. *Environmental Auditing: Fundamentals and Techniques.* Center for Environmental Assurance, Arthur D. Little, Inc., New York, NY, 1985.

International Chamber of Commerce. *Environmental Auditing* [Paris, 1989]. Quoted in David Owen, "Emerging Green Agenda: A Role for Accounting," in *Business and the Environment. Implication of the New Environmentalism*, ed. Denis Smith. New York: St. Martin's Press, 1993.

Lamprecht, James. *ISO 9000: Preparing for Registration.* New York: Marcel Dekker ASQC Press, 1992.

Lamprecht, James. *Implementing the ISO 9000 Series.* New York: Marcel Dekker, 1993.

Lamprecht, James. *ISO 9000 and the Service Sector.* Milwaukee: ASQC Quality Press, 1994.

Lamprecht, James. *ISO 9000 for Small Business.* Milwaukee: ASQC Quality Press, 1995.

Makower, Joe. *The E-Factor: The Bottom-Line Approach to Environmentally Responsible Business.* New York: A Plume Book, 1994.

Rogers, Bryant. "Green Management Equals Profit." *Energy and Environmental Management,* (1995).

Smart, Bruce. *Beyond Compliance: A New Industry View of the Environment.* Washington, DC: World Resources Institute, 1992.

CHAPTER **21**

ISO 14001 for the Environment and Your Bottom Line

Jim Hart
Napier University, Edinburgh, Scotland

Introduction

Achieving ISO 14001 accreditation does not ensure anything other than the ownership of a certificate and an entry in the profit and loss account relating to expenses incurred.

Fortunately, it also is possible to use an environmental management system (EMS) to ensure that the environmental impact of your products is reduced and profitability increased. At least two advantages accrue from pursuing these objectives in parallel. First, linking the environment to the bottom line can bring environmental management issues to the heart of business decision making. Second, continuing to focus on reducing the environmental impacts will enable a company to demonstrate the *continual improvement*[1] required by ISO 14001.

In a recent survey (IEM, 1998) in the United Kingdom, 95% of respondents cited "cost savings and improved management control" as benefits sought from certification to ISO 14001; so it would be natural to include environmental costing in an EMS to promote and monitor progress. In the same survey, 84% were looking to ISO 14001 as a means to "meeting customer expectations." We can assume that organizations could use ISO 14001 for this purpose only by improving their environmental performance.

Environment Focus

Organizations can aim to achieve their objectives in environmental management through addressing the environmental aspects[2] of their activities directly (this section) and through the reduction of costs. The latter topic is explored in more detail in a later section of this chapter. We begin by looking at some key steps to creating an EMS that will deliver environmental improvements.

Environmental Assessment—A Crucial First Step

If an environmental assessment gives an inadequate picture of a company's interaction with the environment, then any environmental management successes that follow cannot be expected to match the effort put into achieving them.

There is no alternative to applying effort and expertise to the assessment. Most EMS software packages include a user interface for the assessment, but this does not save the user from gathering data and making informed judgments about the significance of environmental aspects and impact. These judgments will rely on a good understanding of the interaction between the environment and the organization's input and output. Furthermore, the user must consider this interaction in parallel with the unique local environmental conditions that apply to the organization.

In short, to carry out a successful assessment, much data will have to be collected and analyzed by an environmental expert.

Objectives and Targets

A good environmental assessment assists in setting relevant objectives and targets for improvement. However, managers must be careful to avoid falling into traps such as setting unambitious targets or targets with no consideration of the financial implications.

When setting targets, we must consider the technological, financial, and organizational changes that might be necessary to reduce each environmental impact relative to output.

In many cases, significant financial gains can be made with little organizational disturbance (typically, reducing energy consumption, reducing waste output, or using cleaner technologies to eliminate the need for end-of-pipe treatment). In such cases, we can look for major improvements. In other cases, we have to consider the likely costs and benefits associated with the targets. Undertaking full cost-benefit analyses of each proposed target might be onerous, but we at least should consider what the costs and benefits could be—including some of the wider issues.

Environmental Impact of Products

ISO 14001 requires companies to consider the environmental aspect associated with the organization's "activities, products or services." There is a natural tendency to focus primarily on manufacturing activities, because they are more susceptible to visible day-to-day managerial control than the products themselves. However, as Figure 21–1 illustrates, manufacturing can be the least significant life-cycle stage of a product.

While it may be appropriate for some manufacturers to concentrate exclusively on their activities (the "manufacture" bars in Figure 21–1), others—particu-

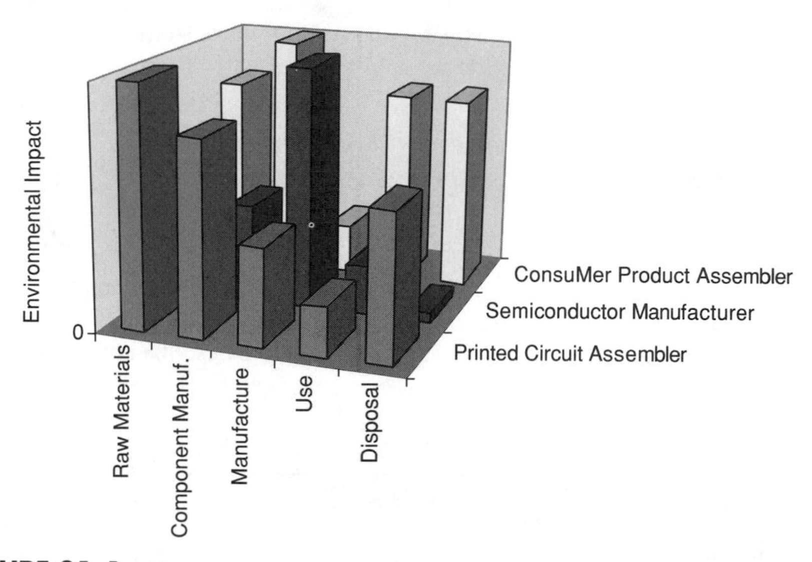

FIGURE 21–1 How manufacturers of different electronic products might view the environmental impact (dimensionless) of the five main life-cycle stages of their products. For simplicity, each bar includes an impact related to the transport of material to that life-cycle stage.

larly assemblers—can address their most significant forms of impact only by reducing the impact from the other four life-cycle stages.

Reducing the Environmental Impact of Products

There are two approaches to reducing the life-cycle impact of a product. The most common method used in EMS is to pressure suppliers into reducing their environmental impact; for instance, by requiring them to go for ISO 14001 themselves. This approach includes an element of buck passing, but it is reasonable to expect suppliers to aspire to the same standards you set for yourself. It is easy to take this approach, but rewards will be correspondingly slight and can relate only to the upstream life-cycle stages.

A more useful approach is to design types of life-cycle environmental impact out of the product. This implies that improving product design for the environment (DfE) should be an integral part of an EMS. Eagan and Pferdehirt (1998) have suggested that the objective-setting stage of the EMS is the appropriate route for DfE into EMS.

We can also set targets for improvements in product design. This would require definition of the environmental impact of our products. Although a full life-cycle assessment of all products would be inappropriate (to say the least), some analysis of the environmental characteristics of the product group would enable us to design a set of environmental indicators for our products. Among others, these might include

- Product weight.
- Percentage of recycled plastic.
- Disassembly time (as one indicator of recyclability).
- Operating power.
- Product lifetime.

Environmental managers would weight the parameters according to their importance and work with designers to set improvement targets in subsequent designs. Some issues relating to one such application are described by Regnier and Hoffmann (1998).

Environmental Costing in EMS

The purpose of integrating environmental costing into an EMS is twofold. First, it is to demonstrate the positive effect of the EMS on the bottom line to those people with influence in an organization. It's no secret that environmental managers have justified their existence by highlighting the financial savings that result from their initiatives. In the electronics industry, for instance, better management of solder paste storage and application by some companies has permitted savings on waste management and on the paste itself. Second, bringing costing into EMS can provide incentive for continual environmental improvements.

Several varieties of environmental costing and accounting have been described, but for the purposes described here, the results of such costing should be expressed in terms of the costs incurred by the company through environmentally damaging activities. Putting a cost on the damage done to the environment and society by the company's activities is not part of this process—such information could only duplicate the environmental assessment, since it relates to environmental impact and not to the bottom line.

Identifying Environmental Costs

Environmental costing within an EMS can take on a number of forms. At a basic level, it is about discovering the expenditure (related to output) on a number of items of environmental consequence, such as

- Energy consumption.
- Waste disposal.
- Cleaning of environmental discharges (including labor and equipment costs).
- Pollution permits and any related monitoring and inspection.
- Likely end-of-life product costs (i.e., the cost of any recycling obligations).

- Reagents (water, solvents, etc.) used in product manufacture but not incorporated into the product.
- Opportunity cost associated with quality failures: rejects generate many costs, which can include raw materials lost, waste management, the production effort invested in the reject (machine time, labor, etc.), and lost sales revenue.
- Transport costs, including distribution and business travel.

At this level, we would decide what costs to include and total expenditure on those items. An objective of reducing this expenditure relative to output could be defined and reinforced with targets relating to each area of significant environmental cost.

Although we can expect a positive correlation between environmental cost savings and reductions in environmental impact, this will not apply to every change that occurs. Because the environmental cost of an item depends on price as much as it does on quantity, a decrease in the energy bill might mask an increase in energy consumption. This is why driving down environmental costs is complementary to the aim of reducing environmental impact rather than an alternative to it.

Environmental Cost Allocation

The approach just outlined can be enlightening, but we may need some assistance in environmental cost management. The key to improving the quality of the information provided is through accurately allocating costs to the products and activities that cause them. Activity-based costing (ABC; Innes and Mitchell, 1998) is the standard-bearer for this task, but we can interpret ABC broadly as a flexible approach toward improved cost allocation.

Traditionally, product costing involves a crude division of production and administrative overhead among the products in question. Often, this fails to take account of the differing quantities of resources demanded as overhead by different products and processes. This is an important point, because environmental costs generally are included in production or administrative overhead.

A mechanism for allocating environmental costs to products is shown in Figure 21–2. We start by dividing environmental costs among various cost pools of activities or groups of activities; for instance, waste management costs might be divided according to the proportion of total waste that arises from the activities in each cost pool.

This accomplished, we transfer the costs from the cost pools to the products by identifying cost drivers for each cost pool. A cost driver shows the demand that products make on the activities in a cost pool. For instance, machine time per unit of output might be seen as the best way of allocating costs from a group of manufacturing activities to products, whereas the number of purchase orders generated by each product might be seen as a fair indication of the costs coming from a pool of administrative activities.

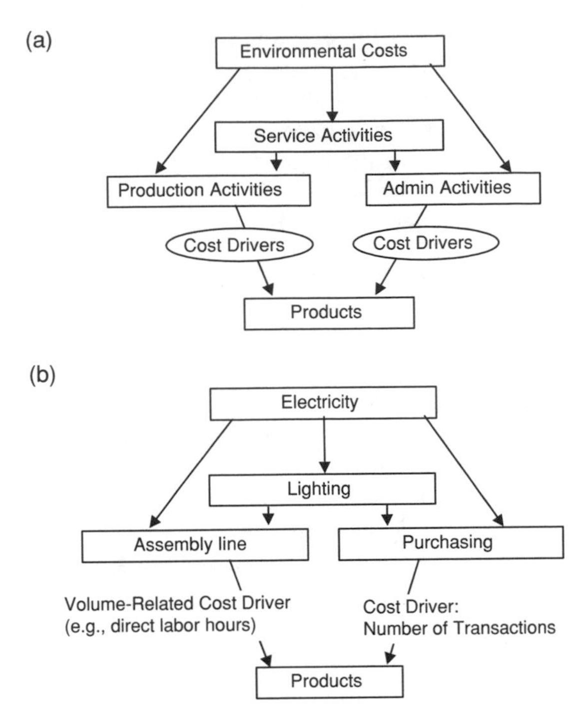

FIGURE 21–2 The allocation of environmental costs to activity-based cost pools and then to products: (a) the general case, and (b) the example of electricity consumption and just three of the many possible cost pools. Note that costs can be allocated to cost pools by way of other cost pools, such as "lighting" in (b).

Using Improved Costing Data

Information from allocating costs to activities can be used to highlight the sources of environmental costs and to find ways of reducing these costs. We can aim for improvements by focusing on the environmental aspect and impact that incurs the greatest costs, or we can focus on the environmental costs themselves by setting cost reduction targets for any activities where this is appropriate.

Allocating activity costs to products provides improved product costing data. Therefore, a relevant EMS objective might be to gather enough data to review the costs of manufacturing each product. From that point, one can make decisions as to whether the prices charged customers and, therefore, the budgeted output are appropriate.

If, in a tool factory, for instance, we discover that chain saws are being cross-subsidized by pitchforks, any price change to correct the imbalance should affect demand in such a way that there is a switch toward producing more pitchforks and fewer chain saws. An automatic cut in the environmental cost per dollar of turnover will follow as well as an increase in profitability. Any price corrections arising from ABC analysis should reduce overall environmental costs per unit of output.

Limitations to Cost Allocation

Introducing ABC switches attention from one imperfect system to another. We cannot precisely allocate all costs to products; some uncertainty always will continue over key issues such as the selection of cost pools and drivers.

The organization must determine whether ABC is appropriate to its situation and implement it to the extent that fulfills its needs. One study (Cobb, Innes, and Mitchell, 1992) found that most firms implementing ABC use the system primarily for cost management; many did not implement a system for product costing. This limited approach would be enough to facilitate the monitoring and control of environmental costs and still would be in the spirit of an EMS.

EMS and Decision Making

If an EMS has become part of a company's culture, then environmental managers will play a role in capital investment decisions and strategic thinking. Decision making in most companies is dictated by factors that demonstrably and quantifiably influence the balance sheet and cash flow; analysis of less tangible environmental costs and benefits is likely to be of secondary interest. Therefore, the first task for environmental managers is to reveal the quantifiable environmental costs that might be hidden from others involved in the decision-making process. It is important to take a realistic view of future costs and benefits and their present value. Environmental managers usually will want to argue against the use of a high interest rate in such analysis, as high interest rates tend to count against projects that require investing now to achieve benefits in the future.

Second, environmental managers must decide whether to quantify intangible environmental costs, such as

- Public relations value—the effect on future sales and recruitment.
- Costs associated with expected environmental legislation.
- Clean-up costs that might occur in the future either through normal operations or as a result of accidents.

Even when these costs reduce profitability in the short term (e.g., when consumers desert a polluter following bad publicity), the scale of the costs will not be predictable; and many such costs will be impossible to anticipate at all (e.g., accidents).

In other words, environmental managers should back up their arguments for change with an outline of the possible costs and benefits in this category and be ready to suggest scenarios in which environmentally damaging decisions might incur costs in the future. However, in the early years of an EMS, at least, detailed financial projections may not be worth the effort, since any numbers presented will be debatable.

The Future

Getting an EMS to the state outlined in this chapter is just the start. A company that gets this far will have become more ecoefficient, but sustainability still will be some way off.

An approach to sustainability can come only through rapid and continual improvement in the environmental profile of products and services, and these improvements can come only through innovation. If this evolution is to be assisted by an EMS, then it will need to be dynamic, increasingly acting to foster innovation in product design, materials, logistics, and marketing techniques.

In this chapter, I have not advocated costing "externalities," but in the future, governments may increasingly see it as their role to charge companies for their external costs through the tax system (e.g., through a "carbon tax"). If such a trend does evolve, then companies will need to investigate full environmental costing, as actions that cause environmental impact—by definition—also will have an impact on the bottom line.

Notes

1. ISO 14001 does not define environmental standards that an organization must achieve. Instead, organizations must set their own targets that will enable them to achieve continual improvement in their relationship with the environment.
2. Environmental aspects are those elements of an organization's activities, products, and services that can interact with the environment; the impact is the resulting changes to the environment.

References

Cobb, I., J. Innes, and F. Mitchell. *Activity-Based Costing—Problems in Practice*. London: CIMA, 1992.

Eagan, P., and W. Pferdehirt. "Using the Objectives Development Process of an Environmental Management System as an Opportunity to Achieve Design for the Environment." Proceedings of the 1998 IEEE International Symposium on Electronics and the Environment, Oakbrook, IL, pp 186–189.

IEM. "ISO 14001 Survey Results." *Journal of the Institute of Environmental Management* 5, no. 4 (October 1998).

Innes, J., and F. Mitchell. *A Practical Guide to Activity-Based Costing*. London: CIMA, 1998.

Regnier, E., and W. F. Hoffmann, III. "Uncertainty in Environmentally Conscious Design." Proceedings of the 1998 IEEE International Symposium on Electronics and the Environment, Oakbrook, IL, pp 207–212.

CHAPTER **22**

Beyond ISO 14000: ST Microelectronics as a Case Study in Environmental Leadership

CAROL BROWN
ST Microelectronics

Nearly a decade ago, the leadership of ST Microelectronics, then known as SGS-Thomson, made a fateful commitment to include the protection of environmental quality as one of its primary business principles. This single decision propelled the company into an uncharted, difficult, and ultimately rewarding journey into a new way of doing business. The commitment meant that, while the rest of the industry was dreaming about green engineering, ST Microelectronics already had put its plan into action. When ISO 14000 was still in its charter stages, ST already had adopted the 16 principles for environmental management of the ICC business charter for sustainable development and was well on its way to reach the goals laid out in its decalogue, its ten commandments of environmental sustainability. In fact, the meeting of the requirements for ISO 14000 was a side effect, a by-product, of meeting these internal goals. The other, even more surprising by-product of these efforts was a significant increase in productivity and profitability.

It was not the easiest of all possible routes. ST set for itself much more rigorous standards than those required for full compliance with *all* national and international regulations, in *every* country its manufacturing facilities were built. With 17 main factories in eight countries on four continents, the body of rules that must be followed is so complex that they often create a confusing, heterogeneous, and sometimes contradictory scenario. This means that if, for example, Germany has the most stringent regulations on packing of goods and requires the adoption of fully recyclable boxes, ST will adopt the same recyclable boxes throughout the company, even in those countries where nonrecyclable boxes still are acceptable.

Experience has shown that it was the right choice. A leading corporation must set an example as a responsible citizen in respecting the right of everyone to a safe environment.

The Bottom Line

More to the bottom line, companies that independently and voluntarily make their own activities conform to increasingly stringent environmental protection standards have an advantage over those who do so only when they are forced to by the law. Moreover, environmentally friendly technologies and processes also are leading-edge ones as well as more efficient and less costly.

Amazingly enough, economic and ecological concerns are not mutually exclusive. From a pragmatic perspective, the sole scope for any business enterprise is that of creating wealth; that is, it must operate as a resource amplifier. It's as simple as that: You feed in a certain amount of resources and the output must be greater than the input. If this is not true, then it is not a business enterprise, it is a parasite. Therefore, a business must amplify the financial resources given by shareholders, by making the best use of them, through a complex industrial process that includes other resources, both material and human.

Within this economic reality, caring for the environment is not only compatible with business objectives but also yields a competitive advantage. Moving beyond a fix-it-right-before-it-breaks mode to anticipate national or local regulations will move ST farther and faster in the direction of becoming a company that is "environmentally neutral."

In a recent speech, Pasquale Pistorio, president and CEO of ST, put it this way:

> To do this, we are adopting inside our corporation a set of specific norms that are tougher than those imposed by external authorities. Once again, in choosing this strategy we are fully convinced that this is the right thing to do, not just for ethical and social reasons but also because, in anticipating the inevitable evolution of environmental legislation, we can certainly be rewarded by an additional competitive advantage.

Show Me the Money

Throughout the years that ST has been working to green the environment, its efforts consistently have added "green" to its bottom line. For example, investment in energy conservation technologies has cut power consumption from 680 kWh per thousand dollars of revenue to 550 kWh today. Water consumption was reduced by 11.3 cubic meters per thousand dollars, to 7.8 cubic meters. Finally, in terms of waste, the amount sent to be dumped was cut from 71% to 35%, and total corporate paper consumption has fallen from 1,200 tons to 800 tons a year.

Taking What's Been Learned

The most important lesson learned is that fighting pollution has to be taken seriously. When faced with this kind of problem, a solution cannot be imposed;

rather, it's a process of making suggestions and encouraging people to get involved. Initiatives may come from the board, the CEO, or the stockholders, but the work is done by the staff, the employees, the managers. Corporate headquarters does not, and cannot, control everything. The priority becomes encouraging local initiative and creating a network to ensure unity among all sites. Environmental champions are chosen from each site to develop exchanges between the sites, entities, and groups, so that solutions can be shared and knowledge broadened.

And Running with It

To further this exchange, ST intends to set up a database via the company's intranet and open forums so that people can exchange skills, knowledge, and experience. A steering committee is being created for this purpose. Currently, the company is identifying the issues presented by our "global" culture when faced with the environmental question.

Consistent with the total quality management principles of continuous improvement, the environmental mission of the company is "To eliminate or minimize the impact of our processes and products on the environment, maximizing the use of recyclable or reusable materials and adopting, as much as possible, renewable sources of energy, striving towards a sustainable development."

Rust Never Sleeps

Another thing that ST has learned is that continuous improvement also means one cannot retire as the granddaddy of corporate environmental champions and rest on one's awards. Now that most of the goals have been reached, what's next? What's next is a second version of the decalogue, committed to the goals of the first, but adapted to the years 2000–2010. Future local and global restraints such as climatic change and water-related issues will be taken into account.

One of the changes will involve global-warming gas emissions. Carbon dioxide emissions will be measured to reduce them fivefold compared to 1990 by the year 2010. Likewise, a tenfold reduction in emissions of PFCs used in front-end processes is planned, compared to 1994. Alternative energy sources such as wind power, photovoltaics, and fuel cells should represent 15% of ST's energy resources by 2010. As for waste, 80% of packaging should be recycled or reused by the year 2000 and 95% in 2005. Finally, an "environmental accounting" system will be developed to have all the necessary objective information for calculating how profitable investments will be and to help choose industrial processes.

For example, if the goal is to eliminate emissions of acid gases, gas-washing machines (scrubbers) are needed, which represent an investment, to reduce pollution. All machines are assessed according to their impact on the environment. The same goes for waste treatment.

Overall, ST's goal is to reduce total power consumption 60% by 2010, in relation to production value. In addition, through recycling and substitution as well as by reducing consumption, the consumption of the most frequently used chemicals in the company should be cut 5% a year. Finally, ST aims to maintain the renewal of the EMAS validation and ISO 14001 certification for industrial plants.

Back to the Beginning

From the five-plus years that ST Micro has been "walking the walk," it has learned many difficult and rewarding lessons. Perhaps one of the most important lessons it can share with individuals and organizations considering a green path can be summarized this way: The protection of the environment, the sustainability of a process, and the success of a business are interdependent—an ecological system of sorts. As such, each part must be constantly reevaluated for its impact on the system as a whole. ISO 14000 is simply an excellent measurement and a workable method from without.

Section IV
Visions for a New Future

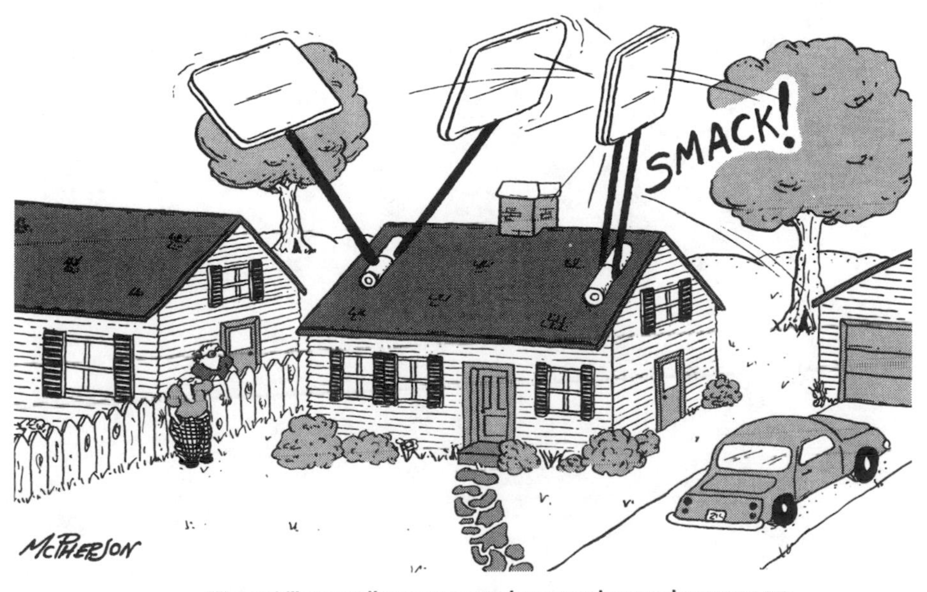

"These kill seven times as many bugs per hour as bug zappers and use only a third the electricity."

Introduction: A Day in the Life . . . Circa 2005

LEE H. GOLDBERG
Chip Center Magazine

Often, it's hard to see the future in facts, figures, and the small details that make up the whole picture. This is especially true with new stuff, things out of our normal realm of experience. Fortunately, engineers usually have good imaginations and need only a few small hints to start scanning the horizon themselves and inventing their own version of a better tomorrow. To get you in the mood for the next section, I'd like to invite you to spend a few minutes visiting one such possible future, set in a time not too far away.

Another Manic Monday

It's a brisk morning in January, and the recently installed rooftop solar panels on the house have just begun to pump power back into the grid as you start the coffee. Your comm-pad has been downloading and stands ready to read you the news and selected e-mail while you fix the kids' breakfast and get ready to head for work. Today is one of the "in-house" days, where you and your design team meet face to face at the design center. You get together like this about once a week to hash out the issues of your latest project that don't lend themselves to teleconferencing between home offices.

With breakfast done and the kids on the way to school, you finish getting dressed. You grab the comm-pad and head for the garage. Once in the car, you punch an access code into the dashboard keypad and wait a couple of seconds for the fuel cells to come up to full power before easing into the street. Before pulling out, you slip the comm-pad into the dash cradle so it can read you the rest of your news and e-mail on the way to the plant.

Not Bad for an Electric

As you reach the highway on-ramp, you punch the accelerator. The hybrid vehicle accelerates sharply as a small set of batteries kicks in to augment the fuel cells' 20-kW output. "Not too bad for an electric," you smile to yourself. Although it didn't cost much more than the mid-sized, steel-bodied gasoline burner you had before, this composite-bodied machine is much quieter, faster, and more comfortable. And it costs a lot less to run. Best of all, this sucker's loaded with electronics.

Your comm-pad jacks directly into the vehicle's local network, allowing you to use the on-board displays and databases. At your command, the pad begins reading you the morning's e-mail and faxes over the car's stereo system. When your mail has an attached graphic, you can choose to display it on the in-dash nav-screen or on the heads-up display in the windshield. While you scan your e-mail, the pad uses the car's cellular link to download your voice mail from work.

By the time you arrive at the plant, the e-mail sent by your teammates has brought you pretty much up to speed. Once parked, you hook your car up to a fuel line and an electrical feed coming out of a small box at the front of your parking slot. You swipe your smart card through a reader in the box and it begins to feed natural gas to your car's fuel cell. The attached cable draws off its steady 20 kW output, feeding it into the local power grid while crediting your account for the wholesale value of the electricity. Your car has begun to pay for itself as you walk into the cafeteria to greet the gang.

Over coffee, everybody quickly reviews the situation. It looks like the full-up simulation of the controller system you're developing has uncovered a few minor software bugs and a compatibility problem with some of its external interfaces. With the whole team in one place today, it should be easy to troubleshoot these problems and start on plans for production.

The pressure is on to get the controller into production. Demand for these new systems is high because of the potential energy savings they achieve in most industrial applications. Thanks to the new global warming legislation, manufacturers are thrice motivated by potential energy cost savings, tax breaks, and the increasing pressure on businesses to report their environmental performance to customers and the public.

Jocks, Weenies, and Greenies

When the team hits the lab, the hardware jocks hunker down with the software weenies and begin a code and electrical debug session on the breadboard unit. Meanwhile, you sit down with the mechanical and packaging group, the manufacturing engineer, and your environmental assurance specialist, otherwise known as a *greenie*, to discuss the issues surrounding tool-up for production. While environmental compatibility is part of everybody's job, the team's greenie acts as an information resource for the rest of the team. She also handles some of the more complicated paperwork that coordinates the environmental and quality-control aspects of the project.

Many of the environmental issues already have been resolved during the first part of the design phase. For example, the unit's case and subassemblies have been through the manufacturability review as well as the recyclability analysis. Although the parts were carefully designed to incorporate the quickest, lowest-cost assembly techniques, the recyclability analysis software fine-tuned them even further, as the "mechs" and greenies made sure the product could be quickly taken apart for salvage at the end of its life. Already, the "green screen" process has cut another three steps and 95 seconds from the assembly process.

Green: Just Part of the Job

Since most of the green, manufacturing, and quality issues were handled as part of the design process, this review is mostly a formality. It's a final check to see that nothing has been missed. The first part of the session does uncover a few things, like a plastic part that does not yet have a molded-in material classification code, an essential feature for recycling.

The mechanical model's first pass through the analysis package verifies that all four types of plastics used in the housing are low-toxicity materials and easily recyclable. The analysis also provides several options for selecting nontoxic, mechanically compatible finishes and EMI coatings that won't interfere with the recycling process. Running the mechanical model through a second part of the software package reveals that two recently changed structural parts now contain mixed materials which cannot be recycled easily. You red flag these items for later action and continue with the review.

Component sourcing is the next topic on the agenda. While cost, availability, and reliability top the list of prerequisites, each component also is screened for criteria like recyclability, energy efficiency, hazardous-material content, and other environmental criteria. This information is fed into a large database, which compiles a multidimensional "environmental index" for the whole product.

The scores from this index give the team, management, and potential customers a rough idea of how closely the product meets the environmental objectives set forth each year, along with the product's sales and revenue projections. You and the greenies carefully review an expanded spreadsheet of each index, looking for "hot spots" that could drag down the overall score.

A materials engineer solves one such problem by specifying a new additive-type manufacturing process for the PC boards used in most of the unit's electronics. The recently developed dry lithographic technique places metal directly on a board only where it's needed, rather than starting with a fully copper-plated board and removing most of the copper with toxic, dangerous acids. The team enters the new values into the database and continues.

The next portion of the "scrub" is not completely automated and takes a couple of hours. Finally, it's over and everybody gets up for a break. You announce that you're buying the coffee.

It's all smiles now. They all know that by finding substitutes for the PCB and a handful of other parts with more "friendly" characteristics, the team has raised the product's environmental index score several points. That design tweak was enough to almost ensure everybody a performance bonus at the end of the year.

A cup of coffee and a stale pastry later, everybody settles back down to work. Most of the electrical and software team is busy testing a couple of power-conservation algorithms they've been developing, while some of the others pin down the last bugs in the I/O section. You grab a chair with the mechanical types again and take notes as they enter the last phase of the component sourcing review.

Mining the Scrap Heap

The unit's power supply and several other basic components have been selected from a preferred menu of standard, prequalified models used across many of the company's product lines. In addition to the economies of scale this affords, it allows the reuse of these components after they're extracted from older products, tested, and reconditioned. As an added bonus, the 10–15% of each unit's mass currently rolled back into other products dramatically reduces the cost of recycling and disposal at the end of the product's life.

While most of the reclaimed power supplies, displays, cooling fans, I/O boards, and the like are destined for use as field-service spares, the company is just beginning to experiment with a process for recertifying them as new. The initial results look good, with a cost savings of over 50%, even with a rigorous reconditioning and screening process. One pilot program under way involves reusing the computer motherboards reclaimed from an earlier top-of-the-line product as a controller subsystem in next year's mid-tier models.

Things roll along until a bit past noon, when the review is pretty well complete. As you stop for lunch, most of the team heads off to the cafeteria for a well-deserved break. Everybody will need to be rested before pushing on into the extended-service-life-plan (ESLP) review.

Most of the afternoon will be spent with a "red team" assembled from management, senior QC people, and selected members of other design teams. Their job will be to take a close look at the provisions you've built into the controller for maintenance and future upgrades. With a minimum service-life target of ten years, they have to be sure the controller can operate reliably for that long. It also must be able to receive upgrades, many of which have not yet been designed. It's going to be a tough afternoon.

Although fairly new, this part of the review process already is having a major effect on profits. Back around 2001, management realized that, rather than concentrate on selling the highest number of units per year, it could do better by keeping existing products in the field longer. Both customer and producer are beginning to benefit from products that easily can be upgraded as the user's needs change. The slight dip in unit sales has been more than offset by the steady stream of upgrade hardware and software, as well as the very lucrative maintenance contracts that often accompany them.

Is It Worth the Trouble?

Relaxing after lunch, you kick back in your seat for a bit and think about the weekend. You look out the atrium windows at the fresh snow in the distant hills and think a cross-country ski outing at the nearby state forest would be nice. Then you remember that when you started working here back in 1999, the mountains were a pretty rare sight. Six years ago, the haze and pollution were pretty thick most of the time. You felt lucky to see the tall buildings at the edge of town less than a dozen miles away. Now, you get to see the peaks about as often as the weather cooperates. "Hmmm . . .", you muse to yourself, "maybe this 'green' stuff is actually making a difference after all?"

It's quite likely that half or more of the things presented in this story will find their way into our everyday lives later than 2005, or perhaps never at all. Nevertheless, it's a good picture of what could happen if we apply a little vision to our market projections and work with regulators to develop a "commonsense" approach to environmental goals. In fact, all the technology described in this piece—including the hybrid-electric vehicle—already is available or under development.

Ideally, the parts of the book you've read so far have shown you what's possible today. The next chapter is intended to open you up to a few of the more interesting and forward-looking ideas I've bumped into over the course of putting this book together.

While some of the things you're going to read next may appear to be less reality based than the short work of science fiction I've just presented, I wouldn't be surprised to find that they have become part of our work, home, or play a decade from now. After all, the real business of engineers is translating dreams into reality.

Acknowledgment

Adapted from *Electronic Design Magazine*'s January 12, 1999, forecast on green engineering.

Part VIII

Wild Ideas and Possible Futures

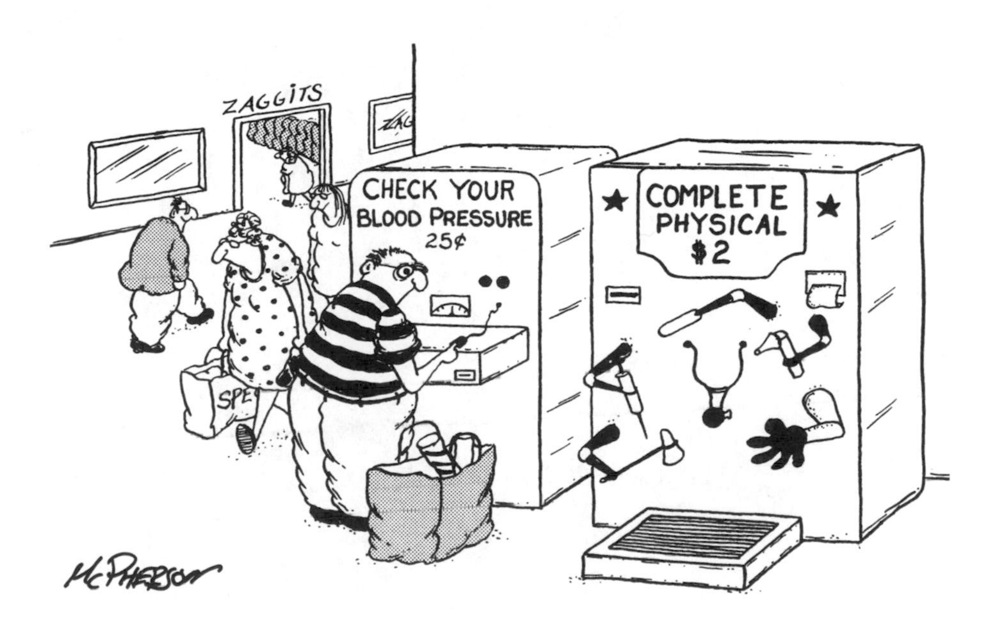

CHAPTER 23

Designing a Better Tomorrow Today with Self-Disassembling Electronics

JOSEPH CHIODO AND ERIC H. BILLETT
Brunel University, Surrey, United Kingdom

Introduction

Industrial recycling is a practice of growing importance. In addition to any altruistic motivations, manufacturers are facing impending take-back legislation in Europe, which most likely will be implemented by 2004, with North America and other regions not too far behind. Today, however, cost constraints limit the number of products that can be recycled. Since the labor for disassembly represents a large fraction of the cost of recycling electronics, the concept of products that take themselves apart is intriguing. If an efficient, inexpensive method of self-disassembly becomes commercially practical, we could significantly increase the volume of recyclable material used in manufacturing new products.

The use of active disassembly using smart materials (ADSM) is an alternative with the potential to be used to enable a wide variety of consumer electronics that could be actively or self-disassembled nondestructively on the same generic dismantling line. The designer can incorporate smart materials early in the design process, ensuring that at its end of life (EOL), perhaps five to ten years later, the product contains all the necessary information and mechanisms to disassemble itself following a single generic triggering event such as heat. It will not be necessary for the dismantler to have a record or plans of the design for the EOL disassembly. In theory, products designed to actively disassemble themselves would need only minor changes to their internal structures to allow releasable fasteners or actuators to be incorporated into their assembly. As we shall see, this novel form of disassembly has shown considerable promise during initial tests on the macro- and subassemblies of consumer electronic products.

Smart Materials

Currently two basic families of smart materials lend themselves to active disassembly: groups of metallic materials known as *shape-memory alloys* (SMAs) and *shape-memory plastics* or *polymers* (SMPs). Below a certain "transformation temperature" (Tx; Gilbertson, 1994a, pp. 2–7), they behave as relatively standard engineering materials and can be used in all normal ways. Above this critical temperature, however, they undergo a very specific shape change that can (if required) be reversible if the temperature is lowered again. This change of shape above a critical temperature can form the basis of active disassembly.

While metals can generate a significant force as they change shape, plastics do not. On the other hand, metals are more expensive at present. Depending on material composition and treatment, Tx can be adjusted within a surprisingly wide range of temperatures. Proper use of different activation temperatures would enable a designer to create a product that could take itself apart sequentially in an orderly manner using a stepped thermal environment.

The smart materials considered in this study are SMA alloys of nickel-titanium (NiTi) and copper-zinc-aluminum (CuZnAl) and SMP of polyurethane composition. These releasable fasteners and actuator devices have the ability to dynamically change shape at specific temperatures and thereby "split" their host candidate products' macro- and subassemblies.

Shape Memory Alloys

A small group of metals made up of two or more metallic elements with particularly remarkable shape-change and force-provision properties. As the temperature crosses or changes across a critical value (Tx), known as *Austenite finishing temperature* (Af; Higgins, 1983), they undergo a large and predictable shape change, the so-called shape-memory effect (SME).

SMAs were invented by the American military and now are used in an increasing envelope of applications, such as glasses wire frames, fighter jet couplings, PCB connector sockets, space station connectors, cell phone antennas, and some medical applications. Prices have dropped and are continuing to fall; therefore, exciting new opportunities exist for inexpensive actuators and connection in common electronic consumer products.

The important qualities of SMA from a design perspective are that they are corrosion resistant and biocompatible materials in many ways resembling stainless steel. They have the mechanical strength to form reliable fasteners, yet on exposure to Af, they will change absolutely reproducibly. The critical temperature can be placed according to the designer's choice between –190 to +190°C (–310 to +374°F). This critical transformation temperature is the point where SME in SMA occurs, As-f. It is best described in Figure 23–1.

The grids represent the crystal structure in a typical SMA, with each square having a uniform mix of the alloy's component metals. The metal deforms easily

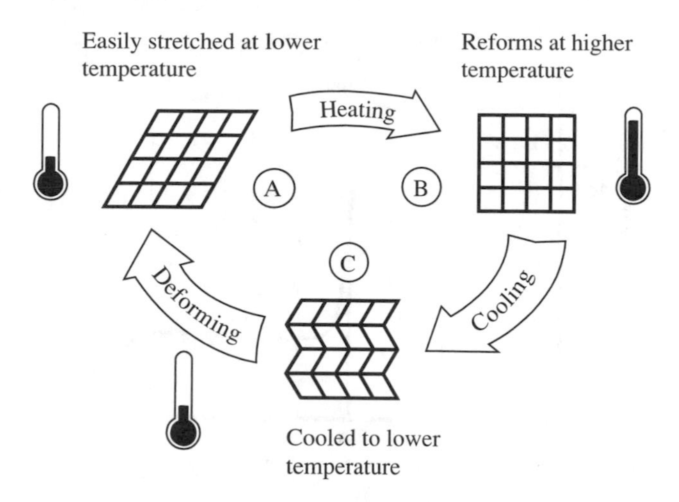

FIGURE 23–1 Mechanics of the SME for SMA.

when below its transition temperature (A) and the crystal's boundaries shift but do not suffer permanent damage. Heating the alloy to above its transition temperature causes the crystals to undergo a phase change and return to their original shape (B); they do this with a large force, several times greater than the force needed to deform them. When again cooled below the transition temperature, the phase change reverses (C) and the metal easily can be deformed once more (Gilbertson, 1994, pp. 1–3).

Shape-Memory Polymers

SMPs (Shirai and Hayashi, 1988; Gordon, 1994) are a very small group of plastics that can be formed by the normal processes, including injection molding and with properties similar to those found in polyurethane, polypropylene, and ABS.

SMP was invented in Japan and became available commercially in the United States only in 1996. It is used in the design of automatic carburetor chokes, utensil handles, medical equipment, and many other applications; more products are surfacing as it becomes commercially exploited.

The SME in SMP is different from that in SMA. The origin of the SME in SMP is not as well understood as in the case of the SMAs. What is known is that, above their transformation temperature or glass transition temperatures (Tg; Walker, 1995, pp. 479–480), SMPs loose their mechanical strength and return to their originally formed shape after external forces are removed (Figure 23–2). Unlike other polymers, SMP has a very narrow Tg range that can be specified within 1°C. It should be noted that, unlike the metals, the plastics provide no significant force accompanying this triggering procedure.

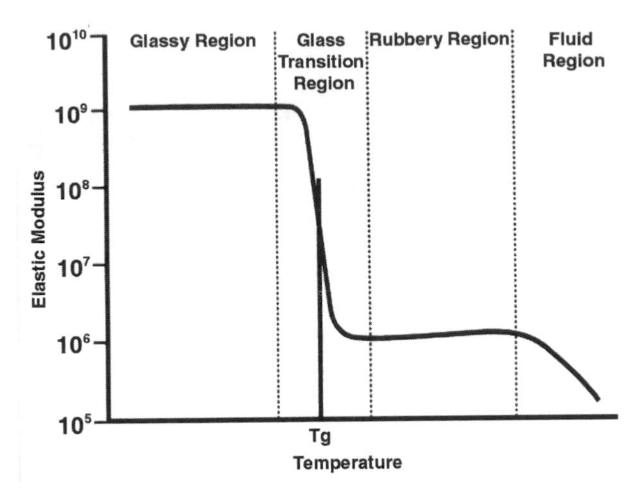

FIGURE 23–2 Glass transition (Tg): Elastic modulus versus temperature (Shirai and Hayashi, 1988).

Shape Memory Effect

SME can be categorized as one-, two-, and multiway SME. The "effect" happens in many different ways and by varying degrees. SMPs generally exhibit a multiway (metamorphic) effect (Spillman, Sirkis, and Gardiner, 1996), while SMAs generally have a one- or two-way effect.

In one-way SME (Tautzenberger, Stockel, and Wayman, 1990, p. 208), materials recover to the original form one or more times after exposure to heat. In one-way effects, the material would have to be forcibly reshaped (Higgins, 1983) to recover again.

In two-way SME (Gordon, 1990), materials can recover many times to the original form and deform again to a secondary form after exposure to a specific temperature or stimulus repeatedly. The SME cyclic values depend primarily on the material, extent of deformation, and exposure to heat.

In multiway SME, the material acts the same as in the two-way states except the material may be formable to more shapes depending on the extent of the external stimuli (heat and force). One could view the variable nature of SME in SMP as metamorphic (Spillman et al., 1996) or it can be considered a "live" material on demand.

These unique characteristics let designers use a single material to create mechanisms that deliver dynamics such as movement and force with a minimum number of parts.

Experiments with Shape-Memory Alloy Actuators

Initial experiments (1996) investigated releasing socketed integrated circuits (ICs) from printed circuit boards (PCBs) and a PCB subassembly. Further experiments attempted the disassembly of product housings. Both one- and two-way SME SMAs were used, and alloys of NiTi and CuZnAl, respectively.

The last set of experiments (1997) tested active disassembly on more than one type of product in the same dismantling facility. The products' self-disassemblies were triggered by a controlled sequence variable temperature regimen, whereby the SMA actuators' Afs were reached. These actuators then actively split apart their host products' assemblies and subassemblies at the appropriate stages.

Initial Tests on Off-the-Shelf Products

A study was conducted to demonstrate the feasibility of using SMA and SMP smart material devices in the active disassembly of consumer electronic products. For this initial investigation, a wide range of ADSM devices were retrofitted to a representative collection of off-the-shelf products, such as computer keyboards, CD players, video games, and telephones. While not all these existing designs lent themselves to easy retrofits for self-disassembly, many of them performed well or even better than expected. Even those that were not completely successful provided valuable and encouraging information for future developments.

Considerable effort was made to fully characterize the ADSM devices prior to insertion into the test articles. Nondestruction of candidate products, cost effectiveness, range of permissible ambient temperatures, and triggering temperatures are considered key parameters in this work and to be optimized in future research. Heat sources (radiation, convection, and conduction) of vector air, steam jet, infrared, and water baths were employed to provide elevated temperatures between 60–225°C (140–437°F) to raise the devices above their triggering temperatures. After the full run of experiments, observations were made detailing outline design guidelines as a starting point to the current work.

Method of SMA Experiments

Generic disassembly experiments were conducted on a very wide variety of products, ranging from cell phones to a small electronic game. The multistage hierarchical temperature experiments were conducted to demonstrate the potential of the sequence controlled self-disassembly of products. Three different design styles in 55 actuators were employed in total. Before the experiments, all the products were disassembled manually without destruction to snap fasteners or product casings. The actuators were strategically inserted into the macro- and subassemblies of the test products (see Figures 23–3 and 23–4).To allow sequential disassembly, lower actuation temperature SMA actuators were placed in the macroassemblies and higher temperature actuators in the subassemblies of the candidate products (see Table 23–1). Also noted in Table 23–1 are Afs, design types, separation techniques required and other comparative data.

On insertion of actuators in the candidate products, the entire sample base was placed in a wooden and glass chamber. The chamber then was heated with air heating

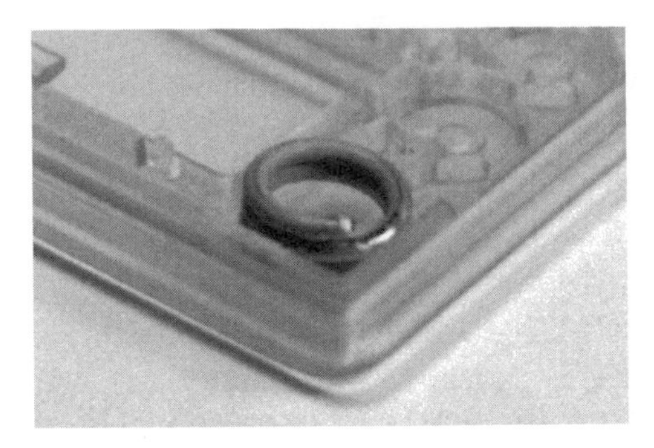

FIGURE 23–3 SMA helical acuator.

apparatus from room temperature, quickly raising the average temperature from 20° to 75°C. The hierarchy in temperature regimen then continued in elevated temperatures of 85°, 100°, and 120°C (Table 23–2). These temperature stages were chosen to surpass the Af of actuators by at least 5°C.

Results of SMA Experiments

Most of the candidate products proved successful in the temperature-hierarchical generic disassembly experiments. Only the A4 (17") CRT monitor, one PC keyboard, and two of the four cell phones were unfit for disassembly as actuator placement proved difficult in the time allotted. Of the 21 products chosen, 4 could not be tested. Of the remaining 17, 12 products were successfully dismantled with 19 SME disassembly occurrences, since some of the products were of a multistage nature. Seven of the products were multistage devices and one, the Kodak S.U. camera (2), was a three-stage device all within the stage of disassembly 2 temperature regimen. The SMA devices in this application successfully dismantled the camera at 70°, 72°, and 73°C. This camera's result exhibits some accuracy potential within an active or self-disassembly system as a generic process. Table 23–1 describes the

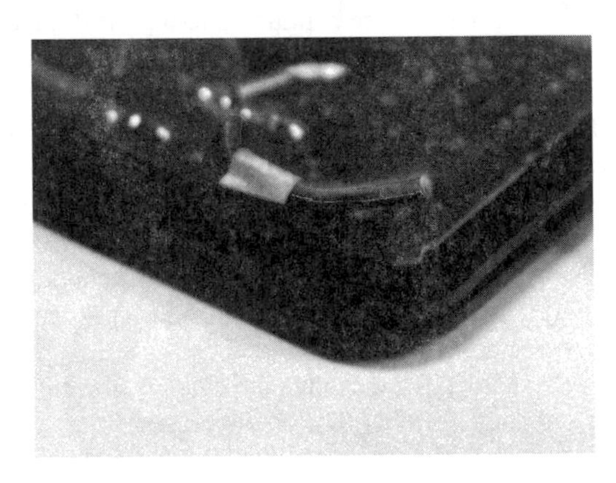

FIGURE 23–4 SMA rod actuator.

TABLE 23–1 Hierarchical Actuator Placement by Product and Results of Generic Disassembly Experiments

Hierarchical Actuator Placement by Product					Results		
Candidate Products	Placement	Af (°C) at Disassembly	Actuator Type	Hierarchy Within Product?	Disassembly Technique	Stages of Disassembly	Fully Successful Disassembly
A4 17" CRT	Attempted at glass seam	N.A.	N.A.	Failed	N.A.	N.A.	
PC keyboard	Attempt on macro-assembly	N.A.	N.A.	Failed	N.A.	N.A.	
Motorola mobile 1	Bottom end	60	Rod NiTi	No	Snap-fit expansion	N.A.	N.A.
Motorola mobile 2	Middle	60	Rod NiTi	No	Snap-fit expansion	N.A.	N.A.
Motorola mobile 3	Attempt on macro-assembly	N.A.	N.A.	N.A.	1	No	
Motorola mobile 4	Attempt on subassembly	N.A.	N.A.	N.A.	1	No	
PC mouse	Center rear	60	Coil NiTi	2 stage	Snap-fit expansion	1	Yes
	Keys, front	73, 73	Coil CuZnAl	2 stage	Snap-fit expansion	2	Yes
Sharp calculator	Top end	60	Coil NiTi	2 stage	Snap-fit expansion	1	Yes
	Middle	85, 85	Coil CuZnAl	2 stage	Snap-fit expansion	2	Yes
Apple adjustable keyboard	Front end	70	Disc NiTi	No	Snap-fit expansion	1	No
Battery charger	Bottom end	68, 70	Coil CuZnAl	2 stage	Snap-fit expansion	2	No
	Middle	100	Coil NiTi	2 stage	Compression-fit expansion	4	No
Kodak S.U.C. 1	Top middle	70	Coil CuZnAl	2 stage	Snap-fit expansion	2	Yes
	Side	70	Coil CuZnAl	2 stage	Snap-fit expansion	2	Yes
Kodak S.U.C. 2	Center bottom	70	Coil CuZnAl	3 stage	Snap-fit expansion	2	Yes
	Top right	72, 72	Coil CuZnAl	3 stage	Snap-fit expansion	2 and 2	Yes
	Top middle	73	Coil CuZnAl	3 stage	Snap-fit expansion	2	Yes
Sung PC mouse 1	Key seats	71, 72	Coil CuZnAl	2 stage	Snap-fit expansion	2	Yes
	Bottom of PCB	85, 85	Coil CuZnAl	2 stage	Compression-fit expansion	3	Yes
Sung PC mouse 2	Bottom of PCB	78, 74	Coil CuZnAl	2 stage	Compression-fit expansion	2	Yes
	Key seats	80, 85	Coil CuZnAl	2 stage	Snap-fit expansion	3	Yes
Brats calculator, round	End	75, 77	Coil CuZnAl	No	Snap-fit expansion	2	Yes
Royal personal organizer	Center	77, 77	Coil CuZnAl	No	Snap-fit expansion	2	Yes
TI calculator	End	76, 75	Coil CuZnAl	No	Snap-fit expansion	2	Yes
Brats calculator, square	Middle	80	Coil CuZnAl	No	Snap-fit expansion	2	Yes
Canon calculator	Ends diagonal	80, 80	Coil CuZnAl	No	Snap-fit expansion	2	Yes
Electronic game	Middle	90, 90	Coil CuZnAl	No	Compression-fit expansion	3	Yes
Adjustable # keyboard	Center rear	100	Coil NiTi	No	Snap-fit expansion	4	No

Legend: N.A.not applicable; Af (°C) = Celsius; Coil = helical coil.
Source: Chiodo et al., 1998.

TABLE 23–2 Hierarchical Temperature Regimen of SMA Actuator Employment by Stage

Actuator Composition	Actual Actuator SME Af	NiTi	NiTi and CuZnAl	NiTi
Actuator design		Rod	Helical coil	Disc
Stages (°C)	(°C)			
1. 70	60	X	X	X
2. 85	68–80		X	
3. 100	80–90		X	
4. 120	100		X	

nature of experiments throughout the four stages of the hierarchical disassembly-temperature regimes.

SMA Experiment Conclusions

Following actuation, the actuators returned in less than 1 second to their previously trained shapes, hence "shape memory." The SME is time independent but takes a noticeable time in the experiment, as heat must be conducted through the entire actuator for it to undergo SME. The experiments made it clear that exposure to ambient temperature was insufficient.

Experiments with Shape Memory Polymer Releasable Fasteners

Numerous experiments were conducted with SMP releasable fasteners, applying them to the active disassembly of various products. These are referred to as SMP *screws* or *devices*. The initial experiments (1996) investigated releasing PCBs and product housing assemblies; that is, BT telephone. The last experiments (1998) tested active disassembly on Philips stereo equipment and Sony entertainment equipment, considering Tg (Walker, 1995) and cost effectiveness.

In these experiments, SMP screws were placed inside the candidate products so that, at Tg, the device exhibits considerable mechanical property loss. This, in effect, is the "letting go" required to actively self-disassemble the product.

Findings include successful active disassembly using novel smart material releasable fasteners of SMP composition. These devices were developed and manufactured specifically for this application, but further SMP releasable mechanism work continues. Successful disassembly triggering was activated at temperatures of >+70 and<+100°C on product macro- and subassemblies. The SMP screws were found to return to their originally molded shape after the active disassembly. This action is the shape-memory effect associated with this smart material that is part of the shape-memory family.

Method of SMP Experiments

The strategy for these experiments was to make minimal changes to the existing design of the products and develop releasable screws (Figure 23–5). Preliminary investigation of these screws suggested they would be effective when incorporated into products.

The experiments consisted of testing products in three temperature sets. To investigate the SMP screws (Tg) holding the consumer products together, three forms of heat transfer were considered to observe the nature of these potential sources on a wide variety of products.

The first experiment tested a Philips clock FM radio on a conveyor system fitted with infrared heaters and air heating guns. Surface temperatures reached 225°C through radiation and convection sources. Subsequent experiments consisted of heat transfer via total water immersion. Here, the same products tested twice in experiments were run at two temperature sets of 70°C and 100°C. Prior to the second set of tests, the products were reassembled with the same SMP screws used where possible.

Product Changes

The candidate products utilized for the experiments are listed in Table 23–3. Some minor changes had to be made to accommodate the experiments. In addition to the conventional screws being replaced with SMP screws, biasing springs were embedded in the vicinity of the fastener enclosures. These spring steel compression springs were placed inside the products for giving evidence of mechanical property loss once Tg was reached throughout the screws. This would take place once the product was placed inside the heated dismantling zone. Once Tg was achieved, the biasing steel springs would propel the product housing apart. Most of the springs

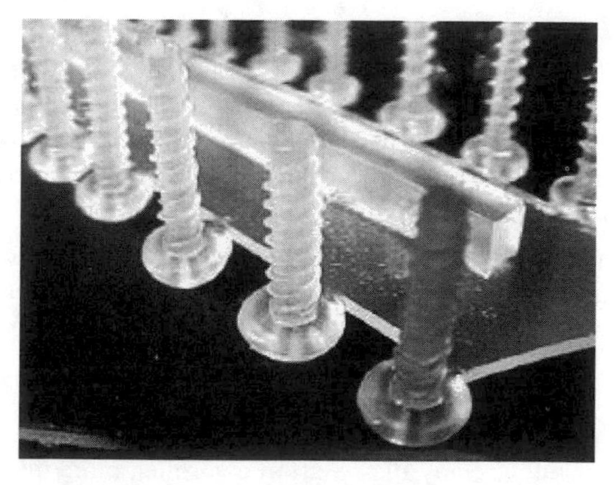

FIGURE 23–5 Novel SMP releasable fastener screws.

TABLE 23–3 Results of SMP Active Disassembly Experiments by Time

	Product					
	Philips AJ3150 FM MW Digital	Philips AJ3150 EasyL clock FM MW	Sony Discman ESP	Sony Play Station, Section 1	Sony Play Station, Section 2	Sony Play Station Controller
Internal product temp. at disassembly	22	22	24	24	24	24
Convection (air jet) and radiation (infrared):						
Trial 1 (225°C)		–180.0*				
Conduction (water bath), times for disassembly						
Trial 2 (–70°C)	25–26		18–92	61–62**	61–62**	–320*
Trial 3 (–100°C)	14		8	8–10**	8–10**	17**

Notes: Temperature accuracy is within ±5°C. Temperatures are in °C. Time is in seconds, within ±0.5 sec.
*Disassembly failed by time.
**Partial disassembly.
Source: Chiodo, Billet, and Harrison, 1999.

were placed encapsulating the screw support posts. Generally, placement of the biasing springs meant carving out the support ribs in the inside of the product housing.

As well as the conventional screws being replaced with SMP screws, snap fits were removed if there were any. This was to allow a clean passage for the separation of product housings during disassembly. Additionally, power cables were removed. In the event of final design and manufacture, snap fastenings and releasable fasteners of conventional or smart material would be considered.

Results of SMP Experiments

In every case but the Sony Play Station controller, more than three bias compression springs were embedded in the candidate products for eventual disassembly.

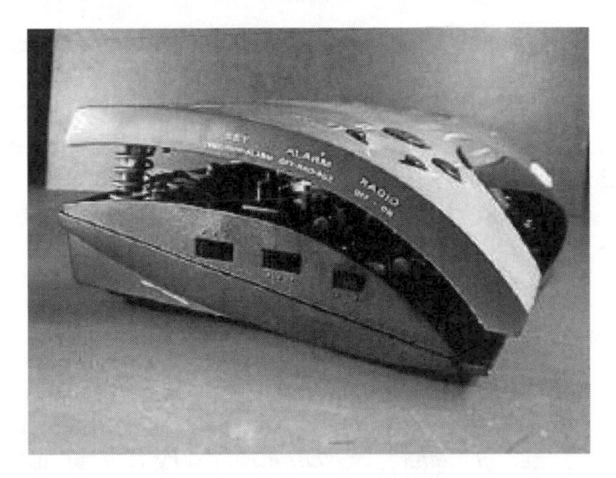

FIGURE 23–6 Successful active disassembly experiment—Philips digital radio.

The Philips audio products were embedded with four biasing springs, as was the Sony CD player. Only the Sony Play Station was embedded with more than four springs.

Within the five products tested, 12 macro- and subassemblies were tested in total. Five assemblies were completely successful, four failed, and three were partially successful. Of the five products, two completely self-disassembled (Figure 23–6 and 23–7). Of the three remaining, only one, the Philips clock radio failed, this was the first conveyor trial.

Within these 12 assemblies were 38 SMP releasable fastener screws, of which 17 (44.7%) failed to allow disassembly while 21 products (55.3%) disassembled successfully. Of these 21 SMP screws, 5 were found to be decapitated after successful disassembly. Remarkably, the remaining 16 SMP screws successfully returned to

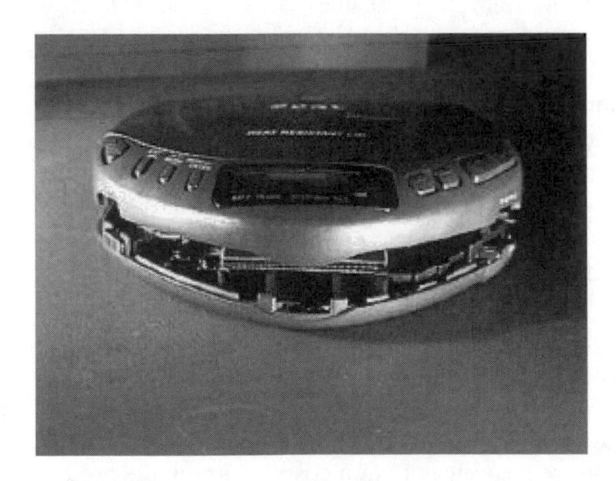

FIGURE 23–7 Successful active disassembly experiment—Sony CD player.

their originally trained shapes with no evidence of ever having been put through the active disassembly process.

Observing data from Table 23–3, trial 1 failed but, we can calculate that in trial set 2 (70°C), the mean time of successful and partially successful disassembly of product assemblies was 60 seconds. In trial set 3 (100°C), the mean time of the same was 12.25 seconds. Of the completely successful experiments in trial set 2, the mean was 59 seconds, while in the same for trial set 3, the mean was 11 seconds.

Conclusions of SMP Experiments

As just stated, 16 of the SMP screws deformed considerably during the active disassembly process but returned to their originally trained shapes; this is what is known as the *shape-memory effect*, or *shape recovery* (Shirai and Hayashi, 1988). The SME occurred despite forced separation in tension from the deflection of the biasing compression springs while surpassing Tg exposure. This could provide a potential means for recycling the SMP fasteners. As elongation at Tg is possible to over 600% (Shirai and Hayashi, 1988), considerable shape flexibility is plausible for the design of a releasable fastener. As the decapitation of the SMP screwheads could be contaminating, a higher Tg SMP with a higher modulus would help solve this. These are currently available.

As SME is temperature dependent, it is crucial that allowances are made in the product sub- and macroassemblies for ambient temperature to allow complete conduction of heat through the SMP devices. This was found also to be the case in SMA active disassembly. In all cases, active disassembly using SMP screws provided the self-dismantling of product housing with no destruction to the host products.

ADSM Conclusions

In both the SMA and SMP devices, most of the ADSM experiments proved successful. We found that a high level of control and predictability was potentially possible with ADSM; in fact, the most successful results revealed a multiple (×3) disassembly sequence ranging within a 1°C margin.

Most of the active disassembly devices are inexpensive and could prove a very valuable investment. Additionally, the smart material actuators and devices are highly reusable, costs too would divide every time the devices are reused. In active disassembly, the cost added to some products may be a few pennies, but most products' costs would not change in volume manufacturing.

One of the most important lessons learned from the candidate products was that active disassembly is much more practical and cost effective the earlier it is incorporated into the design. This work currently is under way with elected manufacturers.

The generic nature of the process would mean that a single dismantling center would accept products from a variety of manufacturers in a single disassembly line. This would minimize the transportation costs returning the products to the manufacturers. This last aspect is very important, as a journey of more than a few miles can consume more resources than are saved by recovering the materials embodied in the product.

Environmental impact reduction and cost reduction or efficiency obviously are the key issues in LCA. As legislation points toward producer responsibility, recycling as an integral part of the life cycle of electronic consumer products becomes a more attractive possibility. Local recycling resources from electrical and electronic equipment would significantly reduce the environmental cost. Active disassembly could provide this and become an important driver to a more environmentally responsible form of product stewardship.

Acknowledgments

Active disassembly using smart materials (ADSM) is the subject of a "Blue Skies" Engineering Physical Sciences Research Council (EPSRC, UK) grant to the faculty of technology, Department of Design at Brunel University. The first phase (one year) of the project was completed in 1997 with such success that further funding has been granted for the second phase, currently under way. This new two-year EPSRC project started in late spring 1998 and is investigating design principles for active disassembly. The research is observing the product design, smart material device design implications, and implementation of ADSM into cell phones.

We thank Brunel University, Runnymede Campus, Design Department, Egham Surey, UK; Dr. David Harrison for his project support; Richard Morris for his camera expertise and photography; and the others at Brunel who have been very helpful. We also thank Tony Anson (Anson Medical, Oxford, UK) for his SMA expertise, generosity of NiTi SMA samples, and support; Tony Micheals (Memory Metals, Ipswich UK) for his generosity of CuZnAl SMA samples; John Dicello (Nitinol Devices and Components Inc., California) for his generosity of NiTi SMA samples; and Shunichi Hyashi (Mitsubishi Heavy Industries Research Center, Nagoya, Japan) for his generosity of SMP samples and literature.

References

Chiodo, J. D., E. H. Billett, and D. J. Harrison. "Preliminary Investigations of Active Disassembly Using Shape Memory Polymers." Eco Design 1999, IEEE International Symposium on Electronics and the Environment, Tokyo, Japan, February 1–3, 1999.

Chiodo, J. D., E. H. Billett, D. J. Harrison, and P. M. Harrey. "Investigations of Generic Self Disassembly Using Shape Memory Alloys." IEEE International Symposium on Electronics and the Environment Oak Brook, IL, May 4–6, 1998.

Gilbertson, R. G. *Muscle Wires Project Book.* San Anselmo, CA: Mondotronics, Inc., 1994.

Gordon, R. F. "Design Principles for Cu-Zn-Al Actuators." *Engineering Aspects of Shape Memory Alloys*. T. W Duerig, K. N. Melton, D. Stockel, and C. M. Wayman, (Eds.), pp. 245–255. New York: Butterworth–Heinemann, 1990.

Gordon, R. F. "Applications of Shape Memory Polyurethanes." First International Conference on Shape Memory and Superelastic Technologies, Pacific Grove, CA, March 7–10, 1994.

Higgins, R. A. *Engineering Metallurgy*. London: Edward Arnold, 1983.

Shirai, Yoshiki, and Shunichi Hayashi. "Development of Polymeric Shape Memory Material." Mitsubishi Technical Bulletin No. 184, Nagoya Research and Development Center, Technical Headquarters, Mitsubishi Heavy Industries, Ltd., Nagoya, Japan, 1988.

Spillman, W. B., Jr., J. S. Sirkis, and P. T. Gardiner. "Smart Materials and Structures: What Are They?" *Smart Materials and Structures* 5, no. 3 (June 1996), p. 248.

Tautzenberger, P., D. Stockel, and C. M. Wayman. *Engineering Aspects of Shape Memory Alloys*. New York: Butterworth–Heinemann, 1990.

Walker, P. M. B., Ed. *Larousse Dictionary of Science and Technology*. (Edinburgh and New York: Larousse Kingfisher Chamber Inc., 1995.

CHAPTER **24**

Ultralight Hybrid Vehicles—Principles and Design

Timothy C. Moore
The Hypercar Center, Rocky Mountain Institute, Snowmass, Colorado

Introduction

The technical feasibility of superefficient family cars has been demonstrated, but most prior designs typically have compromised vehicle performance, safety, cost, manufacturability, or marketability. This is because industry experimentation has tended to focus on improving performance or implementing hybrid-electric drive systems in essentially conventional vehicles, reducing mass and drag, or on improving safety—but few attempts have been made to concurrently optimize all of these factors using whole-system engineering practices. A whole-system engineering design is essential to move toward commercial viability.

Simulations and performance modeling provides evidence that it is possible to produce automobiles that would be three to four times more fuel efficient than today's, with emissions approximating the California proposed equivalent zero emission vehicle requirement for hybrids (~0.1 × ultralow emission vehicle requirements). Such vehicles could have safety, performance, and marketability surpassing that of many current automobiles.

The commercial success of such designs depends on the concurrent optimization of numerous parameters, with emphasis on tractive- and accessory-load reduction and component and control development. Platform optimization is of primary concern, because only tractive-load reduction (e.g., vehicle mass and drag) makes hybrid drive systems commercially viable. Therefore, the artful combination of hybrid-electric drive with lightweight, low-drag platform design appears requisite to the cost-effective optimization of efficiency, emissions, performance, and safety for production worthy and marketable automobiles.

Design Criteria

Industry design criteria for efficient vehicles have tended to focus on limiting compromises in performance rather than on improving it. The Rocky Mountain Institute's analysis suggests that efficient designs could yield generally improved acceleration, handling, braking, safety, and durability. The following criteria (based in part on similar criteria developed by the U.S. Partnership for a New Generation of Vehicles) appear essential for the U.S. market and were assumed for this analysis (all improvements are relative to current touring-class production sedans):

- Acceleration from 0 to 100 km/h in 8.5 sec at test mass (half-full fuel tank; two 68-kg occupants), and 12 sec at gross mass (five 68-kg occupants; 91 kg luggage).
- Gradability sufficient to maintain 105 km/h on a 6.5% grade at test mass, and 90 km/h at gross mass for 20 min. Acceleration also should be reasonable on grades to facilitate safe merging on steep highway entrance ramps, suggesting 0 to 100 km/h acceleration in ~15 sec at gross mass on a 5% grade.
- Improved handling, maneuverability, tire adhesion, antilock braking, and traction control.
- Improved crashworthiness, interior safety features, and ease, speed, and safety of postcrash extrication.
- Combined urban/highway range of 640 km.
- At least equivalent ride, handling, and control of noise, vibration, and harshness.
- Carrying capacity for the gross-mass load and occupants with equivalent comfort and cargo space.
- Useful life of 320,000 km, maintenance of original performance and emissions specifications for at least 160,000 km, improved service intervals, and comparable reliability and refueling time.
- Equivalent or improved customer features, such as climate control and entertainment systems, and total real cost of ownership.

Propulsion Systems

Efforts to meet California's zero emission vehicle and ultralow emission vehicle or similar mandates have spawned major advances in propulsion systems; for example, motors and controllers with high specific power and system efficiencies well over 90% for much of their usable range (Eriksson, 1995; West, 1994; Cole, 1993a; Blake and Lawrenson, 1992; Lovins and Howe, 1992; Hendershot, 1991) and load-leveling devices (LLDs) capable of meeting real-world hybrid vehicle requirements with careful systems integration (Burke, 1995; Rudderman, Juergens, and Nelson, 1994; Post, Fowler, and Post, 1993; Trippe, Burke, and Blank, 1993). These advances enable auxiliary power unit (APU) technologies (such as gas turbines, Stirling engines, thermophotovoltaic burners, and fuel cells; Moore and Lovins, 1995) that aren't well suited for conventional cars but work well in hybrids when accompanied by efficient electric drives.

Most of these technologies have been around for decades but until recently were not sufficiently developed or were not enabled by other key technologies for automobiles. Many would still be overly complex, bulky, and probably cost prohibitive if applied to conventional cars or heavy-battery electric cars.

Conventional, Battery, or Hybrid-Electric Drive?

Conventional automotive drive systems based on an internal combustion engine (ICE) mechanically coupled to the drive wheels through a multispeed transmission are limited by the inflexibility and mechanical systems and the inability to recover braking energy. To provide ample power for acceleration and gradability, a conventional vehicle's ICE must be oversized to roughly ten times the 100-km/h, level-ground requirement and three to four times the 100 km/h, 6% grade requirement set by the U.S. Partnership. Unfortunately, the engine can't be optimized for all the speed and load range combinations under which it must operate. Efficiency is diminished and emissions are elevated for many segments of the engine operating regimen map.

Gross oversizing of the engine results, both because it must cover the peak load and because peak power occurs at a fixed engine speed that would be available only at all wheel speeds with a continuously variable transmission ratio.

While electric-only may be appropriate for some applications, the electric storage capacity required for even a modest range would preclude meeting many of these design criteria, limiting marketability. Combustion-free range also would be unnecessary under proposed equivalent zero emission vehicle (EZEV) standards (CARB, 1995). Battery Electric Vehicles' (BEV) problems center on performance, range, and cost. BEVs such as the GM EV-1 easily satisfy requirements for acceleration and gradability but not load-carrying capacity, interior space, or range requirements. While the cost for mass-produced versions of such BEVs eventually might be acceptable, it isn't clear whether batteries with low enough replacement cost or long enough life under deep discharge conditions are feasible. As designs move toward acceptable range and performance, the mass of the battery snowballs until almost every component and structure in the vehicle becomes bigger, heavier, and costlier than desirable. Furthermore, as batteries are added to increase range, much of the energy in the batteries is required simply to transport the batteries themselves. So like conventional cars, BEVs waste much of their performance and energy storage potential on transporting their own mass.

Flywheels and ultracapacitors have the high specific power needed for performance but only enough specific energy capacity to function as LLDs that might extend battery life in a BEV. (Energy storage capacity in flywheels is similar to that of mid-range batteries, but higher unit cost precludes installing numerous flywheels.)

The fundamental advantage of Hybrid Electronic Vehicles (HEV) over BEVs is the 10^2 times higher usable Wh/kg of fluid fuels over current batteries. An HEV's performance and efficiency is not impaired by massive batteries nor is its range limited by electrochemical energy storage technology.

However, HEVs easily can suffer from compounding size, mass, cost, and added complexity if care is not taken to optimize the design for low mass from the start (Moore and Lovins, 1995; Lovins, 1995). Ultralight design is the key to a successful Electronic Vehicle (EV), but the EV must be an HEV to be ultralight.

Purpose-built series HEVs, however, can be less mechanically complex than conventional vehicles, particularly with a solid-state APU such as a fuel cell or thermophotovoltaic burner. Since electric motors are mechanically simple, expenditure on machined parts can be lower than for conventional cars.

Hybrid drivetrain systems can be classified in two broad categories: parallel and serial. Parallel systems have separate mechanical inputs to the drive wheels from the battery storage system and the APU. Serial systems have no mechanical connection between the APU and the driven wheels, necessitating the energy from the APU and the storage system to utilize a single path. As we shall see, each approach has its advantages and drawbacks.

Parallel Hybrid Drive Systems

Parallel HEVs theoretically are more efficient at cruise because a well-designed mechanical drive to the wheels can have less energy loss than the electromechanical conversion process. However, they can tend toward mechanical complexity by trading a multispeed transmission for one with multiple input shafts or some sort of four-wheel-drive arrangement. A single, fixed-ratio gear set for each input is possible but requires a control strategy that runs the APU only at high speeds. This increases the dependence on battery range for urban driving, which reintroduces mass-, power-, and cost-compounding problems.

An alternative parallel hybrid drive system design (Figure 24–1) has the potential for improved highway fuel economy. It would function as an on-off series

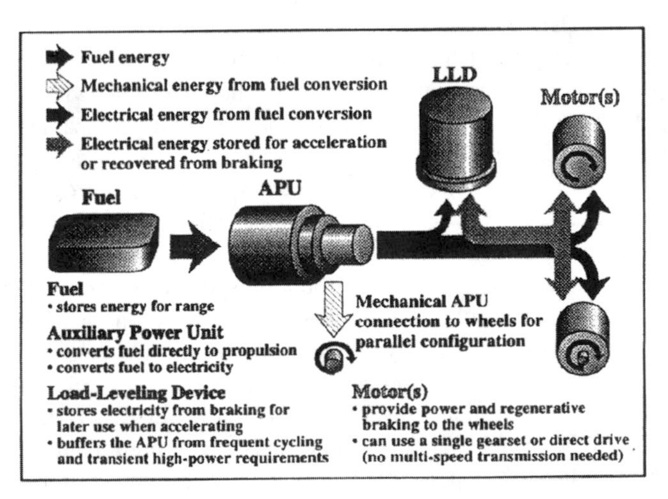

FIGURE 24–1 Series and dual-mode parallel HEV schematic.

hybrid under low-speed urban conditions and as a power-assist parallel hybrid for highway driving. This would allow the potentially more-efficient mechanical connection (a trade-off between avoided energy conversion steps and increased APU map and possibly additional mechanical losses) of the APU to the drive wheels for highway use. A small LLD could replace the large, heavy batteries typical of many parallel hybrid designs. The electric portion of the drive system might be slightly smaller, depending on the APU control strategy.

Trade-offs relative to series HEVs would be increased complexity (adding cost), higher emissions and fuel use for some APU technologies, and cumbersome transition to solid-state APU technologies.

Series Hybrid Drive Systems

Series HEV drive systems (with no mechanical connection of the APU to the driven wheels) appear to have only the advantage of regenerative braking but all the disadvantages of multistage conversion (Figure 24–1). Series HEVs have significant efficiency, emissions, and power-plant-sized advantages over conventional vehicles, even if the APU is an ICE. Volvo concluded that series HEVs are considerably more efficient than parallel HEVs (Lovins, 1995). The power unit output needs to pass through the LLD only to the extent required by controls to maintain a target state of charge (SOC) and an optimal load range for the APU itself.

Many advantages stem from decoupling the APU from peak power requirements and vehicle speed with an LLD and electric drive system. The LLD minimizes the load range or engine map. APU peak-power requirements for a series HEV thus are determined more by gradability than acceleration (which, given our design criteria, would require ~75% more power without an LLD). Cutting peak-power requirements toward average loads allows a smaller APU, which can then operate closer to wide-open throttle (if ICE), reducing pumping losses. Decoupling the APU from wheel speed means maximum continuous APU power for hill climbing can be extracted at any speed.

Vehicle Design to Reduce Tractive and Accessory Loads

The synergistic combination of reduced tractive loads and optimized hybrid drive systems can improve fuel economy three to four times or more while making performance criteria more readily attainable. Without extreme measures, constant-speed tractive loads on level ground can be reduced by about 60% (Figure 24–2). Also, load reduction might incur little or even negative net manufacturing expense if reduced driveline size and complexity saved more than reduced platform drag cost.

Mass Reduction

While HEV fuel economy may be less sensitive to mass reduction than to other variables, such as APU efficiency, the requirement for high acceleration and

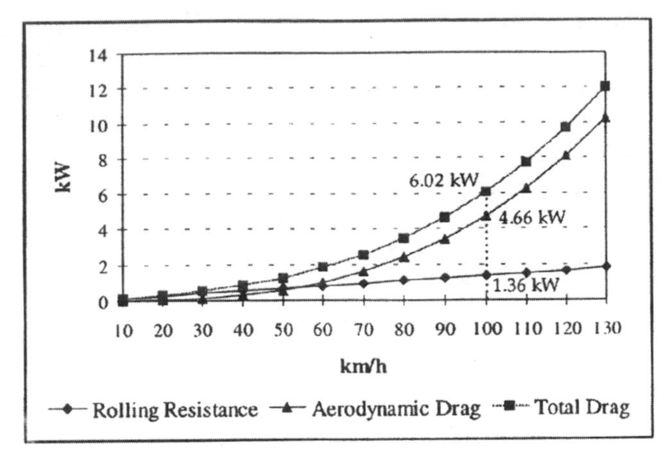

FIGURE 24–2 Reduced tractive loads on level ground.

braking performance while maintaining reasonable drive-system component costs and packaging may lead to greater mass reduction.

Even though made less important by efficient drive systems, regenerative braking, and low-rolling-resistance tires, mass reduction still contributes significantly to fuel economy. It contributes directly by lowering rolling resistance and power required for acceleration and hill climbing. It is important, however, to apply a systems approach to mass optimization: The ratio of fuel economy improvement to mass reduction should exceed the ~1:2 achieved by treating mass as an isolated variable.

Mass reduction indirectly aids HEVs' fuel economy by allowing much smaller APU and traction-motor maps. The control strategy turndown ratio (peak-to-lowest-power operation) can be better matched to the APU's highest efficiency.

Mass Decompounding

Mass decompounding is nonlinear, discontinuous, complex, and inadequately captured by automakers' rule-of-thumb ~1.5 multiplier. For a given payload capacity, the primary and secondary units of mass saved tend to converge over recursive reoptimizations and more rapidly as payload mass becomes a relatively larger factor than curb mass. One of the most significant discontinuities in the mass decompounding curve is the threshold at which mass reduction allows an economical series hybrid-electric drive system with fewer mechanical parts and smaller components (Williams, 1993). If material substitution were used to cut body-in-white (BIW) mass by 50% and other components downsized accordingly, with no recursions, 40% curb mass reduction might be challenging. If, however, substitutions are applied to all components, which in turn require less structure, and the process is repeated several times, 45–55+% curb mass reduction appears feasible.

System optimization can lead not only to downsizing but also potentially to displacing components, saving further mass and cost. Recursive optimization uncovers many linked opportunities for mass and cost savings. Accelerating less mass cuts drive-system output, reducing driveline and associated structural support requirements. The reduced power requirements may even displace all gears with low-speed, high-torque motors. Smaller, lower-power drive components require smaller cooling systems, resulting in less coolant mass, smaller air inlets, and reduced aerodynamic drag. This decompounding in turn reduces drive-system energy and power requirements, making those components smaller and lighter yet. With gross vehicle mass equal to the curb mass of today's subcompacts, power steering and power brakes also might be eliminated as they were in the Ultralite, cutting costs and improving high-speed control without sacrificing performance or low-speed maneuverability. Ultimately, the point at which mass reduction minimizes vehicle cost and complexity should be determined before the design is locked into particular structural materials and component choices.

Mass Contribution to Peak Power

Mass is the single largest contributor to both intermittent and continuous peak power requirements. For this reason, mass determines the size, and often cost, of the drive-system components. Maintaining 90 km/h at gross mass on a 6.5% grade requires 3.3 times as much power at the wheels (20 kW as modeled) as all level-ground tractive loads at test mass combined. The average power needed for acceleration from 0 to 100 km/h in 8.5 sec at test mass is ~1.6 times larger still (39 kW). Reducing curb mass 10% lowers the power required to maintain 90 km/h on a 6.5% grade at gross mass by ~4% (or ~6% for five-occupant vehicles with a curb mass of ~1,000 kg) and the power required for 8.5-sec 0 to 100 km/h acceleration at a test mass by ~8.5%. Thus, payload dilutes the effect of the curb mass reduction.

Body-in-White Structure: Materials and Mass Reduction

Technologies for mass saving and parts consolidation with high-strength and carbon steel, and for producing and fabricating aluminum and polymer or metal-matrix composites, contribute to the potential for 40–55% curb-mass reduction without downsizing (Moore and Lovins, 1995; Masscarin et al., 1995; Gjostein, 1995a; Sherman, 1995; Eusebi, 1995). The American Iron and Steel Institute (AISI) claims that, with a "holistic" approach to design, vehicle curb-mass reductions of up to 40% can be achieved (AISI 1995). Porsche Engineering Services, commissioned by AISI, calculated the "realistic achievable potential" for BIW mass reduction using steel to be 15–20%, with a theoretical maximum around 30% (AISI, 1994). Ford's 199-kg Taurus AIV (aluminum-intensive vehicle) BIW is 47% lighter than the standard Taurus BIW. This was accomplished without even taking full advantage of mass decompounding from downsizing the engine and chassis components. The aluminum BIW for Volvo's five-seat hybrid ECC (environmental-concept car) also weighs ~200 kg, has sufficient strength to carry 350 kg of batteries plus its payload, and includes extensive provisions for crashworthiness (Volvo, 1992). Composites offer advantages in both vehicle design and production. High specific-material strength and stiffness along with very high fatigue resistance allow significantly reduced mass while maintaining or even improving component strength and durability and vehicle stiffness. The engineering properties and degree of isotropy of polymer composites are controllable over a wide range (Eusebi, 1995). With proper design, specific crash-energy absorption can be two (Eusebi, 1995) to five (Kindervater, 1994) times that of steel. Assembly steps, finish processes, and tooling can be reduced by an order of magnitude through parts consolidation and lay-in-the-mold finish coatings, potentially eliminating material cost penalties (Mascarin et al., 1995). Industry analysis shows potential for ~60–67% BIW mass reduction using carbon-fiber-reinforced composites (Gjostein, 1995b). These materials, however, do face manufacturing-engineering challenges.

Decoupling Mass From Size

Using lightweight materials for the BIW largely decouples vehicle mass from size, allowing substantial mass reductions without downsizing. This is particularly true for polymer composites, with their exceptionally high specific strength.

Design and Materials for Safety

Lightweight vehicle design, while presenting new challenges, does not preclude crashworthiness. Using proven technologies for energy absorption, force-limiting occupant restraints, and rigid passenger-compartment design, light vehicles can surpass the safety of today's cars in many types of collisions (Moore and Lovins, 1995; Eusebi, 1995; Kindervater, 1994; Hobbs, 1995; Niederer et al., 1993; Seal and Fitzpatrick, 1982). High-speed head-on collisions with, and side impacts from, significantly heavier collision partners, might be effectively dealt with through innovative and careful design, such as force-limiting restraint systems, large crush zones with multiple stages of increasing stiffness, and dedicated polymer-composite energy absorbing structures (Moore and Lovins, 1995; Eusebi, 1995; Kindervater, 1994; Hobbs, 1995; Niederer et al., 1993; Seal and Fitzpatrick, 1982). A similar strategy could be used for the rear and side. Intrusion prevention, restraints such as airbags, and interior bolsters should be emphasized for side impacts where crush space is limited. These are illustrated in Figure 24–3.

To avoid rejection by consumers, light hybrid vehicles should provide at least equivalent safety when colliding head-on with vehicles of average or higher mass at the time of introduction. This may require absorption of several times the static fixed-barrier crash energy in a collision with a vehicle weighing twice as much.

Low-Mass Vehicle Dynamics

Improved handling, maneuverability, tire adhesion, and braking are possible with low curb mass, new tire compounds, and HEVs' potential for ultraresponsive four-wheel ABS and traction control. High specific-strength materials allow very stiff passenger compartment designs improving suspension performance and ride

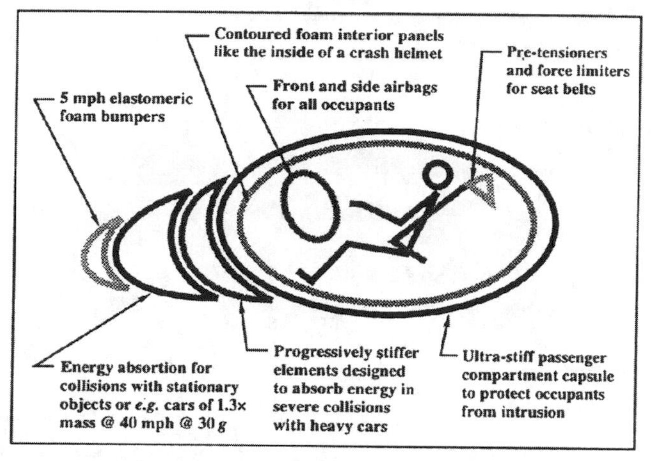

FIGURE 24–3 Multistage energy-absorption schematic.

without excessive mass. Ultralight wheels (perhaps a carbon-fiber composite over a magnesium skeleton for graceful failure), aramid-belted tires, hub carriers, and brakes (with metal-matrix calipers and carbon/carbon-silicon-carbide rotors) can keep the spring-to-unsprung-mass ratio high enough (>10:1) for excellent ride and suspension performance. Locating brakes inboard on driven axles can further reduce unsprung mass, while improving aerodynamics. Fully electric power steering can be provided only as needed at low speeds, high gross mass, and in tight turns.

Rolling Resistance and Tires

Rolling resistance is the product of vehicle mass times the coefficient of tire rolling resistance (r_0), plus parasitic losses from wheel-bearing and brake drag. The power required to overcome it rises linearly with vehicle speed. Rolling resistance reduction of ~50–70% from average appears desirable to meet industry goals and our design criteria (Volvo claims a rolling resistance reduction of 50% using tires from Goodyear on its 1,580-kg hybrid ECC, a noteworthy accomplishment, given that the ECC is ~130 kg heavier than average midsize sedans).

Aerodynamics: Frontal Area

Assuming that the vehicle must seat five in a sedan format (two seating rows), the practical limit for the frontal area (A) of the interior space is ~1.65 m^2. While roof and floor sections need not add significantly to this dimension, the practical limit, and perhaps equally important the marketable limit, for the cross-sectional area of the doors, including interior bolsters for side impacts, is ~0.1 m^2 each. Roof curvature adds another ~0.05 m^2. So an appropriate practical-limit dimension for A in a four or five-occupant design would be ~1.9 m^2 (~0.23 m^2 less than the 1995

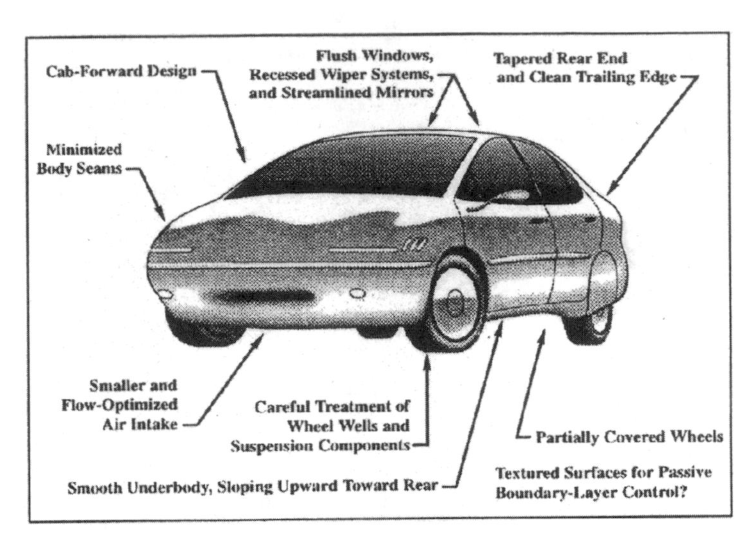

FIGURE 24–4 Marketable aerodynamic design.

Ford Taurus). Despite or perhaps because of these constraints, the resulting vehicle design can be attractive as well as functional (see Figure 24–4).

Aerodynamics: Drag Coefficient

Aerodynamic drag varies as velocity cubed and is the largest load at highway speeds on level ground. For an average 1995 model cruising at 100 km/h, aerodynamic drag typically consumes well over twice the power of rolling resistance. Given the limits of frontal area (A) of the interior space, ~1.65 m^2, lowering the drag coefficient (C_D) is the principal way to reduce this load. The C_D results from combined form, interference, induced, surface, and internal-flow drag.

Cab-forward design with a smooth underbody (from the start of design to avoid the mass, cost, and complexity of add-on panels) that tapers toward the rear and has clean trailing edges can substantially reduce form drag. Cutting surface drag would depend on reducing skin friction with specially textured surfaces that provide passive boundary-layer control. While textured surface finishes might pose marketing challenges on the upper body, underbody flow still could be improved. Internal-flow drag can be minimized by smoothing internal flow paths and downsizing cooling inlets for the reduced cooling loads from lower tractive loads and an efficient drive system. HEVs also have fewer and smaller components, which otherwise could complicate smoothing the underbody for maximum drag reduction.

Many small (two- to four-seat) prototypes have demonstrated $C_D \sim 0.18$–0.19. If, however, traditional appearance and stylistic flexibility take precedence, C_D might bottom out around 0.20.

Glazing and Accessory Loads

Reducing accessory loads becomes important at low tractive loads. Spectrally selective glazing, insulative body panels, breathable seat materials, photovoltaic-powered automatic ventilation fans, and other design options all can reduce cooling and heating loads, which reduces the mass, bulk, and power requirements of the HVAC system. Careful system integration can cut the fuel, weight, and cost penalties of interior heating and cooling by ~50–75% or more (Hopkins, Rubin, and Arasteh, 1994; Diekmann and Mallory, 1991; Gawronski, 1992). As modeled, a 250 W reduction in accessory loads improves fuel economy 8% on the Federal Urban Driving Simulation (FUDS) × 1.3 driving cycle.

Modeling

To explore these ideas quantitatively, the Rocky Mountain Institute developed parametric spreadsheets for use in combination with SIMPLEV, a second-by-second component-matrix-based model (Cole, 1993b), for a relatively comprehensive modeling of vehicle performance, fuel economy, and emissions; details are available from the author.

Summary of Modeling Inputs

Occupants: 4–5	(2 × 68 kg @ M_{test})	$A_{frontal}$	1.9 m^2
M_{curb}	585 kg	C_D	0.19
M_{test}	721 kg	$r_{0 \text{ tires (SAE)}}$	0.0056
M_{gross}	1016 kg	$r_{0\text{+road \& toe-in}}$	0.0062
$I_{rotational}$	11.0 kgm^2	r_1	1.6 E^{-5} sec/m
$M_{test\ effective}$	858 kg	$\mu_{\text{brks \& bearings}}$	1.36 Nm
$\text{Ratio}_{\text{sprung:unsp.}}$	10:1	$P_{\text{HVAC \& access.}}$	500 W

APU: Stirling Thermal Motors, Ann Arbor, Michigan.
Input matrix: Engine/generator η & emissions @ % load.
Power: 26 kW continuous @ STP.
Efficiency: 40% peak at shaft, 35% average at DC out.
APU Mass: 47 kg w/custom auxiliaries, some MMCs.

LLD: Pb-A: Bolder Tech., Wheat Ridge, Colorado.
Input matrices: V & IR @DOD; *C* rating and Peukert construction.
Specific power: 800 peak W/kg from 10–70% DOD.
Specific energy: 30 Wh/kg @ 25*C* (30 A), 36 Wh/kg @ *C*/2.
Pack voltage: 300 VDC nominal.
Peak power: 28.8 kW @ 300 VDC.
Energy capacity: 1.3 kWh (450 80-g, 2-V, 1.2-Ah cells).
Mass: 42 kg including l connector.

Motor: PM: Unique Mobility, Golden, Colorado.
Input matrices: η @ torque cel& speed; torque @ speed.
Starting torque: 226 Nm.
Gradability power: 22 kW (continuous @ 6,000–8,000 rpm).
Peak power: 48 kW (maximum for acceleration).
Mass: 37.5 kg (scaled to 90% of 53 kW).

Motor controller, digital: Unique Mobility, Golden, Colorado.
Input matrix: η @ motor torque and speed.
Voltage range: 200–400 VDC
Maximum current: 300 A (starting-torque limit).
Mass: 13.6 kg (scaled for use with APU and LLD).

Motor controller, transaxle: Based on data for Chrysler ETV-1.
Input matrix: η @ torque AND speed (η + 2% ≈ 0.95 average).
Gear ratio: 6.6:1 fixed ratio (single-stage reduction).

SIMPLEV modeling correlates closely with vehicle test data (Burke, 1995) and shows very slightly worse fuel economy than CarSim (Cuddy, 1995), a proprietary HEV simulator developed at AeroVironment (Monrovia, California) for GM.

The U.S. federal urban (FUDS) and highway driving cycles were simulated, along with versions of those cycles with all second-by-second input velocities multiplied by a factor of 1.3 to represent more realistic driving patterns (see Table 24–1). This is somewhat more conservative than the EPA correction factors applied to fuel economy results, and has the advantage of simultaneously correcting power, energy-storage, and emissions parameters.

The performance and SIMPLEV modeling results were as follows:

For 0 to 100 km/h,
Acceleration at test mass: 8.6 sec.
at gross mass: 11.6 sec.
at test mass on a 5% grade: 10.4 sec.
at gross mass on a 5% grade: 15.4 sec.
Starting grade at gross mass: 30%.
Velocity on a 6.5% grade,
at test mass: 104 km/h.
at gross mass: 86 km/h.

TABLE 24–1 The U.S. Federal Urban and Highway Driving Cycles

Driving cycle	km/l	1/100 km	mpg	55% City/ 45% Hwy	HC	CO	NO_x
FUDS	44.7	2.24	105	46.5 km/l	0.0002	0.009	0.024 g/km
Highway	48.7	2.05	115	110 mpg	0.0002	0.008	0.022 g/km
FUDS × 1.3	38.7	2.58	91	38.2 km/l	0.0005	0.011	0.026 g/km
Highway × 1.3	37.6	2.66	88	90 mpg	0.0008	0.016	0.025 g/km

Regenerative braking from 40 km/h,
at test mass: 0.31 *g*.
at gross mass: 0.23 *g*.
Max. Δv for frontal crush, frontal crush,
at test mass and 30 *g*: 65 km/h.
0.55 m at 30 *g*, 0.3 m at 40–50 *g*: 88 km/h.
Offset strike of 50% crush area,
at test mass and 15 *g*: 47 km/h.
0.55 m at 15 *g*, 0.3 m at 20–25 *g*: 62 km/h.

Conclusions

Although not quantitatively definitive, this analysis demonstrates the value of combining lightweight, low-drag, thermally efficient platform design with efficient hybrid drives. The technology fusion substantially improves fuel economy and emissions without compromising safety, performance, and marketability.

While not contributing much more fuel economy per change in load fraction than the drive system per change in efficiency, tractive load reduction stands out as the largest untapped source of fuel economy improvement. Because the required drive-system power output is reduced, vehicle emissions necessarily decrease at least in proportion to tractive load reduction.

Acknowledgments

This research was supported by The Compton, Nathan Cummings, Energy, W. Alton Jones, Joyce, and Surdna Foundations and Changing Horizons Charitable Trust. Travel was sponsored by Mitsubshi Electric America and Mitsubishi Motor Sales America. Many thanks to my colleagues and numerous advisors in the field.

References

American Iron and Steel Institute. “Holistic Design with Steel for Vehicle Weight Reduction.” Southfield, MI: American Iron and Steel Institute, February 1994.

American Iron and Steel Institute. “Steel’s Potential to Meet the PNGV Goals.” Southfield, MI: American Iron and Steel Institute, 1995.

Anderson, Catherine, and Erin Pettit. 1995: “The Effects of APU Characteristics on the Design of Hybrid Control Strategies for Hybrid Electric Vehicles,” SAE 950493. Warrendale, PA: Society of Automotive Engineers Inc., February 27, 1995.

Bennethum, James E., Thomas D. Laymac, Lennart N. Johansson, and Ted M. Godett. "Commercial Stirling Engine Development and Applications," SAE 911649. Society of Automotive Engineers Inc., Warrendale, PA: August 2–5, 1991.

Blake, R. J., and P. J. Lawrenson. "New Applications of Very Large and Small Switched Reluctance Drives." Proceedings of the Power Conversion and Intelligent Motion Conference, Nürnberg, Germany, April 1992.

Burke, Andrew F. "Electric/Hybrid Super Car Designs Using Ultracapacitors." 30th International Electric Car Engineering Conference, Orlando, FL, August 1995.

California Air Resources Board (CARB). "ARB Staff Proposal to Allow Hybrid-Electric Vehicles to Receive Zero-Emission Vehicle Credit." El Monte: California Air Resources Board, April 10, 1995.

Cole, G. H.: "Comparison of the Unique Mobility and DOE-Developed AC Electric Drive Systems," Idaho Falls: EG&G Idaho, Inc., January 1993a.

Cole, G. H. "SIMPLEV: A Simple Electric Vehicle Simulation Program." Idaho Falls: EG&G, Inc., April 1993b.

Cuddy, Matthew. "A Comparison of Modeled and Measured Energy Use in Hybrid Electric Vehicles." Society of Automotive Engineers International Congress and Exposition, Detroit, National Renewable Energy Laboratory, 27 February–3 March 1995.

Diekmann, John, and David Mallory 1991: "Climate Control for Electric Vehicles," SAE 910250. Warrendale, PA: Society of Automotive Engineers Inc., February 25, 1991.

Eriksson, Sture. "Drive Systems with Permanent Magnet Synchronous Motors." *Automotive Engineering* (February 1995).

Eusebi, E. "Composite Intensive Vehicles: Past, Present and Future" Vice President's Symposium on Structural Material Challenges for the Prototype Next-Generation Vehicle, Washington. DC, February 22–23, 1995.

Gawronski, Francis J. "Natron Reinvents HVAC for the 90's." *Automotive Industries' Insider* (May 1, 1992), p. 3.

General Motors. "Impact: Goodyear Designs Special Tires for the GM Electric Car." Press release, General Motors, 1990.

Gjostein, N.A. "Technology Needs Beyond PNGV." Conference on Basic Research Needs for Vehicles of the Future. New Orleans, January 5, 1995a.

Gjostein, N. A. "PNGV Material R&D Roadmap." Vice President's Symposium on Structural Material Challenges for the Prototype Next-Generation Vehicle, Washington, DC, February 22–23, 1995b.

Hendershot, James R., Jr. "A Comparison of AC, Brushless & Switched Reluctance Motors." *Motion Control* (April 1991), pp. 16–20.

Hobbs, C. Adrian. "Dispelling the Misconceptions About Side Impact Protection," SAE 950879. Warrendale, PA: Society of Automotive Engineers Inc., February 27–March 2, 1995.

Hopkins, D., M. Rubin, and D. Arasteh. "Smart Thermal Skins for Automobiles." Proceedings of the Dedicated Conference on Supercars (Advanced Ultralight Hybrids), International Symposium on Advanced Transportation Applications, Aachen,Germany, October 31–November 2, 1994, pp. 667–674.

Kindervater, C. M.: "Crash Resistance and Strength of High Performance Composite Light Vehicle Substructures." Proceedings of the Dedicated Conference on Supercars (Advanced Ultralight Hybrids), International Symposium on Advanced Transportation Applications, Aachen, Germany, October 31–November 2, 1994, pp. 741–751.

Lovins, Amory B. "Supercars: Advanced Ultralight Hybrid Vehicles.," In *Encyclopedia of Energy Technology and Envirionment*. New York: Wiley-Interscience, 1995.

Lovins, Amory B., and Bill Howe. "Switched Reluctance Motor Systems Poised for Rapid Growth." Tech Update, E Source. Boulder, CO (November 1992).

Mason, William T., Jr., and Urban Kristiansson. "Hybrid EVs versus Pure EVs: Which Gives Greater Benefits?" SAE 94C017. Warrendale, PA: Society of Automotive Engineers, Inc., October 17–19, 1994.

Mascarin, Anthony E., Jeffrey R. Dieffenbach, Michael M. Brylawski, David R. Cramer, and Amory B. Lovins. "Costing the Ultralite in Volume Production: Can Composite Bodies-in-White Be Affordable?" Advanced Technologies and Processes, Proceedings of the International Body Engineering Conference, Detroit, October 31–November 2, 1995, pp. 56–69.

Moore, Timothy C., and Amory B. Lovins. "Vehicle Design Strategies to Meet or Exceed PNGV Goals," SAE 951906 (also in *Electric and Hybrid Vehicles: Implementation of Technology*, SAE SP 1105, pp. 79–121). Warrendale, PA: Society of Automotive Engineers, Inc., 1995.

Niederer, Peter F., Felix H. Walz, Robert Kaeser, and Anton Brunner. "Occupant Safety of Low-Mass Rigid-Belt Vehicles," SAE 933107. Warrendale, PA: Society of Automotive Engineers, Inc., November 8–10, 1993.

Post, R., T. Fowler, and S. Post. "A High-Efficiency Electromechanical Battery," *Proceedings of the IEEE* 81, no. 3 (March 1993), pp. 462–474.

Rudderman, M.A., T. Juergens, and R. Nelson. "A New High Rate, Fast Charge, Sealed Lead Acid Battery," Proceedings of the Dedicated Conference on Supercars (Advanced Ultralight Hybrids), International Symposium on Advanced Transportation Applications, Aachen, Germany, October 31, 1994, pp. 121–127.

Seal, M. R., and M. Fitzpatrick. 1982: "A Proposal to Design and Build Viking 21: A Solar/electric CNG Hybrid Car." Vehicle Research Institute, Western Washington University, Bellingham.

Sherman, A. M. "Future Research for Aluminum Vehicle Structure." Conference on Basic Research Needs for Vehicles of the Future, New Orleans, January 5, 1995.

Stirling Thermal Motors. "Engine Performance Test Data." Ann Arbor, MI: Stirling Thermal Motors, 1995.

Trippe, Anthony P., Andrew F. Burke, and Edward Blank. "Improved Electric Vehicle Performance with Pulsed Power Capacitors," SAE 931010. Warrendale, PA: Society of Automotive Engineers, Inc., March 1–5, 1993.

Volvo Car Corporation 1992: "Volvo ECC: A Volvo Environmental Concept Car", press literature (Goteborg, Sweden).

West, John G. W. "DC, Induction, Reluctance and PM Motors for Electric Vehicles." *Power Engineering Journal* (April 1994), pp. 77–88.

Williams, Robert H. "Fuel Cells, Their Fuels, and the U.S. Automobile." First Annual World Car 2001 Conference, Riverside, CA, 1993.

CHAPTER **25**

The Environment and Nanotechnology

VINCENT F. DI RODI
Electronic Recyclers Inc., Shrewsbury, Massachusetts

The arrival of the new millennium presents us with many opportunities. As a benchmark in history, the millennium allows us the opportunity to meditate on humanity's successes. It also gives us an opportunity to reconsider our failures. The exploding size of human population has resulted in increasing levels of human activity. This level of activity is having a negative impact on the global cycling of carbon, nitrogen, phosphorous, and sulfur, the basic building blocks of life. At an accelerating rate, ecosystems have been subject to change, decline, fragmentation, and simplification from these cyclical changes. These continuing shifts in the balance of biochemical cycles will continue to produce unpredictable and devastating environmental results, according to Beck, Boyack, and Berman (1998). A major challenge in the next century will be to use the strength of our emerging technologies to confront the environmental consequences of an exploding human population.

Only recently, through fields of study such as industrial ecology, have we begun to make a conscious effort to consider the consequences of our activities. Industrial ecology is a field of study that crosses over many academic disciplines. It focuses on the relationship between human needs and the cycles and needs of nature. Similar to nature, industrial ecology attempts to provide closed-loop systems to industrial processes and products. These industrial systems are designed to lessen, if not eliminate, impact of manufactured products on natural cycles. Working under the umbrella of industrial ecology, we currently use tools such as DfE and life-cycle assessment (LCA) in developing products that use the latest technologies in an environmentally friendly manner, as shown by Graedel and Allenby (1995).

But, are these current technologies and those under development consistent with the principles of industrial ecology? Could newly emerging technologies be matured in a manner that addresses environmental issues in the developmental stages? As we explore into the new millennium, we should not overlook exciting alternate futures. Although the rate of technological change cannot be determined, current work in the emerging technology on the nanoscale allows us the opportunity to explore.

Nanotechnology is technology controlled at the level of the individual molecule. One of its primary goals is to manufacture and ultimately assemble objects one molecule at a time. Current methods of manufacturing employ a top-down approach. This top-down approach requires the use of macroscale tools and techniques to manipulate bulk quantities of resources. Nanotechnology presents us with a new paradigm, a bottom-up approach to manufacturing.

Techniques currently are being developed to precisely assemble molecules into nanostructures such as motors and numerical control systems for computations, according to the *Foresight Update* (Peterson 1998). The use of these bottom-up techniques and the resulting components may lead to the presence of tools at the nanoscale. These tools may evolve into self-replicating molecular assemblers for use in manufacturing. In theory, this first will be accomplished at the nanoscale and eventually lead to the manufacture and assembly of macroscale objects.

The application of this emerging technology presents us with endless possibilities. Envisioning the future, nanoscale objects will be built to exact engineering specifications, possibly through self-replication. Nano objects also will be constructed using more basic and benign raw materials. This will result in these products being produced at much lower manufacturing costs, according to Drexel (1986). Although these are visionary projections, the science of nanotechnology today is on the road to being a reality.

Current work in the field of nanotechnology has resulted in "nanolasers" (Gourley, 1998) and the "tiny wheel," developed by IBM and the French National Center for Scientific Research, Phelps (1998). According to Peterson (1998), "With nanotechnology being funded by the National Science Foundation, bragged about on IBM's home page, conferred on by the US Army, and favorably featured in *Business Week* the field has clearly gone mainstream."

Along with its applications in medicine, computation, and manufacturing, nanotechnology has the possibility of greatly influencing the environment. If the principles of industrial ecology are incorporated into the basic research of nanotechnology, then a significant positive interaction between human needs and the needs and wants of the environment will occur. Some of the benefits to the environment are

- Reduced resource consumption through dematerialization.
- Reduced chemical pollution through material substitution.
- Products, present and future, never reaching an end of life.
- Conversion of current waste into new resources.
- Enabling recycling to be performed at the consumer-household level.

Looking at the first of these predictions, the application of nanotechnology would allow our products, both nano and eventually macro in size, to be made much more precisely. The result will be great advancements in dematerialization. Current macromanufacturing methods are crude and imprecise. The clumsy manipulation of raw material ends up as waste. This waste stream is caused by our orchestration of material using comparatively crude, bulk methods of extraction and manufacture with equally large quantities of disorganized energy. We take millions of atoms, bond, grind, and manipulate them into objects. The results of these processes are millions of other atoms labeled as manufacturing scrap. Nanotechnology would allow us to use only what is needed and place it exactly where it belongs. The assembly of products at the molecular level, the ultimate in device scaling, should result in objects designed and assembled with near zero tolerances and complete purity of materials.

This would almost eliminate our current manufacturing waste stream and may result in absolute dematerialization. Also, this application should produce dramatic reductions in resource consumption, possibly in energy and certainly in raw material consumed. As the field of nanotechnology matures, it could render current parameters for operational tolerances obsolete. Through changes in physical properties, efficiencies of usage may be greatly increased. From a material point of view, raw material produced or extracted through nanotechnology would be much stronger, lighter, and purer than current materials.

This would make the resulting products stronger, lighter, smarter, and cheaper to manufacture, according to Nelson and Shipbaugh (1995) and Merkle (1993). For example, the power trains of vehicles could be designed with manufacturing tolerances that would result in dramatic reduction in friction, allowing vehicles to consume much less energy. Also, the purity of the raw materials used to make the vehicles might allow for size and weight reduction. Nanofabrication techniques also could allow the materials to be assembled into stronger configurations, which should allow for new material substitution possibilities. These substitutions may lead to products using fewer, if any hazardous, materials. Because of the presence of nanotechnology, the need for use of toxic elements such as lead and mercury could be reduced. Hazardous manufacturing processes, through the evolution of this technology, could become inert.

Microscopic living organisms have designed systems that rid themselves of unwanted waste. This waste then is the feedstock of other organisms. Similarly, industrial ecology tries to utilize manufacturing waste as resources in other operations. The possibility exists to develop this emerging technology, not only to assemble new products but also to disassemble existing waste (inert and biological) one molecule at a time. These molecules could then be reassembled into new resources and products. In theory, this cyclical approach, if designed into the system, would allow all products and by-products, past, present, and future, to never reach an end of life.

In spite of industrial waste prevention and municipal recycling, most material extracted or manufactured still ends up as waste in landfills or dispersed in our environment. In today's society, landfills and hazardous waste sites are viewed as a liability; with nanotechnology, the possibilities emerge of mining these sites for necessary resources. This may be accomplished in two ways. First, molecules of particular elements or compounds in landfills would be recognized as a feedstock by a nanostructured system. This system initially may be a biological microorganism (artificial cell) or subcellular organelle that has been tamed by nanotechnology to provide a service. The nanostuctured system would be programmed to seek out and consume certain types of landfill waste, recognizing it as a feedstock. The landfill waste would be either collected as a resource for human consumption or converted into the nanostructure's own waste, which then would enter nature's environmental cycles. The second method requires that the nanostructure be programmed to recognize certain elements or compounds as waste within its own environment. The nanostructure then would be programmed to remove this material, in essence collecting it for reuse. Through this process of molecular demanufacturing, toxic wastes could be disassembled and recycled back into their inert elements.

Nanotechnology may make it possible someday to produce, repair, and recycle within our own homes. Similar to the way we produce meals in our kitchen to fill our need for hunger, we may be producing other objects in our basements to fill other basic needs and desires for wealth. It is possible to envision a tub that contains all the molecules necessary to assemble a list of products. The consumer would add the instructions, maybe bioengineered software, to assemble the product needed. This product, when it is no longer needed, would not have yet reached its end of life. Instead of being disposed of in a landfill, the consumer would throw the product back into the tub to be disassembled. Using bioengineered software instructions and nano-sized disassemblers, the product would be recycled back to the original molecules. A new set of bioengineered software then would be added to assemble a new product the consumer needs. When developed to this level, nanotech could allow the individual consumer the opportunity to perform both manufacturing and recycling in his or her own home. In theory, this mechanism would allow industrial, government, and consumer waste to be reused, recycled, and remanufactured absolutely and infinitely.

With the new century, it may be wise for humanity to review our long-term strategies and partnerships. One effective way to promote a sustainable future would be to view the natural environment as humanity's customer. As with any customer, a symbiotic relationship exists in which the need or want of an entity is filled by a product or service. The consumer provides a form of payment for which satisfaction or displeasure is realized. Through the centuries, we have extracted energy, water, and mineral resources from the environment, a form of payment. In return, our customer has received only the value of our by-products. Now is the time to apply the basic principles of industrial ecology to developing nanotechnology to provide satisfaction to our customer, the environment. By utilizing this new technology as part of a strategy to build a new relationship with the parent ecosystem, we are working toward ensuring our long-term sustainability.

References

Beck, D., K. Boyack, and M. Berman. *Industrial Ecology Prosperity Game*. Scandia Report SAND98-0643. Albuquerque, NM: Scandia Laboratories, 1998.

Drexel, K. E. *Engines of Creation*. Garden City, NY: Doubleday Books, 1986.

Gourley, P. "Nanolasers." *Scientific American* (March 1998).

Graedel , T. E., and B. R. Allenby. *Industrial Ecology.* Englewood Cliffs, NJ: Prentice-Hall, 1995.

Merkle, R. C. "Molecular Manufacturing: Adding Positional Control to Chemical Synthesis." *Chemical Design Automation News* 8, nos. 8–9 (1993), p. 1.

Nelson, M., and C. Shipbaugh. *The Potential of Nanotechnology for Molecular Manufacturing*. Santa Monica, CA: RAND, 1995.

Peterson, C. "Inside Foresight." *Foresight Update* 34. Palo Alto, CA: Foresight Institute, 1998.

Phelps, L. "Finally, a True 'Tiny Wheel'." *Foresight Update* 34. Palo Alto, CA: Foresight Institute, 1998.

"Unbounding the Future: The Nanotechnology Revolution." Palo Alto, CA: Foresight Institute, 1997.

Part IX

Case Studies, Resources, and Contact Information

APPENDIX **A**

A Case Study: A Printed Circuit Assembly with a No-Lead Solder Assembly Process

William Trumble

Retired from Nortel Networks, Nepean, Canada

Introduction

In 1995, Nortel Networks Business Development's Environmental Affairs Department reviewed the environmental issues of greatest concern to the electronics industry and found that the lead (Pb) content of electronic products was one of the most important environmental issues for the industry. Furthermore, Nortel Networks realized that a program to eliminate lead not only would be good for the environment and public health but also was a task over which the company could have real control (vis à vis suppliers).

Since 1991, Nortel Networks in Harlow, United Kingdom, had been evaluating various alternatives to lead solder. Research by Ruth Billington, of the Materials and Design Technology Group, developed an excellent selection matrix and evaluation program to select lead-free solders (See Table A–1). Based on these criteria, the number of suitable lead-free solders was reduced to two: 99.3% Sn-0.7% Cu and 96.5 Sn-3.5%Ag. Due to the cost of the SnAg solder and some preliminary solder test results, the SnCu solder became the one of choice.

After the review of a variety of solder tests, the decision was made to apply the solder to a Nortel Networks product, removing the lead from the component lead, the solder, and the board finish—creating a printed circuit assembly with no lead in the interconnect. It was assumed at this early stage that the endeavor would not produce a drop in replacement SnPb solder across the entire Nortel Network product portfolio. However, the technology was sufficiently mature to implement in an appropriate area within the three tiers of products the company offers: customer

TABLE A–1 Lead-Free Solder Selection Criteria

Solder Formulation	Issues
42Sn/58Bi:	Rejected. Has slow melting point. Lead must be mined to produce Bismuth.
77.2Sn/20In/2.8Ag:	Rejected. Three part alloy has non-eutectic melting point. Indium(In) is expensive and rare.
85Sn/10Bi/5Zn:	Rejected. Has poor wetting characteristics and is, non-eutectic. Three part alloy is tricky to formulate.
90Sn/7.5Bi/2Ag/0.5Cu:	Rejected. Four-part alloy is tricky to formulate. It is a non-eutectic alloy, and lead has to be mined to produce Bismuth (Bi).
91Sn/9Zn:	Rejected. Has poor wetting characteristics.
96.3Sn/3.2Ag./0.5Cu:	A possible candidate, but it is a three-part alloy and costs twice as much as 63Sn/37Pb solder. It has a non-eutectic melting point with only a 1 degree range.
95Sn/3.5 Ag/1.5 In:	Rejected, due to cost. The three part alloy uses Indium (rare/ expensive).
96.2Sn/2.5Ag/0.8Cu/o.5Sb:	Rejected. This four part alloy has big ratios of metal and a non-eutectic melting point. Uses antimony (Sb) – a toxic material.
96.5Sn/3.5Ag :	One of the prime candidates. This stable binary alloy has a eutectic melting point, but silver doubles the cost/cubic inch of solder over a 63Sn/37Pb alloy.
98Sn/2Ag:	Rejected. It has a non-eutectic melting point, and the alloy is not universally available.
99.3 Sn/0.7Cu	Nortel's prime candidate, along with 96.5Sn/3.5 Ag passed all tests performed by consortium in U.K. It is a binary eutectic stable alloy that has several suppliers. Has a higher melting point than 63Sn/37Pb but is consistent with higher equipment operating temp.
95Sn/5Sb:	Rejected. This non-eutectic binary alloy raises concerns about the toxicity and long term availability of of Antimony (Sb).
91.7 Sn /3.5Ag. /4.8 Bi:	Rejected. This three-part alloy is non-eutectic. Also, bismuth is recovered through lead mining. Does not have a long history.

Note: There are other solders these were available for our evaluation in 1994.
Note: We were very critical in our selection because it is very expensive to do this research very often.
Note: Cu = copper, Zn=Zinc, SB=Antimony, Ag= silver, In=Indium Sn=Tin, Pb=Lead, Bi=Bismuth

handsets, customer switching equipment (PBXs, etc.), and central office equipment. These three tiers can be described as follows:

- *Customer terminals (consumer products)* are residential or business desktop telephones. These products have a product life of five–seven years, operate in benign environments, at room temperature, at few high speeds, and contain intelligent electronic devices and few outside interconnects.

- *Customer switching equipment (PBXs, business products)* includes small switching devices, with a product life of 10–15 years. They are more sophisticated products, operating at higher speeds than desk sets. Such equipment must operate at higher temperature and in a generally more stressful environment than terminals.
- *Central office equipment (Telco products)* operates like a mainline computer with high-capacity switching of a very-high-frequency signal in a very stressful environment. The expected product life of these products is 20 years or more with a requirement for very low expected downtimes during the product's life.

The lead-free project team decided to start with the telephone and escalate up through the portfolio, adding tests as the program progressed until SnPb was replaced in all equipment.

The Program Mantra

A lead-free project team was assembled, comprising individuals from Nortel Technology in Ottawa, Canada, and Harlow, United Kingdom, with Nortel Corporate Business Development's Environmental Affairs Department as the project sponsor.

In the United Kingdom, European-model Meridian phones were assembled at Nortel's manufacturing site in Cwmcarn, Wales. These phones were virtually free of lead in the interconnection. Due to time constraints and supply logistics, it was impossible to procure all components with lead-free finishes. However, all the solder used was SnCu while the solder protection coating was ENTEK 106 n on FR-4 boards.

In Canada, the team was determined to assemble a board with a completely lead-free assembly. The team was aware that there would remain some Pb inside of the components but this was presently outside the influence of Nortel Network's mandate for a lead-free interconnect. To accomplish the goals of the program, the team instituted some functional rules:

- There will be no lead on the board finish.
- There will be no lead on the component finish.
- Billington's reports recommended the solder to be used, 99.3% Sn (tin) + 0.7 % Cu (copper).
- All forms of solder assembly will be used—reflow, solder wave, and hand (paste, bar, wire).
- Nortel Networks-approved outside sources for assembly will be used to reduce experimental bias.
- All efforts will be focused on using the solder equipment (ovens, placement, etc.) used on SnPb solder to determine if any additional capital costs would be involved to assemble parts.
- Deliberate programs will be instituted to attain early and continuous involvement of outside suppliers of services and materials.

- The team will have no hierarchy with regards to activities directed at attaining the goals.
- No matter what the turmoil, keep the "bow upstream."
- The circuit board design used on the project will be that used on an existing large volume product, which will make electrical and functional testing easier and the results less ambiguous.
- The team will answer the project's central question: What kind of solder joints will be formed?

Some problem issues that needed to be resolved before the experiment included the following ones.

The SnCu solder's melting pint is 227°C, requiring a reflow temperature of 242°C. There was concern that the temperature would adversely affect the FR-4 circuit board and board components, but a check of Nortel's standards revealed that the minimum temperature that components should withstand is 260°C.

Previous experiments indicated that the solder joints on some types of lead did not pass inspection due to appearance and shape. This was brought to the attention of the Multicore Corp., which responded by committing to provide a solder paste formulation suitable to Nortel's needs.

The Canadian team encountered the same supply difficulties as the European team in acquiring lead-free finishes on components. To keep the project moving, the team decided to pursue the acquisition of the lead-free component finishes from commercial sources but at the same time retin the available components with the SnCu solder. Thus, the components used were either retinned with SnCu or tinned with some other lead-free finish.

The last issue to resolve was whether the components could be assembled using the lead-free assembly system but on the usual SnPb solder assembly equipment. This and other assembly questions were referred to Ron Pratt of IEC Electronics Corp., the assembly partner. His studies demonstrated that Nortel Networks could use standard equipment and successfully solder the assemblies providing it used nitrogen blanketing in the solder oven atmosphere.

Finally, enough questions were answered to begin the experiment and rebuild the telephone's boards using a completely lead-free interconnection.

The Experiment

First the teams were organized. The Ottawa Nortel team consisted of Murray Hamilton, director, corporate liaison; Bill Trumble, advisor, materials, project leader; David Bilton, manager, manufacture, PCP consultant; and Jane Brydges, project manager, coordination of component supply and manufacturing schedules.

The Ottawa supplier team was composed of Ton Hamel, Corfin Industries, component retinning; Derek Sellen, Multicore Canada Inc., solder; Ron Pratt and Barb Peters, IEC Electronics Corp., reflow solder assembly; Tom Sullivan, Multicore Solder Inc., solder wave assembly.

Two hundred boards in 2 × 2 panels were ordered from Hadco to be coated with ENTEK 106. The boards were inspected and sent to IEC.

The components to be retinned with SnCu were ordered from Nortel Networks Corporate Supply Management, inspected, and sent to Corfin to be retinned. The component suppliers were pressed to ship lead-free finished components quickly.

Multicore compounded the bar SnCu solder and sent some to Corfin for retinning. The paste was sent to IEC for reflow assembly while the wire solder went to Nortel Networks for manual assembly.

After Corfin retinned the components, it sent them to IEC for reflow assembly. Out of the 200 boards, 153 were successfully assembled on first pass. None of the dropouts were due to the solder process but rather due to part placement problems. Dr. Pratt examined the joints on several boards and pronounced all of them to pass current standards.

The reflow assembled boards were sent to Multicore to be wave soldered. Of the 145 boards submitted, 132 were successfully assembled.

Of the 135 boards received by Kanata, 20 were completed by hand soldering. Ten were sent to Nortel Networks Global Manufacturing Technology, Calgary, Canada, for reliability testing and ten boards were installed into phones for demonstration purposes. Ten boards were assembled using these lead-free finished components and SnCu solder. Five of these boards were assembled into phones for demonstration and five were sent to Calgary.

All the circuit assemblies (completely SnCu and lead free) passed Calgary's electrical and functional tests for telephone reliability.

A six-part project seminar was held for suppliers of components, materials, and services. All pledged to support our program. We had 100% support from suppliers.

Conclusions

This project has given Nortel much valuable information about how SnCu solder assembly can be used to fabricate a reliable printed circuit assembly for consumer products. It has shown that SnCu assembly can be accomplished using present-day SnPb equipment in a SnPb assembly facility with the addition of nitrogen atmosphere shielding. We also are confident that there is a potential cost reduction through the end of life of the products.

References

ASTM Metals. *Metallography, Structures and Phase Diagrams*, vol. 8, eighth ed. ASTM Metals, Philadelphia, PA, 1973.

Bader, W. "Dissolution of Au, Ag, Pd, Pt, Cu and Ni in a Molten Tin-Lead Solder." *Welding Journal*, Research Supplement, 48, no. 12 (1969), pp. 551s–557s.

Fretterolf, T. "99C Wavesoldering Evaluation with No Clean on Copper/Entek." Multicore Laboratory Report 609012, 1996.

Nortel Networks. "Acceptability of Electronic Assemblies." IPC-A-610B, Kanata, Canada, 1994.

Nortel Networks. "Lead-Free 8009 Manufacturing Assembly Trials." EC30, Kanata, Canada, 1996.

Nortel Networks. "Workmanship PCBA Surface Mount." Nortel Workmanship Standard 150.09, 1996.

Porter, D., and K. Easterling. *Phase Transformation in Metals and Alloys.* New York: Van Nostrand Reinhold, 1981.

Pratt, R. "Fracture and Deformation Behavior of Eutectic Pb-Sn Solder Joints." MS thesis, University of Rochester, 1991.

Pratt, R. "The Effect of Noble Metal Contamination on the Mechanical Properties of Eutectic Tin-Lead Solder Joints." Ph.D. thesis, University of Rochester, 1994.

Pratt, R. "Bell Northern Research A0649450 Lead-Free Assembly Process Details." IEC Technical Report RP-25-96, August 1996.

Pratt, R. "Mircrostructural Analysis of Eutectic Sn-Cu Alloy Solder Joints." IEC Technical Report RP-26-97 (August 1997).

Pratt, R. "Microstructural Analysis of Eutectic Sn-Cu Alloy Solder Joints after 2000 Thermal Cycles, 0°C–100 C." IEC Technical Report RP-28-97 (September 1997).

Pratt, R. "Microstructural Analysis of Eutectic Sn-Cu Alloy Solder Joints after 4000 Thermal Cycles, 0°C–100 C." IEC Technical Report RP-01-98 (January 1998).

Pratt, R., E. Stromswold, and D. Quesnel. "Effect of Solid-State Intermetallic Growth on the Fracture Thoughness of Cu/63Sn-37Pb Solder Joints." *IEEE Transactions on Components, Packaging, and Manufacturing Technology—* Part A, 19, no. 1, CHMT-19 (1996), pp, 134-141.

Romig, A., et al. "Physical Metallurgy of Solder-Substrate Reactions." In *Solder Mechanics: A State of the Art Assessment.* TMS Publications, 1991. [[AU: Please add the names of all the authors of the chapter, the name(s) of the editor(s) of the volume, and the city of publication.]]

Smith, W. *Principles of Materials Science and Engineering.* New York: McGraw-Hill, 1989.

Stromswold, E., R. Pratt, and D. Quesnel. "The Mechanical Properties of Cu/96.5Sn-3.5Ag Solder Joints with Comparisons to Cu/63Sn-37Pb Solder Joints." SAND93-7102, Sandia Laboratories, White Sands, NM, 1993.

Trumble, W., and J. Brydges. "World's First Lead Free Circuit Telephone." IPCWorks '97, October 5–9, 1997.

Warwick, M., and S. Muckett. "Observations on the Growth and Impact of Intermetallic Compounds on Tin-Coated Substrates." *Circuit World* 9, no. 4 (1983).

APPENDIX **B**

Case Study: A Search for Chromate Conversion Coating Alternatives for Corrosion Protection of Zinc-Plated Electronic Shelves

William Trumble and Pat Lawless
Nortel Technology

Introduction

Hexavalent chromium oxide has been used for at least 60 years as a corrosion preventative for painted and unpainted aluminum, zinc, and other metal surfaces used for cabinets and shelves for electronic equipment. The shelf essentially serves as a faraday cage for the electronics within, which emanate a broad spectrum of electromagnetic interference (EMI) and in turn are sensitive to EMI, even between shelves. Until recently, the electromagnetic-interference shielding requirements of these electronic shelves were such that the contact and surface resistivity of the chromate coating provided sufficient performance. As signal speeds and amplitudes within equipment have increased, they require coatings that have higher electrical conductivity to form more effective connections between shelving elements.

Nortel became increasingly aware of the environmental and electrical issues in the use of hexavalent chrome and decided to search for alternatives in 1994. A program was initiated to explore conductive paints, zinc alloys, and new conversion coatings to provide an alternative to the hexavalent chromate coating as a metal protectant and EMI shielding gasket interface.

Program Approach

To focus an effective search for an alternate conversion, a set of criteria was laid out. The criteria for the program are

1. The process will not involve materials that are as environmentally threatening as the chromate process.
2. The application process will not present undue danger to the operation.

3. The application process shall not involve a large number of process steps to apply.
4. The conversion coating process shall not require high energy input or a arcane processes to apply—KISS.
5. The coated product is to show no white corrosion or red rust for up to 96 hours of exposure to a salt fog environment, as per ASTM B117. The selected conversion coating shall be exposed to the following test conditions. A suitably clamped sandwich of the plate-coated samples shall be exposed to 10 days of a 85°C/85% RH environment, then exposed for 1,000 hours to a Battelle Class IV environment. The surface resistance of the individual samples shall not vary more than 10% from initial readings and the contact resistance of the sandwich shall not vary more than 10%.
6. The surface resistivity and the contact resistance of the test sample of the new conversion-coated zinc-plated mild steel sample shall be less than 50% of that of the chromated samples.
7. Cost will not excessively exceed that of chromate.
8. The surface of the finished part will be of uniform texture.
9. The surface will have an esthetic pleasing appearance.
10. The conversion coating shall be commercially accessible.

Search for Alternative Conversion Coatings

Nortel conducted an in-depth search of periodicals and research papers to discover a suitable alternative conversion coating. Most coatings failed the criteria of electrical conductance. Finally, a series of journal articles described the performance of a molybdenum phosphate conversion coating in experiments conducted by Torbin Tang of the Polytechnical Institute of Denmark. The journal articles convinced Nortel that this process was the candidate for our application and Tang was contacted. Subsequent negotiating resulted in Nortel acquiring the formula for experiments.

Concurrently, information generated from the NCMS report "Alternates to Chromate for Aluminum" revealed that some formulations from the Bulk Chemicals Corp. would likely be a secondary candidate. All necessary materials were collected and the experiment was organized. Both coatings were reviewed and found to be of the best environmental process.

Experiment

The following base samples were used:
Alkaline zinc-plated mild steel.
Cyanide zinc-plated mild steel.
Stainless steel.
Zinc nickel on mild steel.

The following conversion coatings were applied:

Alkaline zinc	Yellow chromate	Cyanide zinc	Bulk 923
Cyanide zinc		Zinc nickel	
Zinc nickel		Alkaline zinc	Bulk 923x
Alkaline zinc	Molybdenum phosphate	Cyanide zinc	
Cyanide zinc	Formula 66	Zinc nickel	
Zinc nickel		304 stainless-steel base	
Alkaline zinc			

Sample Description for Exposure Tests

The tests used

2" × 2" steel coupons, both perforated and unperforated, for a salt fog test.
3/4" × 4" double steel coupon for an 85/85 Battelle Class IV (unprotected) test.

Tests used five devices for each coating sample. Each metal wafer was stamped with an identifying number and broken into appropriate groupings for each test profile (e.g., alkaline zinc yellow chromate). Most samples were plated and conversion coated according to the instructions appropriate to that plating or coating by Alexander Hastings of Zincon Inc. The cyanide zinc plating was provided by Technospec of Montreal and the zinc-nickel-plated samples were provided by Newtech Plating and Process.

All the coating and plating processes, with the exception of the molybdenum phosphate and bulk 923 and 923x, were performed on a regular process-plating line to ensure the process would be as close to the actual uninterrupted production process as possible. The molybdenum phosphate and bulk 923 and 923x were applied on a small plating line to the manufacture's specifications by Zincon.

Nortel arranged to have a commercial plater involved in all experiments to ensure standard commercial practices were applied and could be repeated when the research was successful.

The range of colors on zinc with molybdenum was from light blue to yellow. The desired color for Nortel's purpose was a light violet. This was easy to achieve on all samples, except for the edges of the holes in the stamped perforated samples. The residual stress allowed more permeation and reaction between metal and conversion coating. The samples were dried and allowed to complete the reaction.

The samples then carefully were packaged and sent out for testing and analysis as previously designed with Newtech Plating and Processing. Nortel used as many commercial facilities as it could to conduct this research so that when the program was successful, the technology would not suffer from culture to culture.

As the test progressed, N. Satar of Newtech submitted reports describing the red rust and white rust of the samples exposed for 96 and 300 hours to salt fog (ASTM-B117). Progress reports were given for all samples exposed to the Battelle Class IV test.

Newtech provided SEM analysis of the treated samples as they emerged from the test. The SEM analysis was performed to try to relate changes in electrical behavior to change in material composition of the surface of the test sample.

Conclusions

Molybdenum is a viable alternative to chromate for Nortel's design purposes. Molybdenum provides no corrosion protection of yellow chromate but meets the Nortel and Bellcore requirements.

The tests demonstrated that an alkaline zinc plate coated with molybdenum performed equally to that of cyanide-plated zinc; therefore, efforts will be made to move the cyanide process out of Nortel products.

The molybdenum coating provides a uniform blue violet color that gives an esthetically pleasing appearance to Nortel products.

Using commercial outside sources to complete the various tasks of the research was successful in that all participants showed enthusiasm for the impending change.

Most of the samples using molybdenum on zinc displayed better electrical conductivity than those coated with chromate. The electrical conductivity was stable throughout the Battelle Class IV test. These results indicate that molybdenum would provide a better gasket interface in faraday cages than that of chromate.

The coating is applied easily if the process conditions are stable. The perforated sample gave erratic results but perforated samples always do on first experiments.

Other Design and Environmental Benefits

EMI tests demonstrated that, because of the superior conductivity of the molybdenum phosphate, the expensive copper beryllium gasket is not needed to ensure electrical contact between elements of the shelf. A flexible gasket in contact with the conversion coating suffices. This situation removes the need to plate any gasket with tin lead plating, as was done with the copper beryllium gasket.

The molybdenum phosphate coating is resistant to the high heat of the powder coating of baking cycle. The more environmentally friendly, lower-cost powder coating could be applied to product, which could not be done with chromate.

What Next?

Nortel is committed to changing its conversion coatings from hexavalent chrome. Tests demonstrate that molybdenum phosphate is the alternate conversion coating to develop into a Nortel process, and the molybdenum system will be tested on aluminum and metal surfaces exposed to the outdoors.

APPENDIX **C**

Case Study: "Butterfly," an Application of DfE Principles to a Telephone

William Trumble

Retired from Nortel Networks, Nepean, Canada

Background

As part of Nortel Networks' commitment to the environment, a Green Design research project was initiated to review the use of energy, resources, materials, and waste associated with all stages of manufacture, use, and disposal. The project aims to explore sustainable design and production practices that decrease the environmental impact and provide a competitive edge in the global economy. A key aspect of this project is the creation of a "concept" telephone to demonstrate leading environmental features such as Nortel Networks lead-free interconnection technology, fewer parts, and a reduction in the number of materials for ease of recycling.

Nortel Networks strives for design leadership through a focus on both business and environmental value. Its experience shows that strong environmental performance can lead to cost reduction, enhanced brand image, new sources of revenue, and market growth. By applying business principles to environmental projects in the portfolio, the company obtains estimates of the true value of environmental performance. The innovative solutions produced add value to Nortel Networks while reducing the corporation's impact on the environment.

The company continually seeks to move beyond compliance with environmental regulations to minimize resource consumption, waste, and the adverse environmental impact from its products, operations, and business activities. Nortel Networks is taking responsibility for the environmental impact of its products throughout their life cycles from design to final disposition. This is driven not so much by regulatory pressures as by market pressures, which take the form of customer requirements, the

ISO 14000 series of environmental management system (EMS) standards, and ecolabels.

Design for Environment

Design for environment (DfE) adds environmental values to the typical design criteria of functionality, cost, and aesthetics. In response to emerging environmental need, DfE stimulates innovate designs that

- Use fewer materials and avoid those that are toxic or nonrenewable wherever possible.
- Increase energy efficiency throughout the product's life cycle.
- Use cleaner production practices and less packaging.
- Extend product life.
- Provide for easy disassembly to recover and recycle materials and components.
- Reduce parts by integrating functions.

From a business perspective, DfE can reduce the cost of producing, distributing, and owning a product and can lead to increased revenue by meeting emerging customer needs and enhancing a producer's brand image. At the same time, DfE reduces the environmental impacts associated with these activities.

Recent examples of DfE within Nortel Networks include the development of the world's first lead-free telephone, an environmentally preferable replacement for chromate conversion coating of metal parts, and DfE guidelines to identify and promote an environmentally responsible design approach for all Nortel Networks' products.

All DfE initiatives must be carefully analyzed to ensure they actually prevent pollution. Pollution often is displaced from one media to another; for example, air to water or water to soil. Pollution liabilities also can be transferred across the economy, from a manufacturing site to its suppliers or to customers.

Life-Cycle Assessment

Environment Canada, the Canadian government's environmental department, provided funding toward Nortel Networks Green Design research project for an in-depth review of the energy, resources, materials, and waste associated with all stages of manufacture, use, and end of a product's life. A life-cycle assessment (LCA) was conducted on a consumer business telephone set due to its commercial availability, consumer applicability, and technology level. Also, the telephone in question has been manufactured for ten years and was selected due to the availability of useful information on it.

This initiative is the first time the government of Canada and private industries have teamed up to examine an entire produce life cycle.

Making It Happen

Nortel Networks plan was to incorporate as many environmental features into the model as possible to create a concept telephone demonstrating the value of design for environment. The model would include such features as

Thin wall plastic construction.
Maximization of recycled plastic content.
New keypad technology.
Elimination of labels.
Use of alternative fasteners (no metal screws).
New product packaging.
Material recyclability and compatibility.
Lead-free solder assembly.
Nonhalogenated flame retardant board.
Integrated mechanical design.
A smaller speaker and microphone.

Nortel Networks sought out the best available talent to help realize these objectives. The response from its business partners was tremendous, with their ideas exceeding its expectations. A general specification was created, and each objective was assigned a coordinator from among Nortel's internal experts and external business partners.

Green Concept Telephone

The design of the green concept telephone (see Figure C–1) was completed by one of Nortel Networks' most experienced industrial designers. The team's vision was to create a telephone that was both environmental and aesthetically pleasing to customers.

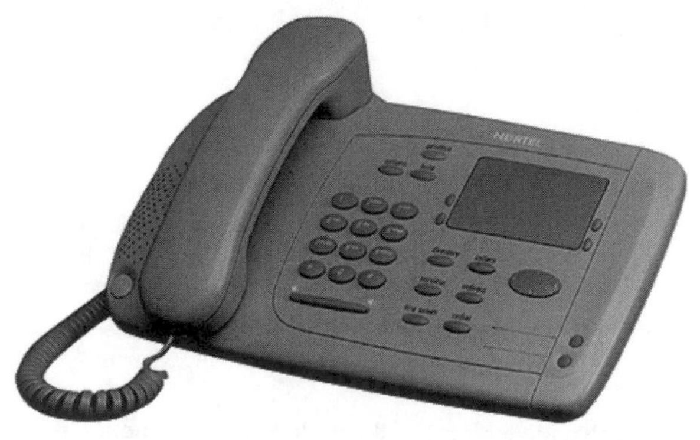

FIGURE C–1 Predictive model image.

The features explored for the "concept" telephone are driven by DfE but encompass other areas, such as design for assembly, disassembly, and installation or DfX (design for efficiency). Another initiative pursued and incorporated in the design was z-axis assembly. The environmental features of the "concept" telephone fall into two broad categories: materials reduction and compatibility and toxicity reduction.

Materials Reduction and Compatibility

Using materials that were compatible and reducing the variety of materials used make for easier assembly and recycling at the end of the product's life. Also, reducing the number of parts in the construction reduces assembly time and labor costs. The amount and variety of materials used to manufacture a telephone were targeted for reduction in the design of the "concept" telephone.

Plastic Housing

The main function of the plastic housing is to protect the internal electronic components. To reduce the amount of plastic used for the telephone housing, a variety of initiatives and technologies were investigated, including reduction of plastic through industrial design, thin-wall plastic, and maximized recycled content.

Plastic Reduction Through Industrial Design

Rather than having the largest component in the telephone dictate the thickness of the entire telephone, the plastic was minimized by designing around the components. This is illustrated in Figure C–2 with the speaker.

The base telephone included a bracket that could be rotated for desk or wall mounting. For the "concept" telephone, this piece was eliminated to reduce the amount of material. Also, customer demand for the mounting business telephone

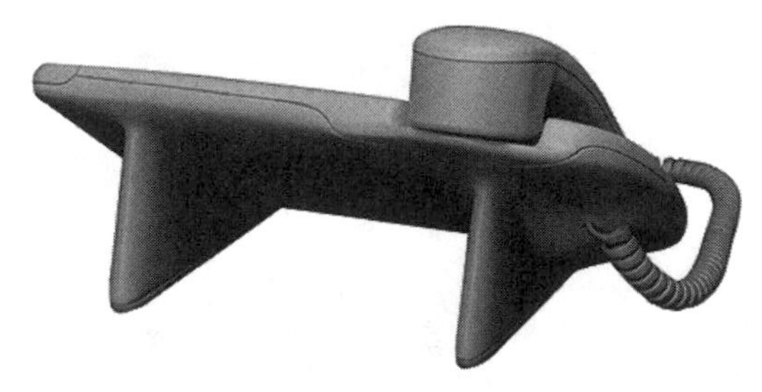

FIGURE C–2 Predictive model image, illustrating plastic reduction through industrial design.

sets is approximately 10%. Therefore, the team proposed to design a separate bracket that could be purchased by customers requiring a wall mounting.

Thin-Wall Plastic The base telephone has a wall thickness of 3 mm using acrylonitrile-butadiene-styrene (ABS). With the new advancements in thin-wall technology, Nortel saw an opportunity to apply these principles to its green telephone with the input from General Electric Plastics.

By using the modular properties of the plastic rather than the bulk properties of the plastic, the wall thickness in the concept phone was reduced, resulting in materials savings. The material used for the design was a blend of polycarbonate (PC) and ABS.

Additionally, asymmetric and other customized fillets around bosses, gussets, and the like strengthen the plastic housing in the critical cantilever area. Research demonstrates that we could use opposing forces in the two housing parts to further strengthen the finished shell. Furthermore, the component attachments are configured so that the installation itself will reinforce the structure in the housing. All edges and corners are designed to eliminate stress concentration for impact (drop) tests.

The key advantages to using a thin-wall plastic technology are materials savings and productivity improvement due to decreased cycle times.

Maximized Recycled Content The thermoplastic scrap produced during the molding process (i.e., runner and sprues) for this telephone can be reused in the molding process to a maximum of 25%. Using regrind in the plastic housing minimizes the amount of waste generated during the molding process.

Elimination of Labels

The paper as well as the adhesives contribute to contamination during the recycling of the plastic housing. Labels can be eliminated with alternatives such as laser etching, embossing, and in-mold decorating. The plastics also are labeled in accordance with International Standard Organization (ISO) standards.

Alternative Fasteners

The base telephone is held together with six metal screws. Fasteners are a major barrier to efficient assembly, repair, and disassembly. Also, metal screws are small and could be accidentally mixed with the plastic, which would contaminate the batch. Some alternative fastening techniques investigated include snap fit, plastic hinges, and plastic screws.

Other

To overcome the involuntary movement of the telephone due to its light weight, a nonskid design will be used on the feet.

Handset

The handset is smaller in size than traditional Nortel Networks handsets. First, the handset uses a smaller speaker and microphone than the traditional handset. Second, the plastics have been reduced in size as well as in wall thickness.

Keypad Technology

The keys and keypad for the base telephone consist of 93 pieces of five different types of materials, which make separation and recycling at the end of the product's life difficult. Reducing the number of pieces aids in making the telephone easier to assemble and repair.

The new membrane keypad technology eliminates many of these pieces and makes the keypad easier to assembly and disassemble. The membrane keypad was developed and proven by True North Printed Plastics Inc.

Also, the base business telephone set has 12 keys for repeated dialing. To eliminate the quick dialers, a menu driven display was incorporated. This initiative helped reduce the number of pieces during the assembly of the telephone.

Packaging

Addressing the growing concern of packaging material, Nortel Networks examined new packaging for the green telephone. The key issues considered include enhanced recycling of materials, increased recycled content in packaging and reduced materials in transport.

The amount of packaging for transport is reduced by integrating the structural properties of the product with the packaging. The optimum size of packaging, to get as many telephones on a pallet as possible, was investigated.

Toxicity Reduction

Using toxic materials in the construction of telephones poses environmental and safety concerns. Reducing toxicity helps eliminate the risk of toxic substances entering the environment and makes the assembly line a safer place for employees. Some of the new initiatives pursed by Nortel Networks include the lead-free interconnection technology and nonhalogenated flame retardant.

Lead-Free Interconnection Technology

Lead, although the long-time industry standard for solder, is a heavy metal that can pose significant threat to human and environmental health. The alternative solder equivalent or better in cost than tin-lead was tin-copper.

In January 1997, Nortel Networks announced that it manufactured the world's first lead-free telephone. Not only was it a historic milestone for Nortel Networks but a breakthrough for the environment.

Nonhalogenated Flame Retardants

A halon is a chemical compound comprised of bromine, fluorine, and carbon (USEPA, 1996). Until recently, halons have been widely used as fire extinguishing agents. They may be incorporated into a system, such as the coating on a printed circuit board, or be contained in portable fire extinguishers. Although effective as flame retardants, this group of chemicals can have a negative impact on human and environmental health.

Using the technology developed by Isola, Germany, and experience from Siemens, Nortel Networks procured a nonhalogenated printed wiring board FRN (Duraver 150) in replacement of the standard FR-4 laminate.

Conclusions

Design for environment offers a powerful way for Nortel Networks to improve resource productivity, environmental performance, shareholder value, and customer value. By minimizing material and energy consumption and maximizing reuse and recycling, Nortel Networks can reduce the environmental impact of the corporation's products and services.

The Green Design project sets an example of leadership in environmental design. The "concept" telephone is used as a vehicle to implement and educate the value of DfE throughout the corporation and set a standard for the industry to change.

References

Bergendahl, C. G., P. Hedemalm, and T. Segerber. *Handbook for Design of Environmentally Compatible Electronic Products, an Aid for Designers.* The Swedish Institute of Production Engineering Research, Molndal, October 1995.

"Life Cycle Management by Design." Pittsfield, MA: GE Plastics, 1996.

Smith, M. T., R. Roy, and S. Potter. "The Commercial Impacts of Green Product Development." UK: The Open University, Design Innovation Group, Milton Keynes, UK, July 1996.

APPENDIX **D**

Resources

Publications

Allenby, B. "Testing Design for the Environment—Should Lead Solder Be Used in Printed Wiring Board." *Semiconductor Safety Association Journal* (December 1992).

Hawken, Paul. *The Ecology of Commerce.* New York : HarperCollins Publishers, 1993.

Kartha, S. "Fuel Cells: Energy Conversion for the Next Century." *Physics Today* 47 (November 1994), pp. 54–61.

Lamprecht, James L. *ISO 14000: Issues and Implementation Guidelines for Responsible Environmental Management.* New York: Amacom, 1997.

Lave, L. "Recycling Decisions and Green Design." *Environmental Science and Technology* 28 (1994).

Pacey, Arnold. *The Culture of Technology.* Cambridge, MA: MIT Press, 1983.

Pitts, G. et al. "Implementing Cleaner Technologies in the PWB Industry: Making Holes Conductive." Microelectronics and Computer Corp., 1996.

Pitts, G. et al. "PWB Pollution Prevention and Control Technology Survey." Microelectronics and Computer Corp., 1996.

Sayre, Don. *Inside ISO 14000: The Competitive Advantage of Environmental Management.* Delray Beach, FL: St. Lucie Press, 1996.

Stellman, Jeanne Mager, ed. *Encyclopedia of Occupational Health and Safety,* vol. 3, fourth ed. Geneva, Switzerland: International Labor Organization, 1998.

Weissman, S. "Environmentally Conscious Manufacturing—A Technology for the Nineties." *AT&T Technical Journal* (November 1991).

Websites

Computer recycling projects. At www.learner.org/sami/computer-recycle.shtml.

OSHA Website on semiconductors. At www.osha-slc.gov/sltc/semiconductors/index.html.

Recycling links. At www.dnr.state.oh.us/odnr/recycling/litter/links.html.

Semiconductor safety references. At www.umich.edu/~oseh/semiref.html.

Scientific American. At www.sciam.com/exhibit/052796exhibit.html.

Organizations

ECP News, IBM Engineering Center for Environmentally Counscious Products, FXLB/061, 3039 Cornwallis Road, Research Triangle Park, NC 27709-2195.

EPR2 Update, National Safety Council/Environmental Health Center, 1025 Connecticut Avenue, NW, Suite 1200, Washington, DC.

E-Source, Inc., 1033 Walnut Street, Boulder, CO 80302; Website at www.esource.com.

Hypercar Center, 1739 Snowmass Creek Road, Snowmass, CO 81654; phone (970) 927-3851, fax (970) 927-3420, Website at www.rmi.org/hypercar/dox/center.html.

IEEE International Symposium on Electronics and the Environment, c/o IEEE Travel and Conference Management Services, 445 Hoes Lane, Piscataway, NJ 08855-1331; phone (732) 562-3875, fax (732) 981-1203.

LCD PS Team R&T Update (life-cycle design), 248 Baker Systems, 1971 Neil Avenue, Columbus, OH 43210.

Microelectronics and Computer Corp. (MCC), 3500 W. Balcones Center Drive, Austin, TX 78759; phone (512) 338-3400, Website at www.mcc.com/env.

PPIC (Pollution Prevention Information Center) U.S. EPA, 401 M Street SW (7409), Washington, DC 20460. Website at www.ipc.org/html/ehstypes.htm#design or www.epa.gov/dfe.

Rocky Mountain Institute, 1739 Snowmass Creek Road, Snowmass, CO 81654; phone (970) 927-3851, fax (970) 927-3420, Website at www.rmi.org.

Sandia Labs, *Sandia Lab News*, Website at www. sandia.gov/LabNews/LN3-15-96/intell.html.

APPENDIX **E**

Author Contact Information

By Chapter and Section

Book Introduction

Lee Goldberg, 202 Mather Avenue, Princeton, NJ 08540, USA, PH (609) 720-0015, Email: prestomeco@home.com, lgoldberg@chipcenter.com

Section I Introduction

Amory Lovins, Rocky Mountain Institute, 1739 Snowmass Creek Road, Snowmass, CO, 81654-9199, USA, PH (970) 927-3128, FAX (970) 927-4178 Email: ablovins@rmi.org

Chapter 1

Gary Smerdon, Advanced Micro Devices, Network Products Division, One AMD Place Sunnyvale, CA 94088, USA, Email: gary.smerdon@amd.com

Chapter 2

Radim Vishinka, Motorola s.r.o., B.Nemcove 1720, Roznov pod Radhostem, 756 61, Czech Republic, PH 420.651.667.175 FAX 420.651.652.099 Email: r28108@email.mot.com

Chapter 3

Ondrej Pauk, Motorola s.r.o., B.Nemcove 1720, Roznov pod Radhostem, 756 61, Czech Republic, PH 420.651.667.171 FAX 420.651.652.099 Email: r24529@email.sps.mot.com

Petr Lidik, Motorola s.r.o., B.Nemcove 1720, Roznov pod Radhostem, 756 61, Czech Republic, PH 420.651.667.171 FAX 420.651.652.099

Chapter 4

Aengus Murray, Analog Devices Inc., Motion Control Group, 831 Woburn Street, Wilmington, MA 01887 PH (781) 937-1697 Email: Aengus.Murray@analog.com

Chapter 5

Pitipong Veerakamolmal, Laboratory for Responsible Manufacturing, 334 SN, Department of MIME, Northeastern University, Boston, MA 02115, USA, PH (617) 373-7635 FAX (617) 373-2921 Email: pitipong@usa.net

Surendra M. Gupta, Laboratory for Responsible Manufacturing, 334 SN, Department of MIME, Northeastern University, Boston, MA 02115, USA, PH (617) 373-4846 FAX (617) 373-2921 Email: gupta@neu.edu

Chapter 6

Craig Boswell, HOBI International Inc. 5145 Norwood, Suite C, Dallas, TX 75247, USA, PH (214) 951-0143 FAX (214) 951-0144 Email: cboswell@hobi.com

Chapter 7

Dr. Arpad Horvath, Carnegie Mellon University, Department of Civil & Environmental Engineering, Pittsburgh, PA 15213-3890, USA, PH (412) 268-5763 FAX (412) 268-7813 Email: ah3p+@andrew.cmu.edu

Dr. Wolfgang M. Grimm, Robert Bosch GmbH, Corporate Research and Development, Dep. FV/FLI P.O. Box 10 60 50, D-70049 Stuttgart, Germany, PH (49-711) 811-7654 FAX (49-711) 811-7601 Email: wolfgang-michael.grimm@de.bosch.com

Dr. Markus Klausner, Robert Bosch GmbH, Corporate Research and Development, Dep. FV/FLI P.O. Box 10 60 50, D-70049 Stuttgart, Germany, PH (49-711) 811-7653 FAX (49-711) 811-7601 Email: klausner+@andrew.cmu

Chapter 8

Joan Williams, Federal Reserve Bank, 1701 San Jacinto, Houston, TX 77002, USA, PH 713-652-1596 Email: Joan.E.Williams@dal.frb.org

Chapter 9

Sudarshan Siddhaye, UC Berkeley, 131 Hesse Hall, UCB Campus, Berkeley CA 94720, USA, PH (510) 643-6512 Email: siddhaye@greenmfg.me.berkeley.edu

Paul Sheng, UC Berkeley, 131 Hesse Hall, UCB Campus, Berkeley, CA 94720, USA, PH (510) 643-6512 Email: psheng@me.berkeley.edu

Chapter 10

Brian Glazebrook, Ecobalance Inc., 7101 Wisconsin Avenue, Suite 700 Bethesda, MD 20814, USA, PH (301) 548-1752 x1754 FAX (301) 548-1760 Email: ecobalance@compuserve.com

Section II Introduction

Christopher Rhodes, 4229 N. Claremont, Chicago, IL 60618-2905 PH (773) 279-8342 Email: crrhodes@mindspring.com

Chapter 11

William Trumble, 18 McClure Cresent, Kanata, Ontario K2L2H3 PH (613) 592-2068 Email: wtrumble@home.com

Chapter 12

George Yender, 9 Holly Lane, Westford, MA 01886, USA, PH (978) 692-7701 Email: gyseabee@ma.ultranet.com

Chapter 13

John Lott, DuPont Electronic Materials, 14 T. W. Alexander Drive, Research Triangle, NC 27709, USA, PH (919) 248-5046 FAX (919) 248-5341 Email: john.w.lott@usa.dupont.com

Holly Evans, Director of Health, Safety and Environmental Programs - IPC, 14000 Eye St. NW Suite 540, Washington, DC 20050 PH (202) 333-2331 Fax (202) 333-0145 Email: HollyEvans@ipc.org

Chapter 14

William Trumble, 18 McClure Crescent, Kanata, Ontario K2L2H3 PH (613) 592-2068 Email: wtrumble@home.com

Chapter 15

William Trumble, 18 McClure Cresent, Kanata, Ontario K2L2H3 PH (613) 592-2068 Email: wtrumble@home.com.

Section III Introduction

Ted Polakowski, Microelectronics Group, Lucent Technologies Inc., 2 Oak Way, Berkley Heights, NJ 07322, USA Email: tpolakowski@lucent.com

Chapter 16

Jill Matzke, c/o S.S. Moondance, callsign: wcy6324, e-mail: wcy6324@sail-mai.com, formoondance@yahoo.com, Home address: 3328 St. Michael Dr., Palo Alto, CA 94306, USA. OR Apple Computer, 1 Infinite Loop MS 26-ETS Cupertino, CA 95014, USA, PH (408) 974-5912 FAX (408) 974-5377 Email: matzke@apple.com

Chapter 17

Jill Matzke, c/o S.S. Moondance, callsign: wcy6324, e-mail: wcy6324@sail-mai.com, formoondance@yahoo.com, Home address: 3328 St. Michael Dr., Palo Alto, CA 94306, USA. OR Apple Computer, 1 Infinite Loop MS 26-ETS Cupertino, CA 95014, USA, PH (408) 974-5912 FAX (408) 974-5377 Email: matzke@apple.com

Chapter 18

Kelly Weinschenk, Corbet Consulting, 203 Chippendale Court, Los Gatos, CA 95032 Email: CorbetCons@aol.com

Chapter 19

Carsten Nagel, Fraunhofer-Institut for Material Flow and Logistics IML, Joseph-von-Fraunhofer-Str. 2-4, D- 44227 Dortmund, Germany, PH 49.231.9743-362 Fax 49.231.9743-451 Email: nagel@iml.fhg.de

Chapter 20

Jim Lamprecht, 27636 Ynez Road L-7, Suite 275, Temecula, CA 92591, USA, PH (909) 506-9426 Email: liml@pe.net

Chapter 21

Jim Hart, University of Strathclyde, Signal Processing Division, Electronic and Electrical Engineering, John Anderson Campus, GLASGOW G1 1XQ jimh@spd.eee.strath.ac.uk

Chapter 22

Carol Brown, SGS Thompson Microelectronics, 55 Old Bedford Road, Lincoln, MA 01773, USA, PH (617) 259-2519 FAX (617) 259-9423 Email: brownc@stm.com

Section IV Introduction

Lee Goldberg, 202 Mather Avenue, Princeton, NJ 08540, USA, PH (609) 720-0015 Email: prestomeco@home.com, lgoldberg@chipcenter.com

Chapter 23

Joseph Chiodo and Prof. Eric Billet, Cleaner Electronics Institute, Brunel University, Runnymeade Campus, Egham, Surrey TW20 OJZ, UK, PH 44.1784.431.341 (PH in Canada - 9905) 723-8806) FAX 44.1784.472.879 Email: joseph.chiodo@brunel.ac.uk Web address: http://www.brunel.ac.uk/~dtsrjdc/ASDM.html

Chapter 24

Timothy Moore, The Hypercar Center, Rocky Mountain Institute, 1739 Snowmass Creek Rd., Snowmass, CO 81654-9199, USA, PH (970) 927-3851 FAX (970) 927-4510 Email: tmoore@rmi.org or hypercar@rmi.org

Chapter 25

Vincent DiRodi, Electronic Recyclers, 400 Boylston Street, Shrewsbury, MA 01545, USA, PH (508) 842-4208 Email: recyclers@wn.net

---

Additional book personnel

Assistant editor

Wendy Middleton, RR2 Box 221A, Watsontown, PA 17777, PH (570) 742-7193 Email: wendym@pcspower.net

Cartoonists

John McPherson, closetohome@compuserve.com, www.closetohome.com

Fred Sklenar, c/o Sklenar Marketing, 664 College Avenue, Staten Island, NY 10302, PH (718) 876-6092 Email: fsklenar@aol.com

Photographer

Paula Jensen, 122 Silver Lake Road, Blairstown, NJ 07825

Index